D0965734

Carlton E. Munson, PhD

The Mental Health Diagnostic Desk Reference

Visual Guides and More for Learning to Use the Diagnostic and Statistical Manual (DSM-IV)

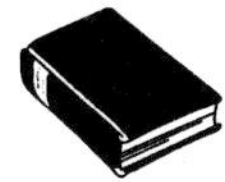

Pre-publication REVIEWS, COMMENTARIES, EVALUATIONS . . .

"Dr. Munson has produced a critically important text for a broad spectrum of practitioners and students in the helping professions. In addition to providing a rich, comprehensive, well-ordered, and richly illustrated body of information that will assist in the complex interdisciplinary process of diagnosis, the volume also contains a wealth of historical material about the search for accuracy in the understanding and subsequent treatment of the range of mental disorders. Related to this, the material on cultural aspects of these disorders will also be of considerable assistance. Even though the text is principally aimed at practitioners, its format and content neatly bridge the professional-lay gap and will be of great assistance to those who wish to, or need to, learn more about the DSM approach to classification."

Francis J. Turner, DSW, CSW
Professor Emeritus,
Faculty of Social Work,
Wilfrid Laurier University,
Waterloo, Ontario
Canada

More pre-publication
REVIEWS, COMMENTARIES, EVALUATIONS . . .

"We live in a time when proficiency in the use of the *Diagnostic and Statistical Manual (DSM-IV)* has become a requirement of contemporary clinical practice in mental health not only in North America, but in other countries as well. The diagnostic language and classificatory scheme of the DSM-IV has gradually been adopted by social service agencies, insurance companies and managed mental health care, and many state and federal health agencies. Unfortunately, training programs in mental health have not always provided students with a meaningful introduction to this taxonomic system. Furthermore, until now there has been no text available with which to accomplish this task. Dr. Munson's book, *The Mental Health Diagnostic Desk Reference,* provides both trainees and less-experienced clinical professionals with a practical and highly readable guide for using the DSM-IV taxonomic system.

The book begins with an informative and detailed chronology of important figures, events, and contributions to our understanding of mental health and illness from antiquity to the present. In the chapters that follow, Dr. Munson reviews the multiaxial system of classification, and proceeds to discuss the vast range of disorders (now numbering 340) that are currently classified in the DSM-IV. An obvious strength of this text is its liberal use of charts, diagrams, and other visuals throughout the book's twenty-three chapters. Furthermore, the author does not shrink back from the task of identifying important philosophical and other controversies surrounding the use of this psychiatric taxonomy, a sine qua non for any balanced and scholarly discussion of the DSM. This is a carefully organized and user-friendly guide for the beginning student and less-experienced practitioner of social work, clinical psychology, psychiatry, or psychiatric nursing, and will be a valuable addition to the literature on clinical assessment of mental disorders."

Jerrold R. Brandell, PhD, BCD
Professor,
School of Social Work,
Wayne State University,
Detroit, MI;
Founding Editor,
Psychoanalytic Social Work

More pre-publication
REVIEWS, COMMENTARIES, EVALUATIONS . . .

"Munson's *Mental Health Diagnostic Desk Reference* will prove to be an invaluable tool for multiple users. The reference utilizes a combined narrative and visual approach, designed to increase understanding of the DSM-IV. Practitioners will be able to more effectively and accurately complete diagnostic work and laypersons will be more able to understand mental illness and the process of mental health evaluation.

Two special features of this reference work will be particularly helpful to practitioners. 'Tip Boxes' are located throughout the chapters to emphasize significant information and give useful suggestions. The final chapter provides definitions and a case illustration of the Outline for Cultural Formulation, providing a useful example for utilizing cultural information in a sensitive and meaningful way to reach a decision on diagnosis and treatment."

Jan Black, MSW
Professor Emeritus,
Department of Social Work,
California State University,
Long Beach

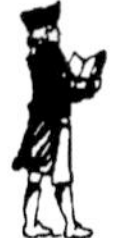

The Haworth Press, Inc.

NOTES FOR PROFESSIONAL LIBRARIANS AND LIBRARY USERS

This is an original book title published by The Haworth Press, Inc. Unless otherwise noted in specific chapters with attribution, materials in this book have not been previously published elsewhere in any format or language.

CONSERVATION AND PRESERVATION NOTES

All books published by The Haworth Press, Inc. and its imprints are printed on certified pH neutral, acid free book grade paper. This paper meets the minimum requirements of American National Standard for Information Sciences-Permanence of Paper for Printed Material, ANSI Z39.48-1984.

The Mental Health Diagnostic Desk Reference

Visual Guides and More for Learning to Use the Diagnostic and Statistical Manual (DSM-IV)

The Mental Health Diagnostic Desk Reference

Visual Guides and More for Learning to Use the Diagnostic and Statistical Manual (DSM-IV)

Carlton E. Munson, PhD

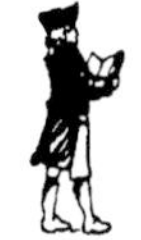

The Haworth Press®
New York • London • Oxford

The Haworth Press, Inc., 10 Alice Street, Binghamton, NY 13904-1580

Cover design by Monica L. Seifert.

Library of Congress Cataloging-in-Publication Data

Munson, Carlton E.
The mental health diagnostic desk reference : visual guides and more for learning to use the Diagnostic and statistical manual (DSM-IV) / Carlton E. Munson.
p. ; cm.
Includes bibliographical references and index.
ISBN 0-7890-1075-5 (hard : alk. paper) — ISBN 0-7890-1076-3 (pbk. : alk. paper)
1. Mental illness—Classification—Handbooks, manuals, etc. 2. Mental illness—Diagnosis—Handbooks, manuals, etc. I. Title: Visual guides and more for learning to use the diagnostic and statistical manual (DSM-IV). II. Title.
[DNLM: 1. Mental Disorders—classification—Handbooks. 2. Mental Disorders—diagnosis—Handbooks. WM 34 M969 2000]
RC455.2.C4 M86 2000
616.89′001′2—dc21

00-020779

CONTENTS

Preface

The classification of mental illness has been a quest of humans since the beginning of time. This search for organization and meaning has not been a purely philosophical or academic effort; the desire to classify and understand mental disorders has a practical and utilitarian purpose. Through understanding the origins of mental problems, we can plan effective treatment and even cures. The history of the study of classification has not always been smooth or consistent. Much chicanery and controversy are associated with this quest. When the history of the study of classification is reviewed, it is apparent that a core evolutionary process has brought us to our present state of knowledge. Over the years, a narrowing of the source of fundamental information related to classification has occurred. For practitioners in the United States and many other industrialized countries, that source is the *Diagnostic and Statistical Manual of Mental Disorders,* Fourth Edition (DSM-IV), published by the American Psychiatric Association. That narrowing of the source of classification has led to more concentrated research and differentiation of classes of mental disorders. This has produced significant refinement in how mental disorders are viewed and treated. Although much controversy still surrounds the DSM classification system, it is the most recognized and most thoroughly researched model available.

Recognizing the connection between diagnosis and treatment has become paramount. Although this connection has always been acknowledged, the research generated by the consolidation of classification into a single system has heightened this connection. It would be very difficult today for a practitioner to begin a course of treatment without the benefit of a thorough assessment and a DSM multiaxial diagnosis. This has not been the case in the past. Any practitioner today who does intervention that is not based on a thorough diagnosis is engaging in risky professional activity. The historic concept of study, diagnosis, and then treatment is more true than ever before. At the same time, the methods for delivery of mental health services have been radically changed. The increased emphasis on brief treatment and symptom relief has generated the need to perform accurate, thorough, differential diagnosis in a brief period. Given the complexity of diagnosis and the wealth of data required to make an accurate diagnosis, the challenge facing the mental health practitioner is to find a way to do this within significant time constraints.

At the same time, mental health services are being delivered by an expanding cadre of mental health practitioners. Until fifteen years ago, the core mental health professionals were generally defined as psychiatrists, psychologists, psychiatric nurses, and clinical social workers. Today, in addition to the core mental health disciplines, numerous other disciplines deliver mental health services. Some of these practitioners receive little or no training in the use of the DSM system. While the core of mental health providers has expanded, the amount and extent of available treatment has decreased. This has led to practitioners in other areas, such as public social services and criminal justice, having to be concerned with mental health issues.

Due to these recent trends, psychoeducation has become much more important in making mental health information available to laypeople. Ironically, but perhaps appropriately, this may create more demand for mental health services in an era of reducing costs by decreasing services. Just as diagnosis is important to the mental health professional planning treatment, knowledge of the condition is also important to the person being treated. In this information age, people with certain mental conditions can find valuable self-help resources outside traditional treatment, but to do so in a safe and effective way, they need accurate information about mental disorders.

These trends were the impetus for writing this book. The book is designed to aid practitioners in making more effective, efficient, and accurate diagnoses. It can also help laypeople better understand mental disorders and how they are diagnosed. This book is written in clear language that explains complex procedures without oversimplifying them. The philosophical and practical controversies regarding the mechanics of the DSM system have caused some people to avoid using it or to limit their use of it. Some complain that the manual is not conceptual; it is not theoretical; the numbering system is inconsistent; the organization is confusing; the structural presentation of disorders is inconsistent; it employs a confusing, unique grammatical construction; and capital letters are overused. Some of these complaints are valid, and some are trivial, but most of them come from a lack of knowledge of the nature, organization, and presentation of the disorders. Explanations can be given for most of the previous complaints. After reading this book, most of these complaints can be understood and overcome by the practitioner. Another complaint is directed toward the lack of sensitivity to cultural issues, but the DSM-IV, Appendix I, which lists and explains how to apply the culture-bound behaviors, is a step toward a more comprehensive view of the role of cultural beliefs and behaviors in mental functioning. This book provides a detailed explanation of how to use the information relating to culture, including an illustration of how to construct a cultural formulation in the context of performing differential diagnosis.

I have tried to explain the essence of the DSM-IV system from beginning to end. I start with a review of the history of classification that I think is crucial to understanding current diagnostic procedures and terminology. I explain the organization of the DSM-IV manual and give a detailed explanation of how to do an accurate and thorough multiaxial diagnosis, which is the heart of the DSM-IV. I cover all the disorders listed in the DSM-IV, disorders undergoing research for inclusion (Appendix B of the DSM-IV), and conditions that may be a focus of clinical attention. The intent is that upon mastery of the content in this book, the reader can make more effective use of the DSM-IV. More details of the organization of the book are provided in Chapter 1. In writing this book, my singular goal has been to make the DSM-IV more understandable for the wide array of people who may need to use it within the context of the current mental health delivery system.

Carlton E. Munson

ABOUT THE AUTHOR

Carlton Munson, PhD, is Professor of Social Work at the University of Maryland—Baltimore and Director of the Washington Area Supervision Institute at Woodstock Forest. A nationally recognized academician and teacher, he was inducted into the National Academy of Practice in 1996 based on his teaching, research, and scholarship related to clinical practice. Dr. Munson is the author of numerous articles and book chapters, as well as four books that have been widely adopted as textbooks in the United States. In addition, Dr. Munson is the founding editor of *The Clinical Supervisor* (Haworth), an interdisciplinary journal devoted to supervision research. He is also the founding editor of the forthcoming publication *The Journal of Diagnosis and Assessment in Mental Health* (Haworth). Focusing on trauma and loss in children, he is also a consultant to a number of child treatment facilities. The recipient of the Education Award from the Maryland Network Against Domestic Violence in 1999, Dr. Munson has trained over 3,500 mental health professionals in the use of the DSM-IV system.

Acknowledgments

It is not possible to list all of the people who assisted in the preparation of this book. So many people contributed in large and small ways to the ideas, preparation, and production to make this book a reality that a complete list would be quite long. I do want to thank my wife, Joan Smith Munson, for her many contributions to this project. She endured much work and activity alone while I was isolated in my study for months preparing this manuscript. She reviewed the entire text and offered gentle, but wise, suggestions on many aspects of the manuscript. Joan has been there for me on every writing project over the last thirty-nine years and has never once complained about the struggles, tasks, and separations that are associated with such undertakings. I can never completely and adequately express my indebtedness to Joan for her contribution to this and my other endeavors.

I want to thank the staff at The Haworth Press for their many contributions to this book. I have been working with The Haworth Press since 1983 and have always been impressed with their helpfulness and pleasant, cooperative, positive, "can-do" attitude. At times when some tasks seemed overwhelming, the Haworth staff would reassure me it was possible and set in motion the necessary actions to get the job done. The assistance of the Haworth staff on this project has been especially commendable because of the unusually large number of complicated illustrations that were essential to the core concept of this book. I want to specifically mention Bill Cohen, President and Publisher of The Haworth Press, for his support, ideas, and guidance. Bill Palmer, Vice President and Managing Editor of The Haworth Press Book Division, facilitated the publication activity in a number of ways, and I deeply appreciate all of his work on this project. I want to thank Sandy Jones Sickels, Vice President of Marketing, for her work in making people aware of this book through use of her talented promotional skills. Margaret Tatich, Haworth Sales and Publicity Manager, also contributed to the marketing and promotional aspects of this project. Margaret was always so responsive to my many telephone calls for advice. Melissa Devendorf, Administrative Assistant in The Haworth Press Book Division, was extremely helpful, as she always is, with the mechanics of the administrative work associated with publishing this book. Patricia Brown, Book Division Production Manager, was very helpful in the many aspects of the production of this book. My appreciation goes to Andrew Roy for his review of the manuscript and for his assistance in the permissions process, which was a crucial part of producing this book. I thank Amy Rentner for her thorough and perceptive editing. I know these are just a few of the many Haworth staff who worked hard to make this book possible, and I am grateful for all of the effort by this dedicated group.

I want to thank the University of Maryland, Baltimore, Administration, for the sabbatical leave granted me during the Fall 1999 semester that made possible the completion of this book. Many years of accumulated material had to be crafted into a coherent narrative, and without the sabbatical leave, I am not sure I would have been able to take the large blocks of time necessary to complete this book.

I appreciate the assistance of my longtime colleague and friend, Dr. Herman Curiel, of the University of Oklahoma, for his review and suggestions regarding the case example in the section on culture-bound syndromes.

I also am appreciative of the research assistantships provided to me by the Graduate School over the last seven years. The graduate assistants did much of the background research for several aspects of this book. I want to thank Denise Pintello, Judy Barnstone, and Steven Wilz, University of Maryland, Baltimore, doctoral students, who served as my research assistants and performed much of the research related to this project. I also want to thank my students and continuing education program participants who provided feedback about my illustrations and my methods of conceptualizing this material. During the last ten years, over 3,500 students and continuing education program participants were exposed to the material in this book. The final content is truly the result of an evolutionary process of refining and honing the material to make it as understandable and concise as possible. My students and workshop participants contributed significantly to the refinement of the book and also served as a major source of motivation and stimulation for the ideas and conceptualizations that are the heart of this book.

Thanks again. I am eternally grateful for being blessed with the support, guidance, and help of all of you!

Disclaimer

This book should not be used to perform DSM-IV diagnosis. Diagnosis should be done only by a qualified mental health professional through use of the DSM-IV manual. Every effort has been made to ensure accuracy of the material in this book. It is possible that some small errors or inaccuracies do exist. Any questions about accuracy of content in this book should be discussed with a qualified mental health professional. Information regarding qualified mental health practitioners can be obtained from state and local medical societies, psychologist licensing boards and associations, and state social work licensing boards. Readers who discover what they believe to be errors or inaccuracies should contact Dr. Munson at:

Dr. Carlton Munson
School of Social Work
University of Maryland, Baltimore
525 West Redwood Street
Baltimore, MD 21201-1777
Telephone: 410-706-3602
E-Mail: cmunson@ssw.umaryland.edu

Chapter 1

Introduction

ABOUT THIS BOOK

This book is about how to use the *Diagnostic and Statistical Manual of Mental Disorders,* Fourth Edition (DSM-IV), published by the American Psychiatric Association in 1994. The manual has expanded and become more complex since the first edition was published in 1952. The current edition has 886 pages containing 340 disorders. About a dozen study guides review the manual and assist practitioners in becoming effective users of the DSM-IV. Most of these guides assume a certain level of preexisting knowledge of the DSM system and its terminology. This book is intended to be different in that it employs a conceptual framework of mastering the organization of the manual through a narrative and visual approach. This book includes eighty-one illustrations that aid in conceptualizing how to perform diagnosis.

I have been doing diagnosis for thirty years, and in 1987, I was required to teach a course in the DSM system at Fordham University in New York City, where I was a faculty member. There I was confronted for the first time with the task of effectively conveying to others how to use the DSM. Since teaching that first class, I have taught over 3,500 students and practicing professionals how to use the DSM. Although I have been teaching this system for twelve years, I still learn something new each time I prepare for a seminar. The complexity of teaching the system led me to develop many visuals to convey the information. Students and practitioners responded favorably to this visual approach and frequently asked for copies of the transparencies. Consequently, I decided to make the visuals into a book. When I sat at the computer for the first time and tried to create narratives to accompany the visuals, I discovered that writing about the visuals was not nearly as easy as talking about them. I did develop a renewed respect for the DSM manual as I was going through it page by page in preparing this book. Although I have been through the manual hundreds of times, and have employed it thousands of times to make diagnoses, I learn something new each time I use the manual.

For those who feel discouraged by the wealth of detail in the DSM-IV and who believe they will never master the system, some solace may be found in the fact that probably not one person in the world has mastered the entire DSM-IV, or knows completely how to use this book as a clinical tool. The DSM-IV was never designed to be mastered in toto, and I believe that is why many professionals have difficulty learning to use it. In school we are not taught to use books as reference tools, but to read them cover to cover and somehow comprehend them as whole documents. The DSM system is not designed that way and cannot be mastered completely. Remember, DSM-IV was designed by a committee. When you assume the reference book stance in relation to the DSM-IV, you are in a position to master it by learning to conceptualize the discrete classes of disorders rather than trying to learn a method that works for the entire manual. The manual was not put together that way. The DSM-IV was compiled by a committee of over 1,600 people! If you do not believe this, look at Appendix J of the manual, which lists all the contributors to the DSM-IV project. I am sure these people did not sit in a room together and work on the manual, but over forty task groups and forty organizations contributed to its production. If you keep in mind the number of persons and groups that contributed to this work, understanding why it is difficult for one person to master this large volume becomes a little easier. For these and other reasons, you cannot expect the DSM-IV to be highly conceptualized from one perspective. It does not represent any theoretical orientation. The numbering system is not completely consistent because it had to be compatible with the International Classification of Diseases System. The organization of the different sections is inconsistent because of the varied nature of the disorders. For example, mood disorders do not lend themselves to the same framework as anxiety disorders, and anxiety disorders do not lend themselves to the same organization as psychotic disorders. For the same reason, the specifiers and subtypes vary greatly from class to class and disorder to disorder. The manual employs a unique grammatical construction and use of words, as well as a unique use of capitalization. You should note that all disorders use capitalization for all words that are key in the diagnosis and the subtypes and specifiers.

This study guide, or any other, for that matter, is not a substitute for using the DSM-IV for doing diagnosis. Whenever making a diagnosis, the diagnostician should always consult the DSM-IV manual. The only goal and function of this guide is to enhance your ability to use and understand the DSM-IV.

Following this introduction, Chapter 2 provides a brief review of the history of classification of mental disorders. Classification of mental illness has a long history, and any person performing diagnosis should have a basic knowledge of this history. Laypeople reading this chapter can be reassured that many mental conditions described in this book have a long history of research and confirmation of effective treatments. Chapter 3 gives an overview of the organization of the manual and explains each section and its relevance to diagnosis. Some basic concepts used in the DSM-IV are explained in this chapter. Chapter 4 describes the multiaxial system of the DSM-IV, including a detailed explanation of the five axes and how to use and understand them. This chapter also has a discussion on treatment planning using the DSM-IV criteria as the basis for intervention. Chapter 5 begins the coverage of the specific classes of disorders in the DSM-IV. Chapters 5 through 20 explain the disorders in the same order as they are presented in the DSM-IV. Chapter 21 describes the conditions in the DSM-IV that can be listed as part of the multiaxial diagnosis, but are not considered full-fledged mental disorders. This section of the DSM-IV is titled "Other Conditions That May Be a Focus of Clinical Attention." Chapter 22 reviews the twenty-six disorders or items that were considered for inclusion in the DSM-IV as full-scale disorders, but that did not quite meet the research criteria for a mental disorder. These twenty-six items were in a group of over 100 disorders considered for possible inclusion in the manual. Based on research findings, the Task Force that prepared the DSM-IV manual decided that the disorders in this section had been sufficiently researched to warrant partial inclusion. Further research that will stem from these disorders being listed in Appendix B of the DSM-IV will determine whether they qualify for full recognition as mental disorders in future editions of the DSM diagnostic system. How to use and correctly diagnose these potential disorders is explained in Chapter 22. The final chapter explains how to use Appendix I of the DSM-IV, which is a new section that takes into account cultural factors that may influence the behaviors and symptoms of a person who seeks a mental health evaluation.

ORGANIZATION OF THE CHAPTERS RELATED TO SPECIFIC DISORDERS

The organization of this book is based on common topical headings used in the chapters that cover specific disorders. Some deviations from the format occur because of the nature of variation in presentation of disorders in the DSM-IV. The headings provided in most chapters are as follows.

Disorders

Each chapter begins with a listing of the disorders in the corresponding section of the DSM-IV. No commentary is included as part of the list. The list is presented as a quick reference for the class of disorders covered in the chapter.

Fundamental Features

This section includes short paragraphs, often with each main point indicated by a bullet. Key words are highlighted in italic or bold type throughout. This section describes the most basic and fundamental information needed to understand the disorders in the corresponding section of the DSM-IV. It also includes a brief conceptualization of the disorders in that section of the manual. Each set of disorders is supplemented with visual representations of the disorders explained in the text. These visuals are central to this book, and the text material is organized around them. The visuals can be studied as overviews of each disorder or class of disorders. The specifics of the organization of the disorder or class of disorders illustrated in the visuals are explained in the chapter's text. "Tip boxes" are presented throughout the chapters to highlight significant diagnosis-related information and techniques that are not in the DSM-IV or that may be difficult to locate in the manual.

Differential Diagnosis

Where appropriate, a section on differential diagnosis lists the other disorders of which the diagnostician should be aware when considering a particular disorder or set of disorders.

Recommended Standardized Measures

For those disorders for which scales and standardized measures are available, I have listed several scales useful in providing objective information regarding that particular disorder. I am familiar with the scales I have recommended and have selected them based on effectiveness, ease of use, brevity of administration, and cost.

Recommended Reading

Most sections have a recommended reading list. Readings have been selected based on relevance to diagnosis and assessment. I have tried to keep each list brief and to select readings that are highly relevant to the disorder rather than providing an exhaustive reading list.

References

The references cited in each chapter are included at the end of the chapter. A master list of all references used in the book can be found at the end of the book, along with multimedia resources available for use in learning the DSM system. The placement of the references both at the end of each chapter and at the end of the book deviates from traditional citation methods, but this was done to facilitate use of the book as a reference guide. The reader does not have to go to the back of the book to find references used in a particular section of the book.

OTHER KEY FEATURES OF THE BOOK

Visuals

The visuals are consistent for the different classes of disorders. They include a brief mention of the disorders' essential features, those disorders included in the class, and those disorders which are in Appendix B and can, therefore, be used for research purposes. The visuals are my representation of how the disorders and the criteria for diagnosis are explained in the DSM-IV text. They include a listing of subtypes and specifiers when they are used for specific disorders. In some visuals I have included supplemental information that can be helpful in understanding the disorders. The graphic presentation of the visuals does vary because of the nature and uniqueness of each class of disorders. The primary intent of each visual is to capture, on one page, an overall image of the organization and conceptualization of all the disorders in a specific class. Other visuals have been included that expand on the information about the disorders. For example, in Chapter 17, "Sleep Disorders," the visuals are related to stages of sleep and age-related patterns of sleep. The text provides explanation of the disorders in each visual. The visuals are designed to be studied and can be used while reviewing the DSM-IV manual. It is recommended that the visuals be used in connection with the DSM-IV because the material in the visuals is summary information, and in-depth understanding can only occur through study of the DSM-IV manual. Where relevant, the page numbers of the DSM-IV that correspond to the visual are included in the visual.

Lay Reader Accessibility

My hope is that this book can aid laypersons who have an interest in understanding mental disorders through reading the DSM-IV manual. People read this manual for numerous reasons. Some may want to learn more about disorders that affect them or family members. Having a diagnosis comes as a relief to some people after years of living with unexplained symptoms. Such relief arises from finally knowing the name for what you have experienced for years, and also from the knowledge that you are not the only person suffering from a particular set of symptoms. Family members can become supporters of an affected relative by reading this guide and developing further understanding of specific disorders; they can come to see that disorders are not always caused by human failures.

This is illustrated by the family of an eight-year-old child I evaluated who had a classic case of Obsessive-Compulsive Disorder (OCD). She had a collection of seventy dolls, stored neatly in boxes, dressed and named uniquely, and carefully cataloged in writing. The catalogs were updated weekly. The child took ninety minutes each morning to groom herself for school. She selected clothes cautiously and combed her hair with five different combs. The parents were supportive and cooperated with treatment, but the grandparents chastised the parents that the child's lack of discipline was the cause of the problem. The grandparents were interviewed and given the content of this book on OCD, as well as other resource material. They changed their view after the meeting and after reading the material. They became supporters of the parents and aided them in the treatment, which was an enormous removal of stress for already stressed parents.

Psychoeducation is a powerful factor in recovery and treatment of many disorders. This book can aid people in seeking understanding. It is not designed, however, to enable self-diagnosis or diagnosis of a friend or relative. The intent is that this book will be read by a layperson who has received mental health intervention and who is attempting to gain more insight into mental disorders.

Abbreviations Used

A number of key abbreviations are used in the text and in the visuals. Visual 1.1 lists these abbreviations.

A FINAL INTRODUCTORY WORD

To experience a mental disorder personally, or through a family member or friend, can be a very difficult and frightening experience. This book is designed to aid mental health practitioners in the diagnosis process so that effective and efficient treatment can be delivered, and to provide laypersons with a basic understanding of mental disorders. Mental disorders requiring

VISUAL 1.1. Abbreviations Used in This Book

Abbreviation	Word or Phrase
ADHD	Attention-Deficit/Hyperactivity Disorder
ASPD	Antisocial Personality Disorder
BRSD	Breathing-Related Sleep Disorder
Dx.	Diagnosis
DFS	Defensive Functioning Scale
ELD	Expressive Language Disorder
GAF	Global Assessment of Functioning Scale
GARF	Global Assessment of Relational Functioning Scale
GMC(s)	General Medical Condition(s)
ICA(s)	Infant, Child, and Adolescent Disorder(s)
ICD-9	*International Classification of Diseases,* 9th Revision
ICD-10	*International Classification of Diseases,* 10th Revision
IP	Identified Patient
LT	Long Term (goal)
MD	Mental Disorder
MRELD	Mixed Receptive-Expressive Language Disorder
NOS	Not Otherwise Specified
OCD	Obsessive-Compulsive Disorder
PA(s)	Panic Attack(s)
PDD(s)	Pervasive Developmental Disorder(s)
R/O	Rule Out
ST	Short Term (goal)
SOFAS	Social and Occupational Functioning Assessment Scale
W/O	Without

mental health intervention are widespread in our society. A study by Kessler and colleagues (1994) found that mental disorders in the United States are extensive, and most people do not receive intervention for these disorders. The study was one of the largest systematic statistical random samples of the U.S. population ever done, and the data were based on lengthy interviews designed to detect mental disorders. The researchers found that 48 percent of the people reported that at some time during their lives they suffered a DSM-diagnosable mental disorder. Over 29 percent of the total sample reported a mental disorder in the last year. Less than 40 percent of the people with a lifetime disorder received any treatment, and less than 20 percent of those with a mental disorder in the last year received treatment. These findings are consistent with the Surgeon General's (Satcher, 2000) extensive survey of mental health research. A summary of the findings of this research is reported in Visual 1.2. These findings provide compelling evidence of the level of mental illness in our society and the need for well-qualified mental health professionals to address the extent of mental problems that people experience in their daily lives. This book was written for that purpose—to contribute to more effective mental health diagnosis and treatment.

VISUAL 1.2. Lifetime and Twelve-Month Prevalence of DSM-III-R Psychiatric Disorders in the United States (N = 8,098)

Disorder	Lifetime (%)	Twelve-Month (%)
Major Depression	17	10
Alcohol Dependence	14	7
Social Phobia	13	8
Simple Phobia	11	9
Substance Abuse	25	11
Anxiety Disorder	25	11
Affective Disorders	20	11
ASPD	3	—
Schizophrenia	0.7	—

Summary of Findings:

- 48 percent reported lifetime history of at least one DSM disorder
- 29 percent reported one or more disorders in the previous year
- 52 percent reported no disorder
- 21 percent reported one disorder
- 13 percent reported two disorders
- 14 percent reported three or more disorders
- Most reported at least two disorders
- Mental disorders concentrated in 14 percent of the population with a history of three or more comorbid disorders
- 40 percent received treatment
- 29 percent received help in the previous year
- 20 percent treated in mental health specialty sector
- 8.3 percent treated in substance abuse facility
- Men more likely to have substance use disorders and ASPD
- Women more likely to have affective and anxiety disorders
- Age: 25-34 most reported age range
- Mental disorders inversely associated with income and education
- Substance use higher in middle-level educated
- Urban/suburban/rural residence showed no significant difference
- Lower incidence of comorbidity in rural areas (disorders more "pure")
- Substance abuse and ASPD higher in the West
- Anxiety higher in the Northeast
- All disorders lower in the South

Source: Kessler, R. C., McGonagle, K. A., Zhao, S., Nelson, C. B., Hughes, M., Eshleman, S., Wittchen, H. U., and Kendler, K. S. (1994). Lifetime and 12-Month Prevalence of DSM-III-R Psychiatric Disorders in the United States. *Archives of General Psychiatry,* 51(1): 8-19.

REFERENCES

Kessler, R. C., McGonagle, K. A., Zhao, S., Nelson, C. B., Hughes, M., Eshleman, S., Wittchen, H. U., and Kendler, K. S. (1994). Lifetime and 12-Month Prevalence of DSM-III-R Psychiatric Disorders in the United States. *Archives of General Psychiatry,* 51(1): 8-19.

Satcher, D. (2000). *Mental Health: A Report of the Surgeon General.* Washington, DC: U.S. Government Printing Office.

Chapter 2

The Historic Heritage of Classification

INTRODUCTION

Learning to do effective and accurate diagnosis that is documented appropriately is often a technical task, one viewed by many as unexciting. The history of classification, on the other hand, is an exciting story of many colorful characters and intriguing events. For example, Alois Alzheimer, who is famous for discovering the histological components of Alzheimer's disease at the turn of the twentieth century, was a nocturnal person. He slept during the day and worked at night in his research lab in Heidelberg, Germany, assisting Emil Kraepelin, the founder of the classification system that is the basis for the DSM system, in an attempt to discover the neurology of dementia praecox (precursor of schizophrenia). He actually discovered the basis of degeneration in senile dementia. In conducting their research, Kraepelin, Alzheimer, and Franz Nissl, a German neurologist, used a small card system to classify patients. Cards with each patient's symptoms were placed in a "diagnosis box" on admission to the hospital. Later, a patient's name would be added to the symptom card after studying the person for a period of time. When the patient was discharged, the "end result" would be noted on the cards. This system became the basis for Kraepelin's grouping of disorders, which reflected his position that classification could be grounded in a common set of symptoms rather than in universal conditions that could be identified and applied to patients (Frances, First, and Pincus, 1995). This simple historical anecdote illustrates how the evolution of classification efforts has contributed to modern diagnosis and continues to serve as a guide for current objective diagnostic activity. Alzheimer's finding—while searching for another disorder—is still pertinent today, as researchers make intriguing new discoveries regarding the nature of this disorder. Alzheimer's finding remains in the DSM-IV in the form of Dementia of the Alzheimer's Type in the section "Delirium, Dementia, and Amnestic and Other Cognitive Disorders." The "diagnostic box" of this research group resembles the assessment, diagnosis, outcome model of intervention used today. This is just one example of the hundreds of historical events in the evolution of classification that have relevance today.

A second more colorful illustration in the history of classification centers around Franz Anton Mesmer. Most people are familiar with the term mesmerized, meaning a person is spellbound or fascinated by something or someone, but do not realize that this term derives from the Austrian-born French psychiatrist once considered a maverick, though he espoused theories that eventually proved irrational. The term mesmerize was once used to mean hypnotize, based on the techniques employed by Mesmer. He married a wealthy widow and had Mozart stage his first opera on the lawn of her mansion in 1768. He plagiarized the work of a famous British physician for his doctoral dissertation and was accused of inappropriately touching a blind female patient, which resulted in him fleeing Austria for Paris. He became a successful practitioner through basing his "animal magnetism" theory on the concepts underlying the recent discovery of electricity. Such reductionism was quite common in the history of mental illness classification and treatment. Mesmer believed that the body contained fluids comparable to magnetic forces. He postulated that mental illness was a manifestation of a maldistribution or deficiency of this "animal magnetism." He treated patients by touching them with a wand while wearing a purple robe. The purple robe was for effect, but the wand was supposed to "correct" the maldistribution of the body's magnetic force. Patients sometimes sat around a covered banquet table holding rods that were placed in holes in the table, which had bottles of chemicals beneath it. Or, patients were placed in an oak barrel while Mesmer moved the rod over it. Because of the settings in which Mesmer conducted these treatments, he is considered one of the earliest practitioners of hypnosis as we know it (Davison and Neale, 1990). Mesmer was subjected to an investigation of his practices, commissioned by Louis XVI, and the commission concluded there was no rational basis for Mesmer's techniques. (As an aside, Joseph-Ignace Guillotin, advocate of the beheading device, and Benjamin Franklin, who was in Paris at the time, served on the commission.) Many well-respected physicians came to Mesmer's defense and presented evidence that many people had been cured by his techniques. Other practitioners argued that they had also successfully used Mesmer's techniques (Stone, 1997). Mesmer symbolizes some of the many varied events that make up the history of classification, and the reader is encouraged to read more about this colorful character.

The details of historical events, such as the contributions of Alzheimer and Mesmer, add life to the long, arduous journey that has brought us to the modern scientific methods of defining and classifying mental illness.

IMPORTANCE OF KNOWING THE HISTORY OF CLASSIFICATION

The importance of studying the history of classification is not simply to be aware of interesting events and developments, but to understand that our current classification system is the result of many years of research. This core set of mental disorders has undergone significant expansion only in recent times. In reviewing the history of classification, one can come to appreciate that little of what we do today with respect to diagnosis, assessment, or treatment is new or novel.

The earliest forms of mental illness were labeled as "wild," "eccentric," or "mad," which became "insane." The term madness dates back 2,500 years. Early written descriptions in the Old Testament of the Bible placed madness in association with "fury and rage." Although no classification system existed, causation was generally attributed to possession by evil spirits. These early singular explanations evolved to a long-standing core classification of mania, melancholia, and dementia. The gradual expansion of this system, with a few diversions, has evolved to include the 340 disorders in the DSM-IV—an unbroken evolution, from the earliest classifications to the present, aimed at sorting and consolidating mental disorders. In my opinion, anyone engaged in diagnosis and assessment must have some basic knowledge of this heritage of classification. I refer to the heritage of classification because I believe a tradition of classification study can be identified, is impressive, and is a common connection for all involved in diagnosis. Visual 2.1 presents an outline of this evolution and serves as the core content of this chapter. Visual 2.2 briefly summarizes the evolution of interventions and illustrates that many of the interventions we use today are far from being new or unique. The remainder of this chapter gives a chronology of the major events in the evolution of the classification of mental disorders.

HISTORICAL SUMMARY

In keeping with the visual and referential intent of this book, I have chosen to present the history in a chronological order in a listed table format. This allows the reader to gain some orderly sense of the vast historical sweep of classification. The following summary lists major events that have contributed to the evolution of the current DSM-IV system of classification. These are brief descriptions, and the reader is referred to the citations given at the end of each for more details on specific items. No citation means the information is general knowledge or no specific source is known. I have limited the list to items that are directly connected to classification evolution, but a

VISUAL 2.1. Evolution and Expansion of Classification Highlights

	2500 B.C. to 100 A.D.	100 A.D. to 1699	1700 to 1849	1850 to 1949	1950 to 2000
General Term in Use	Madness	Lunacy (Relating to lunar cycle)	Insanity	Psychosis Neurosis	Mental Disorder
Specific Categories	Madness	Melancholy Mania Dementia	Melancholy Mania Dementia Paranoia Idiocy Amnesia (Imbecility) Epilepsy	Melancholy Mania Dementia Folie à Deux Circular Insanity Alienation Hysteria Folie du Doute Monomania Nymphomania Refusal of Food General Madness Partial Madness Moral Insanity Weakening of Intellect Pyromania Kleptomania	Mood Schizophrenia Dementia Anxiety Dissociative Infancy/ Childhood/ Adolescence Due to GMC Substance Related Somatoform Factitious Sexual/Gender Identity Eating Sleep Impulse Control Adjustment Personality

Expansion of Disorders

Consolidation of Disorders into Categories

Note: Dates are approximations.

natural consequence was to develop also a list of treatments that accompanied the attempts at classification. Early clinicians and researchers usually developed techniques to accompany the disorders they identified, and it was difficult to disconnect classification and intervention in the historical review. This also illustrates the long-standing connection between classification and intervention. I have limited the mention of techniques of intervention to methods that were directly related to the disorders the person was addressing. For example, some of the people who studied serious mental symptoms attempted institutional and psychotherapeutic reforms and innovations as part of the identification process. In these cases, the interventions have been mentioned, but I have tried to resist the urge to give details of interventions. I have included some mention of interventions because many of the treatments we consider quite modern actually have long, impressive histories. Because the history of interventions is generally unknown, I have listed the major interventions encountered in my research for this chapter in Visual 2.2. No comment is made on these interventions because they are being presented as enlightening information and are not central to the focus of this book.

VISUAL 2.2. List of Historic Interventions

Intervention	**Era**	**Originator (if known)**
Phlebotomy (venesection, bloodletting)	100 B.C.	
Drug hellebore (from white lily)	377 B.C.	Hippocrates
Emetics (enemas)	377 B.C.	Hippocrates
Moderate discourse (psychotherapy precursor)	270 B.C.	Epicurus
Massage	124 B.C.	Asclepiades
Wine tonics	124 B.C.	Asclepiades
Exercise	124 B.C.	Asclepiades
Occupation	124.B.C.	Asclepiades
Theater	124 B.C.	Asclepiades
Relaxation	124 B.C.	Asclepiades
Odoriferous herbs	124 B.C.	Asclepiades
Sleep near temples	124 B.C.	Asclepiades
Music	100 A.D.	Celsus
Induced vomiting	100 A.D.	Celsus
Starvation (diet)	100 A.D.	Celsus
Torture	100 A.D.	Celsus
Flogging	100 A.D.	Celsus
Restraints	100 A.D.	Celsus
Talk in patient's words	100 A.D.	Soranus
Purgatives	1300s	Plater
"Skipping" (free association precursor)	1400s	Abulafia
Incantations	1400s	Tribal
Dreaming	1400s	Tribal
Dream interpretation	1400s	Tribal
Rattles/noises	1400s	Tribal
Symbolic sand painting	1400s	Tribal
Bath therapy (hydrotherapy precursor)	1400s	

VISUAL 2.2 *(continued)*

Intervention	Era	Originator (if known)
Agricultural work (occupational therapy precursor)	1400s	
Healthy diet	1600s	Burton
Increased sleep	1600s	Burton
Confession grief (psychotherapy precursor)	1600s	Burton
"Benign trickery"	1600s	Sydenham
Recreation	1600s	Willis
Water immersing	1600s	Boerhaave
Inducing seizures	1700s	Auenbrugger
Reading layman's guides (self-help)	1700s	
Calming	1750	Chiarugi
Exciting	1759	Chiarugi
Sexual intercourse (sex therapy precursor)	1800s	Reil
Cognitive training	1800s	Reil
Hydrotherapy	1800s	Pienitz
Negotiating	1800s	Jacobi
Isolation	1800s	Ferriar
Moral treatment (interpersonal psychotherapy precursor)	1800s	Daguin
"Tranquilizing chair"	1800s	Rush
"Dunking"	1800s	Rush
"The Swing"	1800s	Cox
Drama therapy	1850s	Browne
"Franklinization"	1850s	Beard
Hypnosis	1850s	Braid
Free association	1900s	Freud
"Rest cure"	1900s	Mitchell
Hydrotherapy	1900s	
Psychodrama	1940s	Moreno
Self-help	1940s	Horney
"Total push"	1940s	Myerson
Group process	1950s	Bion

Note: All dates are approximations. Originators of techniques have been identified in the literature as the source of these techniques, but are not necessarily the only person to use the technique or to have claimed to be the originator.

A series of themes runs through this list of historic events. The following are the most common:

1. The mind and body are viewed in various ways: viewed as separate entities, as a unified whole, and as interrelated.
2. Varied beliefs exist regarding nature versus nurture or heredity versus environment in causing mental illness. Embedded in this theme

is the debate over the role of genetics and biology in causation of mental disorders.

3. One conception is that varied symptoms of mental illness are the result of a small set of core disorders. The opposite view posits a large number of discrete disorders with specific symptoms. These two approaches to classification have been referred to as "lumpers" and "splitters." For example, Kraepelin was a "lumper," and this is illustrated by his view that "catatonia" and "hebephrenia" were varieties of dementia praecox. The "splitters" are illustrated by François Boissier de Sauvages (1706-1767) of the French school of classification, who identified twelve varieties of melancholy (Stone, 1997).
4. Process versus categorical models is another theme. The process model believes that mental illness is a result of a process of events that produce symptoms and difficulties, whereas the categorical model holds that mental illness produces a set of symptoms that can be used to define and diagnose disorders. Freud used a process model, and Kraepelin used a categorical model.
5. The type and quality of care provided the mentally ill and the role of differential care are based on distinguishing the needs of the mentally ill, the mentally retarded, criminals, and the poor.
6. Consideration of who should provide care for the mentally ill is an important theme. One view is that the family should provide the care; the other, that societal institutions should. Initially, care was provided by the family, but the asylum movement shifted care to society's public and private institutions. This pattern has proved cyclical. In the United States, in the 1960s, the development of medications for the chronically mentally ill allowed deinstitutionalization of large numbers of such patients without adequate provision of community-based care. The emergence of managed care has shifted much of the care burden back to families. These events affect classification because family-provided care limits researchers' ability to study the nature and course of disorders.
7. Introduction of new treatments made necessary more accurate diagnosis. For example, the diagnoses of unipolar and bipolar depression require different psychopharmacological interventions.
8. Some treatments have evolved over centuries. For example, water immersing, used by Hermann Boerhaave of Leiden in the 1600s, became "dunking," devised by Benjamin Rush in Philadelphia in the early 1800s, and later emerged as hydrotherapy, practiced in the United States until the 1950s.

9. What some viewed as causative of disorders, others used as treatments. For example, at the beginning of the Christian era, Asclepiades advocated the use of alcohol as a treatment, but Soranus saw it as a cause of distress and wrote, "How can it occur to the mind of any man to dispel intoxication by intoxication?" (Stone, 1997, p. 14).
10. The trend is to identify numerous men as "the father of modern psychiatry," based on their classification achievements and intervention methods. These include Juan Luis Vives for his writings on the soul, Johann Weyer for encouraging humane treatment and his advocacy against women being classified as witches, Benjamin Rush for writing the first medical text on mental illness, and Emil Kraepelin for his categorical diagnostic system that became the basis for the DSM system.

Indicators of these themes can be noted as the reader studies the following historical chronology.

Summary Chronology of Significant Events in the History of Classification

Earliest Times	Conceptualizations of "strange behavior," "unusual personality"; allusions to "madness" attributed to demonic and divine madness.
3000 B.C.	Egyptian Prince Ptahhotep described as suffering from senile dementia (Frances, First, and Pincus, 1995).
2600 B.C.	Sumerian and Egyptian use of melancholia and hysteria terminology (Frances, First, and Pincus, 1995).
1400 B.C.	First attempt to classify mental disorders known as Ayur-Veda occurred in India (Frances, First, and Pincus, 1995).
500-100 B.C.	In Mayan civilization, moon goddess Ixchel was patroness of medicine, and priests and chiefs were the guardians of knowledge and could intervene with the gods on behalf of the people. Disease could derive from knowledge (conscious causation) or from the "inborn and concealed" (unconscious causation). Earth, fire, and water were believed to be free to the tribe so there was no ownership of land (Barton, 1987).

Hippocrates (460-377 B.C.) integrated anatomy, physiology, and temperament by postulating that temperament resulted from combinations of the four "humors" (earth, water, air, and fire). He believed that breathing introduced ether to the brain where movement and sensation were controlled. Phlegm could interfere with this process and cause fits or paralysis. Hippocrates believed dreams were part of the soul and controlled the body during sleep. From an observational perspective, he developed a system of six disorders (phrenitis, mania, melancholia, epilepsy, hysteria, and Scythian disease) and what can be viewed as a second axis set of disorders of four temperaments (choleric, sanguine, melancholic, phlegmatic) based on the theory of humoral imbalance (Frances, First, and Pincus, 1995).

Plato (428-347 B.C.) conceptualized the dualistic view that mind and matter are separate. The soul (mind) was divided into "rational" and "irrational" forms of "madness" (melancholia, mania, and dementia) and emerged when the rational and irrational souls were separated (Stone, 1997). He identified four categories of "divine madness": prophetic, religious, poetic, and erotic. Plato used a rational search for universal conditions to guide his classifications (Frances, First, and Pincus, 1995).

Aristotle (384-322 B.C.) developed the position that the brain condensed vapors originating in the heart. This theory endured into the eighteenth century (Stone, 1997).

10-200 A.D. Celsus (25 B.C.-50 A.D.) embraced the "humor" theory and postulated that "humors" flowed more freely in springtime, making melancholy and insanity more common during this season (one is reminded here of the DSM-IV seasonal affective disorder). He advocated a range of treatments, including restraint, phlebotomy, enemas, induced vomiting, and soft music (Stone, 1997). Celsus coined the word "insania," which was similar to modern conceptions of the term insanity (Barton, 1987).

Caelius Aurelianus identified causes of mental illness: alcohol use, head injury, suppression of menses, exposure to strong sunlight, superstition, excessive preoccupation with philosophy, glory, and greed (Stone, 1997).

Soranus (c. 100 A.D.) introduced the concept of humanistic care of the mentally ill based on service rather than control. He argued against alcohol as a treatment and restraint. He recommended talking to patients in their own language and used techniques similar to modern cognitive/behavioral interventions (Stone, 1997).

Claudius Galenus (aka Galen) (129-199) believed sensation was the basis of human faculties and was controlled by nerve centers, with the brain being the center of psychic functioning (Stone, 1997).

400-900 A.D. Unhammad developed classification of nine types that included melancholia, mania, febrile delirium, manic restlessness, persecutory psychosis, lovesickness with anxiety and depression, disorders of judgment, worry and doubt with obsessions and compulsions (Stone, 1997).

Rhazes (c. 865-925) devised an etiological system based on excess or deficit of the "three souls" (vegetative, animal, and rational) that was a precursor of dimensional classification systems (Frances, First, and Pincus, 1995).

1000-1500 Abū ʻAlī al-Husayn ibn Sīnā (aka Avicenna) (980-1037), masterful diagnostician and therapist, wrote an extensive encyclopedia of medicine, including sections on melancholy and mania. He rejected spirits as causes of mental illness, believing instead it was due to defective temperament (Stone, 1997).

Moses ben Maimon (aka Maimonides) (1135-1204) wrote about diseases of the soul and defined "good" and "wicked" personalities (Stone, 1997).

Abraham Abulafia (c. 1240-1291) of Saragossa developed the technique of "skipping" in which a trancelike state was used to have patients skip from one thought to another until a single thought focused on God was achieved. This technique survived for centuries and was the basis of Freud's technique of free association (Stone, 1997).

Albertus Magnus (1193-1280) wrote about dreams and transformed the view of dreams from suspicion by religious groups to analysis and interpretation by medicine and psychology (Stone, 1997).

In 1205, the founding of the first university was followed by universities in Paris, Naples, Heidelberg, and Prague, leading to independent thought regarding many topics, including mental illness (Stone, 1997).

First asylum built in Hamburg, Germany, in 1375, followed by the famous Bethlem (Maudsley) Hospital in London in 1403 (Stone, 1997). This hospital continues in operation. Prior to this time, most mentally ill were cared for by families in their homes through being locked in rooms, cages, stables, and barns. Asylum care was more available in urban areas. Asylums emerged as facilities for the provision of psychotherapy and physical therapy, but devolved to custodial care before deinstitutionalization closed many facilities in the United States in the 1970s due to development of powerful medications to control behavior (Shorter, 1997).

Aztec physicians shared priests' powers to intervene with the gods whom they believed produced disease when enraged. These "Ticiti" resolved anxieties using mushrooms and herb treatments and dream interpretation. Physicians were responsible for the health of the community and could be put to death if they did not prevent disease. As in Ancient Egypt, women were physicians (Barton, 1987).

1500-1700 The Church gradually withdrew objections to dissection of the body, allowing for research on disease and anatomy (Stone, 1997).

Juan Luis Vives (1492-1540) wrote about the functions of the soul, including intelligence, memory, recall, talent, thought, and will. He defined three groups of emotions: (1) positive (love, lust, desire, goodwill, veneration, sympathy/pity, joy, and pleasure), (2) negative (displeasure, contempt, anger, hatred, envy, jealousy, indignation, vengeance, and cruelty), and (3) despair (sadness, tearfulness, fear, hope, shame, and arrogance). For his work Vives is viewed by some as the "father of modern psychiatry" (Stone, 1997).

Johann Weyer (1515-1588) advocated for women who had been persecuted as witches. He argued that women considered witches were senile or delusional and harmless. Some consider him the founder of modern psychiatry (Barton,

1987). Weyer treated a ten-year-old, religious girl in his home who had become a celebrated community case for having claimed she had not eaten for six months. Weyer housed the girl in the basement and drilled a hole through the kitchen floor to observe. He discovered that the girl's sister, whom she had insisted live in the house with her, was supplying her with food (Stone, 1997). Details of this case have modern parallels in eating disorders and malingering.

Felix Plater (1536-1614), a Swiss anatomist, was a taxonomist of mental illness who used the term "alienation" and developed a classification system based on brain damage. He is given credit for the first attempt to classify mental disease based on symptoms (Stone, 1997).

In 1566, the first mental hospital in North America was established in Mexico City (Barton, 1987).

Thomas Wright (1561-1623), an English priest, devised a new classification system based on emotions (Stone, 1997).

Syphilis emerged in Europe in the 1500s. The disease led to gradual brain degeneration that was labeled general paresis (Stone, 1997).

This era renewed interest in madness associated with frustrated love, based on French literature (Stone, 1997).

Humor theory was giving way to exploration of anatomy and observation of behavior (Stone, 1997).

Edward Jorden (1569-1632), an English physician, represented the emerging view that mental illness was due to life stresses, not evil spirits. He applied this view to the allegations of witchery made against women and served as expert witness in the defense of women, referring to their disorders as "hysterical" (Stone, 1997).

Robert Burton (1577-1640) published *The Anatomy of Melancholy* (1621), in which he provided comprehensive coverage of melancholy, including an unprecedented account of his own mild depression that fits the modern conception of dysthymia (Stone, 1997).

Thomas Sydenham (1624-1689), considered the "father of modern medical thinking," departed from the notion that mental illness had a single root cause and developed the view that each disorder had an independent cause (Frances, First, and Pincus, 1995). He distinguished hysteria and "frank alienation," or psychosis. He used "benign trickery" to cure a man of melancholy by sending him from England to Scotland for treatment by a nonexistent Dr. Robinson. The patient's symptoms remitted on the way to Scotland in anticipation of the intervention, but when he discovered no "Dr. Robinson existed," Sydenham's success in causing the symptoms to remit did not occur to the patient, and during the return to England, the man became enraged at Dr. Sydenham for tricking him (Stone, 1997).

Thomas Willis (1621-1675) coined the term neurology, used the term "psyche-ology," and is considered one of the founders of biological psychiatry. Willis viewed hysteria as a disorder of the nerves and a form of "fit" or convulsion. In 1672, Willis described "madness" that fit the model of dementia praecox (schizophrenia), identified by Kraepelin 200 years later (Stone, 1997).

1523 Henry VIII (1491-1547) established the Royal College of Physicians in London (Barton, 1987).

1645-1692 One hundred witches were executed in England. In Salem Massachusetts, population 4,000, 250 people were accused of being witches and 22 were executed. By 1711, public guilt led to modest financial compensation for the survivors of people executed as witches (Barton, 1987).

1700-1900 George Stahl (1660-1734) advocated specific psychological treatment for the mentally ill (Stone, 1997).

Hermann Boerhaave (1668-1738) introduced "surprise" therapy in the form of dunking patients in cold water. This technique was later used by Benjamin Rush in the United States (Stone, 1997).

William Cullen (1710-1790) coined the term neurosis and defined four types (Stone, 1997).

Leopold Auenbrugger (1722-1809), a musician and son of an innkeeper, applied his knowledge of tapping beer barrels to determine fullness to listening to the chest for sounds of disease. He also successfully treated manic patients by using camphor to induce mild seizures. This treatment was "rediscovered" 150 years later by Ladislaus von Meduna, a Hungarian psychiatrist (Stone, 1997).

Jean-Étienne Esquirol (1772-1840), a leading reformer, coined the term hallucinations. He devised a simple classification of "general madness," "partial madness," "weakening of the intellect," "affective monomania," "pyromania," and "kleptomania" (Stone, 1997). He was the first to use the terms "remission" and "intermission" to describe the course of mental illness (Stone, 1997).

Jean-Pierre Falret (1794-1870) and Jules Baillarger (1809-1890) differentiated mania and melancholy. Falret coined the term "circular insanity." Falret's son, Jules, coined the term folie à deux while working at the Salpêtrière in Paris (Stone, 1997).

Felix Voisin (1794-1872) founded one of the first hospitals for the mentally retarded (Stone, 1997).

Henri Le Grand du Saulle (1830-1886) described the disorder that became the model for schizotypal personality disorder (Stone, 1997).

Benedict-Augustin Morel (1809-1873) was the first to describe the course of the illness, which he named "Demence precoce," that evolved to the disorder schizophrenia (see information on Emil Kraepelin, pp. 11-12, 29) (Frances, First, and Pincus, 1995).

Édouard Séguin (1812-1880) reformed treatment of the mentally retarded in France and later brought his reforms to the United States. He directed the first American private school for the retarded, which was begun by Dr. H. W. Wilbur in Massachusetts in 1848 (Stone, 1997).

1730 In America, the mildly mentally ill were allowed to "roam about" or were cared for at home. The poor insane were cared for in almshouses, and the violently insane were placed in common houses (jails) (Barton, 1987).

1752 Pennsylvania Hospital was the first hospital in the colonies to accept the physically and mentally ill (Barton, 1987).

1806 Thomas Arnold (1742-1816) published text that included a two-category definition of insanity and classified personality disorders similar to the DSM-IV organization (Stone, 1997).

1808 Johann Reil (1759-1813) was a German physician who coined the term psychiatry, which he defined as "treatment of the mind." He described this term in a journal he founded. He utilized many treatments that were innovative and are still used today, such as occupational therapy, and music and drama therapy (Stone, 1997).

Thomas Trotter's (1760-1832) book *A View of the Nervous Temperament,* first published in Europe and reprinted in America, was the first psychiatric book published in America. Trotter believed that mental illness was caused by societal excesses: tea, coffee, work stress, "trashy novels," clothing fashions, and stage plays. He articulated humane treatment for alcoholism (Stone, 1997).

1809 John Haslam (1766-1844), while medical director at Bethlem Hospital, published a textbook that described general paresis and schizophrenia. Haslam is considered to have described the first case of schizophrenia and to have first identified this disorder as occurring in children (Stone, 1997).

1811 At age eighteen, Mary Reynolds suffered prolonged periods of significant personality change characteristic of what we now refer to as dissociation (Stone, 1997).

1812 Benjamin Rush (1745-1813) published the first American medical textbook. He is considered the "father of American psychiatry." He argued that the brain was central to the mind. He did not believe in restraint by chains of the mentally ill, but did use the technique of the "swinging" cure devised by Joseph Cox (1763-1818), in which the patient was placed in a swing-type chair and spun. This was believed to produce harmony of mind and body. Rush used the "tranquilizing chair," which totally immobilized the patient, and he used sudden dunking in water as a technique. Rush coined the term "manicula" for hypomania and "tristemania" for self-persecutory depressive states (Stone, 1997).

1818 Johann C. Heinroth (1773-1843), in his book *Treatise on the Disturbance of Mental Life,* developed a three-part nomenclature. Freud devised an identical one 100 years later (Stone, 1997).

Heinrich Neumann (1814-1884) postulated that unsatisfied sexual drives could give rise to "anxiety."

Gustav Fechner (1801-1887) developed the concepts of "pleasure principle" and "repetition" that became the basis of Freud's "repetition compulsion" (Stone, 1997).

1829 Carl Carus (1789-1869) wrote that biology is regulated by a psychological "plan" that contains a biological "unconscious" (Stone, 1997).

1835 James C. Prichard (1786-1848) coined the term "moral insanity" in a general sense, which later meant antisocial and psychopathological behavior (Stone, 1997).

1838 Jean-Pierre Falret (1794-1870) successfully advocated changing the terms "imbecility" and "furor" to alienation (Stone, 1997).

Franz Mesmer (1734-1815), fascinated by the discovery of electricity and its relationship to magnetism, speculated that mental illness was due to maldistribution of body fluids that could be returned to balance by moving magnetic wands over the body. Mesmer also developed trance techniques that were refined by de Marquis Puységur, James Braid (introduced term hypnosis), Jean-Martin Charcot (1825-1893), and Sigmund Freud (Stone, 1997).

Philippe Pinel (1745-1826) is considered by many to be the father of modern psychiatry. He rejected "humoral" theory for the view that mental illness was the result of heredity or intolerable passions. He rejected the standard repressive treatments for humane treatment based on respect and compassion and used such interventions as exercise, entertainment, and work. He was director of the Bicêtre (for men) and Salpêtrière (for women) hospitals in Paris (Stone,

1997). He developed the classification system of four types (mania, melancholia, dementia, idiotism) that simplified earlier complex systems (Frances, First, and Pincus, 1995).

Isaac Ray (1807-1881) published *Medical Jurisprudence of Insanity,* and he advocated restraint as a cure (Stone, 1997).

1841 The founding of the British Association of Medical Officers of Lunatic Asylums.

Dorothea Dix (1802-1887) began her lifelong devotion to mental illness reforms after conducting religious services for female convicts in a Boston jail (Stone, 1997).

1843 William A. F. Browne (1805-1885) published a four-category classification: idiocy, fatuity, monomania, and mania. He also devised drama therapy in asylums and observed that more insane people lived in America than England because immigration resulted in the "flowing to America" of the "impure and poisoned" (Stone, 1997).

Forbes Benignus Winslow (1810-1874) published *The Plea of Insanity in Criminal Cases,* in which he argued that people could commit crimes during sleep, and the courts should consider this state in determining responsibility for the act (Stone, 1997).

Daniel McNaghten was found not guilty of killing a government official "on the ground of insanity" because he suffered from persecutory delusions that caused him to commit the murder. This ruling set the precedent for a series of court decisions that have defined legal insanity, and these standards are used today (Stone, 1997).

James Braid (1795-1860) published a book using the term hypnosis (Stone, 1997).

1844 Thirteen of the twenty superintendents of the asylums in existence in the United States met in Philadelphia to discuss crowding conditions in their facilities and formed the Association of Medical Superintendents of American Institutions for the Insane. This was the first organized effort in the United States to provide humane care for the mentally ill. Members of this group founded the profession of psychiatry in the United States. This group was the forerunner of the American Psychiatric Association (Barton, 1987).

Jacques Moreau de Tours (1804-1884) declared that madness was the same as dreaming, except it occurred while the person was awake (Stone, 1997).

1848 Phineas Gage, a railroad foreman, suffered a head injury when an explosion caused a steel rod to go through his skull. He survived, but his personality was radically changed, leading to speculation that behavior is controlled by specific parts of the brain (Stone, 1997).

1850 Otto Domrich described "anxiety attacks" (Stone, 1997).

1859 Paul Briquet (1796-1881) described "Briquet's syndrome," which is now referred to as somatization disorder (Stone, 1997).

Charles Darwin (1809-1882) published his book *On the Origin of Species by Means of Natural Selection,* which changed conceptions on the origin of humans (Stone, 1997).

Richard von Krafft-Ebing (1840-1902) studied sexual disorders and discovered a link between general paresis and neurosyphilis (Stone, 1997).

1860 Jean-Baptiste Buillaud (1796-1881) and Pierre-Paul Broca (1824-1880) discovered the brain region controlling speech (Stone, 1997).

1865 Wilhelm Griesinger (1817-1868) was the founder of biological psychiatry and transformed asylum psychiatry to university psychiatry. He viewed mind and body as one and saw mental disorders as somatic disorders. He streamlined nosology and modernized psychiatric language. Griesinger introduced intervention reforms such as elimination of restraints, occupational therapy, baths, medication, conversations, and games (Shorter, 1997; Stone, 1997).

Jean-Martin Charcot (1825-1893) advanced knowledge of hysteria (Stone, 1997).

1874 Carl Wernicke (1848-1905) discovered the sensory speech area of the brain, expanding Broca's speech center. He also clarified psychosis as relating to the internal and external world (Stone, 1997).

Emil Kraepelin (1856-1926) unified nosology and wrote a classic textbook on diagnosis. He defined the categorical approach that became the basis for the current DSM diagnostic system. Kraepelin identified dementia praecox, which became schizophrenia (Stone, 1997). He used the approach of grouping patients experiencing the same disease course and identified the clinical features that were common to patients in each grouping (Frances, First, and Pincus, 1995).

1875 George Miller Beard (1839-1883) published *A Practical Treatise on the Medical and Surgical Uses of Electricity* and coined the term "neurasthenia," which was similar to Robert Whytt's (1714-1766) "nervous exhaustion." Beard used terms such as "franklinization," "voltaic-galvanic stimulation," and "faradic" stimulation to explain his belief that the body could be "recharged." He devised a "faradic machine" to administer the treatments (Stone, 1997).

1879 Henry Maudsley (1835-1918) published *Physiology and Pathology of the Mind,* which was the first book to describe childhood mental illness (Stone, 1997).

1880 Georges Gilles de la Tourette (1857-1904) studied at the Salpêtrière under Charcot and discovered the disorder that is named after him (Stone, 1997).

1885 Hermann Ebbinghaus (1850-1909) published a book that pioneered learning theory and experiential psychology (Stone, 1997).

1887 Hermann Emminghaus (1845-1904) coined the term "psychopathology." He was a renowned child psychiatrist who believed that child and adult disorders should be distinct (Stone, 1997).

Karl Kahlbaum (1828-1899) developed a three-type classification of childhood disorders (Stone, 1997).

Karl Westphal (1833-1890) defined neuroses in the areas of phobias, sexual disorders, and what later would be referred to as obsessive-compulsive disorder (Stone, 1997).

1896 Sigmund Freud (1856-1939) defined psychoanalysis. Freud contributed to the diagnosis of neuroses much as Kraepelin defined the aspects of psychoses. Freud classified anxiety neurosis, depressive neurosis, hysterical neurosis, and obsessive-compulsive neurosis, which are related to the definitions in the DSM system (Frances, First, and Pincus, 1995).

1898 Pierre Janet (1859-1947) published the first of many books on a range of mental disorders that parallel most modern disorders. He developed the concept of "fixed ideas," which corresponds to the current concept of "underlying assumptions" (Stone, 1997).

1903 Alfred Binet (1857-1911) published his research on intelligence (Stone, 1997).

1905 Sigmund Freud published *Three Theories of Sexuality* (Stone, 1997; Gay, 1998).

1906 Alois (also spelled Aloys) Alzheimer (1864-1915) discovered by accident the disease that is named after him while working with Kraepelin to discover the degenerative aspects of dementia praecox. Alzheimer and Franz Nissl were working together to solve the mystery of mental degeneration in dementia praecox (Shorter, 1997; Stone, 1997).

Santiago Ramón y Cajal won the Nobel prize for brain research that served as a foundation for the research that discovered neurotransmitters (Stone, 1997).

1907 Adolph Meyer (1866-1950) and Clifford Beers (1876-1943) started the mental hygiene movement in the United States (Stone, 1997). Meyer introduced the Kraepelinian system to the United States, but eventually devised his own system based on reaction types resulting from individual and environmental stresses (Frances, First, and Pincus, 1995). Meyer aided his wife in devising the label "psychiatric social worker" to describe her work in a New York mental hospital. Meyer's work was instrumental in the development of the DSM-I.

1908 Clifford Beers (1876-1943) published *A Mind That Found Itself,* which gave an account of his psychosis, institutionalization in horrible conditions, and recovery. He led reform efforts and influenced famous psychiatrists such as Henry Phipps and Adolph Meyer (Stone, 1997).

1911 Eugen Bleuler (1857-1939) published a book and coined the terms "schizophrenia," "ambivalence," and "autism." Bleuler identified the four A's as "primary signs" of schizophrenia: autism, association loosening, ambivalence, and affect inappropriateness" (Stone, 1997).

1917 The Committee on Statistics of the American Medico-Psychological Association (became American Psychiatric Association) was concerned about the proliferation of classification systems, as each asylum developed its own classification system to account for patients and plan patient needs. The committee published a list of twenty-two disorders that could be used by all hospitals. This system was based mainly on the Kraepelinian system and was used until 1935 when an updated version was included in the American Medical Association's *Standard Classified Nomenclature of Diseases* (Frances, First, and Pincus, 1995).

1920 Ernest Jones (1879-1958) was founder and editor of the *International Journal of Psycho-Analysis,* which was the first psychoanalytic journal in English. The journal made continuing and concerted efforts to propose psychoanalytic treatments for schizophrenia (Stone, 1997).

1920 Morton Prince (1854-1929) founded and edited the *Journal of Abnormal Psychology,* in which he published an article that described a young woman with "multiple personality." He published prolifically on dissociation (Stone, 1997).

1921 Hermann Rorschach (1884-1922) published his research on inkblot tests (Stone, 1997).

Carl Jung (1875-1961) published *Psychological Types,* in which he used the terms "introvert" and "extravert" (Stone, 1997).

1922 Ernst Kretschmer (1888-1964) published *Body Build and Character* and described "schizoids" (Stone, 1997).

1923 Kurt Schneider (1887-1967) published a work on "psychopathic personalities" using a general, not specific, definition of the term. Schneider's personality types are similar to the DSM-IV personality disorders. He also attempted, without success, to link specific symptoms exclusively to schizophrenia (Stone, 1997).

1926 Jean Piaget (1896-1980) developed a comprehensive explanation of developmental cognitive abilities, first described in *Judgement and Reasoning in the Child* (Kaplan and Sadock, 1998).

1928 First twin study of schizophrenia done in Munich. At this time, schizophrenia was used quite generically in relation to diagnosis of mental illness (Stone, 1997).

1929 Wilhelm Reich (1897-1957) published the *Impulse-Ridden Character,* which included descriptions of the current terminology of borderline personality disorder (Stone, 1997).

1932 The Chicago Psychoanalytic Institute was founded by Franz Alexander (1891-1964), who introduced the German conception of psychosomatic medicine into the United States. Alexander used a vector theory to identify personality types based on psychosomatic features. His views were supported by Flanders Dunbar's (1902-1959) research that formulated personality profiles based on organic diseases. She identified "the ulcer personality," "the coronary personality," and "the arthritic personality," along with many other types (Alexander and Selesnick, 1966).

1935 Leo Kanner published the first child psychiatry textbook in English.

Alcoholics Anonymous was established (Stone, 1997).

1937 Anna Freud (1895-1982) published *The Ego and the Mechanisms of Defense,* in which she described normal and abnormal defense mechanisms (Stone, 1997).

Karen Horney (1885-1952) emphasized the role of culture in giving rise to neurosis in her book *Neurotic Personality of Our Time.*

1938 Burrhus Frederic Skinner (1904-1990) published *The Behavior of Organisms* and argued in a series of writings that neuroses were based on learned behaviors (Stone, 1997).

Lauretta Bender (1897-1987) developed a visual motor gestalt test. She contributed to the knowledge of childhood schizophrenia (Kaplan and Sadock, 1998).

1939 Nathan Ackerman published an article that began his work on classification of family dysfunction to parallel individual models.

Jacob Kasanin coined the term "schizoaffective" (Stone, 1997).

1942 Helene Deutsch (1884-1982) described the "as-if" personality that is not "neurotic or psychotic" in an article titled "Some Forms of Emotional Disturbance and Their Relationship to Schizophrenia ('As If')." The work that culminated in this article was a precursor of borderline personality conceptualizations (Roazen, 1985).

1943 In a paper titled "Autistic Disturbances of Affect Contact," Leo Kanner coined the term "infantile autism" (Kaplan and Sadock, 1998).

1945 The military (Army, Navy, and Veterans Administration) developed systems of classification to address the large number (10 percent) of early discharges due to psychiatric illness. Four classification systems were now in use because the military classifications were in addition to the AMA *Standard Classified Nomenclature of Diseases* (Frances, First, and Pincus, 1995).

Sandor Rado (1890-1972) believed schizophrenia was hereditary and coined the term "schizotype" (Stone, 1997).

1946 Franz Alexander (1891-1964) wrote a book with colleague Thomas French that applied psychoanalysis to a range of mental disorders (Stone, 1997).

1948 World Health Organization (WHO) assumed responsibility for publication of the sixth revision of the *International List of Causes of Death.* WHO renamed the document as the *International Classification of Diseases, Injuries and Causes of Death* (ICD-6) and added a section on mental disorders, which included ten categories of psychosis, nine categories of psychoneurosis, and seven categories of character, behavior, and intelligence (Frances, First, and Pincus, 1995).

1949 J. F. J. Cade published an article reporting some success using lithium with manic patients. This marked the beginning of modern research on medication as a treatment for mental illness (Stone, 1997).

1950 Erik Homburger Erikson (1902-1994) published *Childhood and Society,* which explained his theory of life-span development and conflict resolution.

1951 Rene Spitz identified childhood disorders (especially depression and mental retardation) that can be caused by abandonment, separation, and lack of attachment (Kaplan and Sadock, 1998).

1952 DSM-I was published as a variant of the *International Classification of Diseases,* Sixth Revision (ICD-6) and incorporated ideas of Adolph Meyer.

1953 Harry Stack Sullivan's (1892-1949) lengthy career of publishing culminated with the publication of *The Interpersonal Theory of Psychiatry.* He believed in biological psychiatry, but emphasized the role of the interpersonal in healing. Much of his clinical research was focused on work with schizophrenic patients.

1954 Serotonin discovered in brain tissue.

1959 Selma H. Fraiberg published *The Magic Years,* which related anxiety, neurosis, and child development.

1963 Norman Cameron published *Personality Development and Psychopathology*, a comprehensive review of mental disorders, in which he focused on normal and abnormal functioning and used a developmental approach.

George L. Engel published *Psychological Development in Health and Disease,* which used a developmental approach to mental health and mental illness based on the view that all behavior is based on "biological factors, reality factors, and social factors." The views of Engel and Cameron reflected the emerging comprehensive view of mental health.

Federal government expanded mental health services through launching a broad community mental health program initiative.

1965 Donald W. Winnicott (1897-1971) developed the concepts "transitional object," "primary object," "good-enough mother," "true self," and "holding environment" in relation to normal and traumatic experience (Kaplan and Sadock, 1998).

1967 Otto F. Kernberg published an article on borderline personality.

1968 DSM-II was published. This volume expanded the use of diagnoses and promoted multiple diagnoses for patients.

International Classification of Diseases, Eighth Revision (ICD-8) became effective, with clarification and expansion of psychiatric illness.

1975 *International Classification of Diseases,* Ninth Revision (ICD-9) published and implemented in 1978.

1980 DSM-III was published. Methodological changes included "explicit diagnostic criteria, a multiaxial system, a descriptive approach that attempted to be neutral with respect to theories of etiology." Much effort was made to use empirical research as a basis for disorders and to employ semi-structured clinical interviews (Frances, First, and Pincus, 1995).

1987 DSM-III-R published to correct limitations of DSM-III. Added explicit diagnostic criteria for each disorder and introduced the multiaxial classification format. These changes were based on research efforts started in the 1970s. The specific criteria models used were the "Feighner criteria," which involved inclusion and exclusion criteria, and the Research Diagnostic Criteria (RDC) (Frances, First, and Pincus, 1995).

1992 Stuart Kirk and Herb Kutchins published a book criticizing the use of categorical diagnostic systems, pointing out uses and misuses of the DSM system (Kirk and Kutchins, 1992). The authors have continued their efforts through journal articles and a more recent book (Kutchins and Kirk, 1997) to point out the limitations of an expanding categorical diagnostic system; they have, however, done little to diminish the utilization of the DSM system as the driving force of psychiatric diagnosis in the United States. A number of recent criticisms of the DSM use the themes identified by Kirk and Kutchins. A typical example is a book by Paula Caplan (1995) titled *They Say You're Crazy.*

1993 *International Classification of Diseases,* Tenth Revision (ICD-10) was published. DSM-IV development was underway to make it compatible with the ICD-10.

1994 DSM-IV was published. Changes were mainly in the form of organizational alterations and compliance with research criteria for disorders rather than expert opinion.

The National Association of Social Workers published a classification system for social functioning that was provided as an alternative to the DSM system (Karls and Wandrei, 1994). This system is problem focused and is based on a four "factor" system that includes social functioning problems, environmental problems, mental health problems, and physical health problems. The third factor of mental health problems is made up of the Axis I and Axis II DSM-IV disorders. Few reliability and validity measures of the Person-in-Environment System (PIE) have been taken, and the system has had limited use as an alternative to the DSM system.

2005 Current plans are for the DSM-V to be published.

CURRENT VIEW OF CAUSATION

The evolution of classification of mental disorders has led to many explanations for the causation of mental illness. Much has been learned about causation, but much remains to be learned. Reviewing the summary of classification given here can lead to confusion regarding causation. Whether to provide reference to causation for each disorder in the DSM-IV was debated, and the decision was made to limit causation explanation. Only a few disorders in the DSM-IV have causation associated with them, such as Reactive Attachment Disorder of Infancy or Early Childhood, Mental Disorder Due to a General Medical Condition, Substance-Related Disorders, Posttraumatic Stress Disorder, and the Adjustment Disorders. The Posttraumatic Stress Disorder or the Adjustment Disorders diagnoses require the presence of a traumatic event or an identified stressor. Other disorders do not need identification of causation to be diagnosed. Causation is important to developing intervention plans, and a basic orientation to causation is essential to performing diagnosis and implementing and conducting treatment. The general view is that most disorders have multiple causation or that multiple factors must coalesce for a disorder to occur. Generally, five sources of mental disorders are recognized: (1) genetics, (2) biology, (3) substances/alcohol, (4) stress, and (5) physical and psychological assaults. These sources are summarized in Visual 2.3.

VISUAL 2.3. Major Sources of Mental Disorders

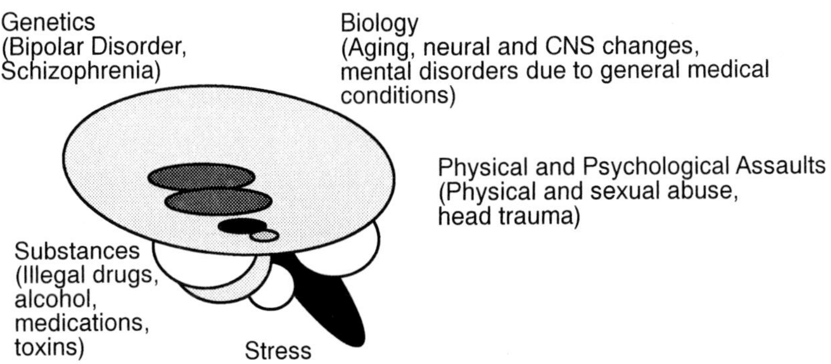

Identification of a traumatic event or stressor(s) is one of the criteria for the diagnosis of Posttraumatic Stress Disorder or Adjustment Disorder in the DSM-IV.

RECOMMENDED READING

Given the long history of classification, the fact that little is written about the topic internationally or within the United States is surprising. Three books served as guides for this chapter and are highly recommended to the reader: (1) Edward Shorter's *A History of Psychiatry: From the Era of the Asylum to the Age of Prozac;* (2) Michael Stone's *Healing the Mind: A History of Psychiatry from Antiquity to the Present;* and (3) Walter Barton's *The History and Influence of the American Psychiatric Association*. Full citations for these books are given in the following reference section.

REFERENCES

Alexander, F. G. and Selesnick, S. T. (1966). *The History of Psychiatry: An Evaluation of Psychiatric Thought and Practice from Prehistoric Times to the Present.* New York: The New American Library.

Barton, W. E. (1987). *The History and Influence of the American Psychiatric Association*. Washington, DC: American Psychiatric Press.

Caplan, P. J. (1995). *They Say You're Crazy: How the World's Most Powerful Psychiatrists Decide Who's Normal*. New York: Addison-Wesley.

Davison, G. C. and Neale, J. M. (1990). *Abnormal Psychology*. New York: John Wiley.

Frances, A., First, M. B., and Pincus, H. A. (1995). *DSM-IV Guidebook: The Essential Companion to the* Diagnostic and Statistical Manual of Mental Disorders. Washington, DC: American Psychiatric Press.

Gay, P. (1998). *Freud: A Life for Our Time.* New York: Norton.

Kaplan, H. I. and Sadock, B. J. (1998). *Synopsis of Psychiatry: Behavioral Sciences/Clinical Psychiatry.* Baltimore, MD: Williams and Wilkins.

Karls, J. M. and Wandrei, K. E. (1994). *Person-in-Environment System: The PIE Classification System for Social Functioning Problems*. Washington, DC: National Association of Social Workers.

Kirk, S. A. and Kutchins, H. (1992). *The Selling of DSM III: The Rhetoric of Science in Psychiatry.* Hawthorne, NY: Aldine de Gruyter.

Kutchins, H. and Kirk, S. A. (1997). *Making Us Crazy: DSM: The Psychiatric Bible and the Creation of Mental Disorders*. New York: The Free Press.

Roazen, P. (1985). *Helene Deutsch: A Psychoanalyst's Life.* New York: Doubleday.

Shorter, E. (1997). *A History of Psychiatry: From the Era of the Asylum to the Age of Prozac*. New York: Wiley.

Stone, M. H. (1997). *Healing the Mind: A History of Psychiatry from Antiquity to the Present.* New York: Norton.

Chapter 3

Organization of the DSM-IV

The DSM-IV has a systematic organization that must be understood to effectively use the manual. Each section of the DSM-IV is discussed in this chapter, followed by a brief explanation of its content. Such an outline is provided to reinforce the importance of reading each section of the DSM-IV in preparation for doing diagnosis.

CONTENTS

Here, all thirty-six sections of the DSM-IV are listed. Eighteen sections include categories of disorders that can be assigned a diagnostic code. Referring to the contents often when learning the DSM-IV will help the reader quickly become familiar with the organization of the manual. The DSM-IV disorders are represented in the manual in the following proportions:

DSM Disorders Class	**Number of Pages**	**Percentage**
Substance	98	15.6
ICA	85	13.5
Mood	75	11.9
Sleep	57	9.1
Anxiety	52	8.3
Sexual	46	7.3
Personality	45	7.2
Schizophrenia/Psychotic	43	6.8
Delirium/Dementia/Amnestic	41	6.5
Somatoform	25	4.0
Dissociative	15	2.4
Impulse Control	13	2.1
Eating	12	1.9
Other Conditions	12	1.9
GMCs	10	1.5
Factitious	5	0.8
Adjustment	5	0.8
Total	**629**	**100.0**

TASK FORCE ON DSM-IV

This section lists the people who served on the DSM-IV Task Force that guided preparation of this edition of the manual. The Task Force was chaired by Dr. Allen Frances of Duke University.

ACKNOWLEDGMENTS

This section acknowledges the more than 1,000 people and organizations that contributed to the preparation of the manual.

INTRODUCTION

This section explains the research focus of the classification system, the historical background of the DSM-IV (some of this background is summarized in Chapter 2), and the relationship of the DSM-IV to the ICD-10 (see Chapter 2). It is important to understand the connection between the International Classification of Diseases system, which is what ICD represents, to relate to payers and statistical reporting requirements. This section also includes the definition of mental disorder that is used in the DSM-IV system. The definition is printed here because of its centrality to the DSM system of classification:

> In DSM-IV each of the mental disorders is conceptualized as a clinically significant behavioral or psychological syndrome or pattern that occurs in an individual and that is associated with present distress (e.g, a painful symptom) or disability (i.e., impairment in one or more important areas of functioning) or with significantly increased risk of suffering, death, pain, disability, or an important loss of freedom. In addition, this syndrome or pattern must not be merely an expectable and culturally sanctioned response to a particular event, for example, the death of a loved one. Whatever its original cause, it must currently be considered a manifestation of a behavioral, psychological, or biological dysfunction in the individual. Neither deviant behavior (e.g., political, religious, or sexual) nor conflicts that are primarily between the individual and society are mental disorders unless the deviance or conflict is a symptom of a dysfunction in the individual, as described above. (American Psychiatric Association, 1994, pp, xxi-xxii. Reprinted with permission from the *Diagnostic and Statistical Manual of Mental Disorders,* Fourth Edition. Copyright 1994 American Psychiatric Association.)

This definition summarizes much of the approach to the classification system of the DSM-IV and reflects the knowledge derived from the long evolution of classifying mental illness described in Chapter 2.

The DSM-IV Task Force points out that when considering mental disorders, one must consider both the "mental" and the "physical." This statement makes the DSM-IV a more medically oriented manual than previous editions, and careful attention has been given to how the person who is not medically trained should approach the use of the manual.

A unit in this section explains the limitations of the categorical approach to human behavior, and another points out the importance of clinical judgment in doing diagnosis. Clinical judgment is a professional ability that cannot be learned through reading a book. This book can aid a person in becoming proficient in the process of accurately recording diagnosis, but no book can substitute for the clinical experience and training involved in performing assessment and diagnosis.

This section includes an important statement about the difference between criteria for a mental disorder in the DSM-IV and those used in the legal system. Any practitioner who works with the legal system should read this information carefully.

Part of this section focuses on ethical and cultural considerations. This discussion covers the appropriate application of diagnosis when working with people from diverse cultures and gives an overview of the cultural variations in clinical presentation of disorders, a description of the culture-bound syndromes, and an outline for measuring and reporting the impact of culture. The details of these areas are contained in Appendix I of the DSM-IV and should be read by all practitioners using the manual. Chapter 23 of this book summarizes Appendix I for the reader.

A brief explanation of the use of diagnosis in relation to treatment is given in this section. In this book I provide a system for linking diagnosis to treatment. Current practice guidelines for mental health professions require that treatment plans be directly linked to the diagnosis. Visual 3.1 illustrates the connection between diagnosis and treatment by listing the steps required to make a diagnosis and formulate a treatment plan with clinical judgment as a key feature. Data collection is done with consideration of duration and frequency criteria and their clinical significance, while ruling out general medical conditions. This process culminates in using clinical judgment to decide if the person meets the criteria for a disorder. If the person does, you continue to the initial treatment planning phase, with periodic review of treatment planning and discharge or termination when the goals or outcomes have been met or cannot possibly be met by the client or practitioner. The reader may want to return to Visual 3.1 after completing Chapter 4, which

VISUAL 3.1. DSM-IV Clinical Judgment and Treatment Planning

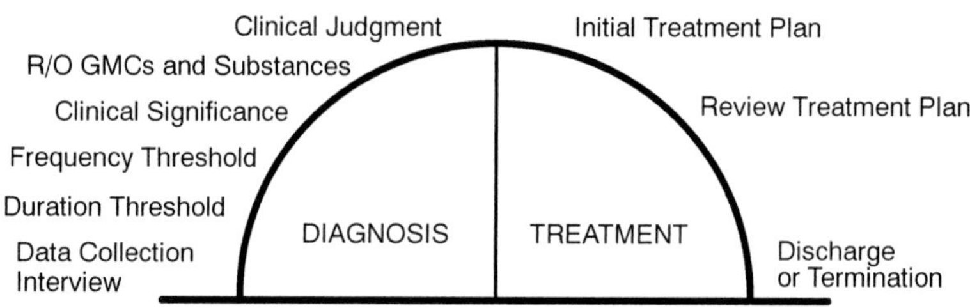

Source: American Psychiatric Association, 1994, pp. xxii-xxv.

provides the details of making a diagnosis. Visuals 3.7, 4.5, and 4.6 relate specifically to treatment planning based on DSM-IV criteria by applying Dysthymic Disorder to a specific diagnosis and generating a treatment plan from the diagnosis.

A brief discussion explains the distinction between mental disorders and physical disorders that are referred to as general medical conditions (GMCs) and reiterates the view of the American Psychiatric Association that no absolute distinctions can be drawn between the mental and the physical.

The section concludes with a brief statement about the organization of the DSM-IV, which includes instructions for use, the listing of the codes and categories, a description of the multiaxial system, the diagnostic criteria for disorders, and ten appendixes.

CAUTIONARY STATEMENT

This one-page statement contains disclaimers about the clinical training needed to use the DSM-IV and the limitations of the uses of disorders in some settings, such as the legal system.

USE OF THE MANUAL

Coding and Reporting Procedures

Diagnostic Codes

The disorders in the DSM-IV have a three- to five-digit code that accompanies the name of the disorder. The number code for each disorder appears to the left of the disorder in the classification section (pp. 13-24), at the beginning of the section that describes each disorder, and in the criteria sets presented in what I refer to throughout this text as the *diagnostic dialogue boxes.* The codes also appear in *Appendix E,* which gives an alphabetical listing of the diagnoses, and in *Appendix F,* which gives a numerical listing of the diagnoses.

Tip: The multiple locations of the codes can be very helpful in locating the code for a particular disorder without referring to the text section for that disorder.

The codes are not sequenced from 1 to 100, nor do they appear in sequence in the text of the DSM-IV. In addition, some disorders have the same number because they are based on the *International Classification of Diseases,* Ninth Revision, codes (see Chapter 2 for details of the ICD system), which many payers for health and mental health services use to reimburse providers. The ICD system consists of physical as well as mental disorders, and the codes range from 1 to 999, with the mental illness codes appearing within that numbering sequence. The ICD system was developed by international agreement before the DSM classification system was implemented.

Tip: Since some DSM-IV disorders have the same code, it is important when recording a diagnosis to list both the code and the name of the disorder. For example: 314.01 Attention-Deficit/Hyperactivity Disorder, Combined Type, since Attention-Deficit/Hyperactivity Disorder, Predominantly Hyperactive-Impulsive Type has the same code number (p. 85).

Subtypes. Some disorders have *subtypes.* Subtypes are discrete subgroups within a diagnostic category. In some cases, these carry a numeric code that is differentiated as a fifth digit. For example, Factitious Disorder has three subtypes:

300.16 Factitious Disorder **With Predominantly Psychological Signs and Symptoms**
300.19 Factitious Disorder **With Predominantly Physical Signs and Symptoms**
300.19 Factitious Disorder **With Combined Psychological and Physical Signs and Symptoms**

Notice the same code for two of the subtypes. Factitious Disorder Not Otherwise Specified also has the code 300.19 (pp. 474-475). Also, some subtype codes must be supplied by the diagnostician. For example, Sleep

Disorder Due to a General Medical Condition requires the diagnostician to supply the GMC as well as the subtype of .52 Insomnia Type, .54 Hypersomnia Type, .59 Parasomnia Type, or .59 Mixed Type (p. 601).

Severity and Course Specifiers

Specifiers are used to refine subgroupings within a disorder and do not indicate difference in type. Some specifiers indicate severity of the disorder (e.g., Mild, Moderate, and Severe) and course of the disorder (e.g., In Partial Remission, In Full Remission, and Prior History). Some disorders require a fifth-digit specifier:

296.21 Major Depressive Disorder, Single Episode, **Mild**

Others permit the diagnostician to enter a comma after the text of the disorder and then write mild, moderate, or severe:

308.3 Acute Stress Disorder, **Moderate**

Visual 3.2 lists the specifiers used in the DSM-IV. This visual can aid the diagnostician in finding the appropriate specifier for a particular disorder.

Some disorders have subtype specifier codes and others do not, due to the relationship between the DSM-IV and the ICD coding system. Some ICD disorders have codes for subtypes and others do not. To add specificity to the diagnoses that do not have these additional codes, the diagnostician can enter them as part of recording the diagnoses.

Tip: A numeric code with an *x* instead of a digit requires the diagnostician to supply the digit. For example, the code 296.2x for Major Depressive Disorder, Single Episode means the diagnostician must supply 1 for Mild, 2 for Moderate, or 3 for Severe and then place a comma after episode and write in Mild, Moderate, or Severe (p. 344).

Tip: On page 2 of the DSM-IV, the generic severity and course specifiers are defined. They are "Mild," "Moderate," "Severe," "In Partial Remission," "In Full Remission," and "Prior History." These specifiers can be added to any disorder that does not have particular specifiers indicated. Severity specifiers have been defined for Mental Retardation, Conduct Disorder, Manic Episode, and Major Depressive Episode. Course specifiers have been defined for Manic Episode, Major Depressive Episode, and Substance Dependence.

VISUAL 3.2. Alphabetic Listing of DSM-IV Specifiers

Specifier	Type	Disorder
Absent	Severity	Schizophrenia (Appendix B)
Acute	Course	PTSD/Adjustment
Chronic	Course	Amnestic/Mood/PTSD
Continuous	Course	Schizophrenia
Depressed	Course	Bipolar II
Due to Combined Factors	Severity	Sexual
Due to Psychological Factors	Severity	Sexual
Early Onset	Course	Separation Anxiety/Dysthymic
Early Partial Remission	Course	Substance
Episodic With Interepisode Residual Symptoms	Course	Schizophrenia
Generalized	Severity	Social Phobia
Hypomanic	Course	Bipolar II
In a Controlled Environment	Course	Substance
In Full Remission	Severity	Mood
In Partial Remission	Severity	Mood
Late Onset	Course	Mood
Limited to Incest	Type	Pedophilia
Mild	Severity	All
Moderate	Severity	All
Mood-Congruent Psychotic Features	Severity	Mood
Mood-Incongruent Psychotic Features	Severity	Mood
On Agonist Therapy	Course	Substance
Other or Other Unspecified Pattern	Course	Schizophrenia
Prior History	Course	All
Recurrent	Course	Transient Tic/Mood/Sleep
Severe	Severity	All
Severe With Psychotic Features	Severity	Mood
Severe Without Psychotic Features	Severity	Mood
Sexually Attracted to Both	Type	Pedophilia/Gender Identity
Sexually Attracted to Females	Type	Pedophilia/Gender Identity
Sexually Attracted to Males	Type	Pedophilia/Gender Identity
Single Episode	Course	Transient Tic
Single Episode In Full Remission	Course	Schizophrenia
Single Episode In Partial Remission	Course	Schizophrenia
Sustained Full Remission	Course	Substance
Sustained Partial Remission	Course	Substance
Transient	Course	Amnestic
Unspecified	Type	Mood
With Atypical Features	Type	Mood
With Behavioral Disturbance	Severity	Dementia/Alzheimer's

VISUAL 3.2 *(continued)*

Specifier	Type	Disorder
With Catatonic Features	Severity	Mood
With Delayed Onset	Course	PTSD
With Depressive Features	Type	Mood
With Full Interepisode Recovery	Course	Mood
With Gender Dysphoria	Type	Transvestic Fetishism
With Generalized Anxiety	Severity	Anxiety
With Good Prognostic Features	Severity	Schizophreniform
With Impaired Arousal	Type	Substance-Induced Sex. Dysf.
With Impaired Desire	Type	Substance-Induced Sex. Dysf.
With Impaired Orgasm	Type	Substance-Induced Sex. Dysf.
With Manic Features	Type	Mood
With Marked Stressor(s)	Severity	Brief Psychotic
With Melancholic Features	Severity	Mood
With Mixed Features	Type	Mood
With Obsessive-Compulsive Symptoms	Severity	Anxiety
With Onset During Intoxication	Course	Substance/Substance Induced Psychotic/Substance Induced Sleep/Substance-Induced Sex. Dysf.
With Onset During Withdrawal	Course	Substance
With Panic Attacks	Severity	Anxiety
With Perceptual Disturbance	Severity	Cocaine Intoxication
With Physiological Dependence	Severity	Substance
With Poor Insight	Severity	OCD/Hypochondriasis
With Postpartum Onset	Course	Brief Psychotic/Mood
With Postpartum Onset	Course	Mood
With Prominent Negative Symptoms	Severity	Schizophrenia
With Rapid Cycling	Course	Mood
With Seasonal Pattern	Course	Mood
With Self-Injurious Behavior	Severity	Separation Anxiety
With Sexual Pain	Type	Substance-Induced Sex. Dysf.
Without Full Interepisode Recovery	Course	Mood
Without Good Prognostic Features	Severity	Schizophreniform
Without Marked Stressor(s)	Severity	Brief Psychotic
Without Physiological Dependence	Severity	Substance

Note: In the disorders column at the right, the disorders have been described only with key words to save space. In some instances, only the class of the disorder has been listed. The word disorder has been deleted to save space. The distinction between a severity and type specifier is at times difficult to make. In some instances, these terms can be considered to be interchangeable.

Recurrence

Recurrence of a disorder after a period of full remission or recovery can take several forms, and the diagnosis of a recurrence is a matter of clinical judgment. There are three options for indicating recurrence: (1) if the symptoms constitute a new episode of a disorder, this can be diagnosed as current or provisional, even before the full criteria for the disorder are met; (2) if the symptoms are clinically significant, but do not clearly indicate a recurrence of the previously diagnosed disorder, the appropriate Not Otherwise Specified category can be used; or (3) if the symptoms are not clinically significant, the term "Prior History" can be noted after listing the disorder.

Principal Diagnosis

The principal diagnosis is the condition that is the basis for the admission of a person to an inpatient setting, or the main reason for the visit of the person to an outpatient setting, and it is the main focus of clinical attention with respect to treatment. The principal diagnosis is always recorded as the first diagnosis on Axis I. If multiple Axis I diagnoses are made, the others are listed in priority order in regard to focus of clinical attention. If Axis I and Axis II diagnoses are present, the principal diagnosis is assumed to be on Axis I unless the Axis II diagnosis is followed by the phrase "(Principal Diagnosis)." Visual 3.3 illustrates how to record a principal diagnosis.

Provisional Diagnosis

The specifier provisional is used when the diagnostician is reasonably certain the person will meet the full criteria for the disorder, but needs more information before the diagnosis can be made. Provisional diagnosis is indicated by writing the word "(Provisional)" after the diagnosis code and description of the disorder. Visual 3.3 illustrates how to record a provisional diagnosis.

Not Otherwise Specified Categories

Each class of disorders has at least one Not Otherwise Specified (NOS) category. This category is at the end of the section for that disorder, and this designation is used when the person has some features of the disorder or unique features that do not precisely fit the class. If one of the following

VISUAL 3.3. Illustration of Principal and Provisional Diagnosis

		Diagnosis 1: Principal Diagnosis on Axis I
Axis I:	300.6	Depersonalization Disorder
	307.1	Anorexia Nervosa, Binge-Eating/Purging Type
Axis II:	V71.09	No Dx.
		Diagnosis 2: Principal Diagnosis on Axis II
Axis I:	300.15	Dissociative Disorder NOS
	303.90	Alcohol Dependence, With Physiological Dependence
	305.60	Cocaine Abuse, Prior History
Axis II:	301.83	Borderline Personality Disorder **(Principal Diagnosis)**
		Diagnosis 3: Provisional Diagnosis
Axis I:	304.30	Cannabis Dependence, Without Physiological Dependence
	300.4	Dysthymic Disorder, Late Onset **(Provisional)**
Axis II:	799.9	Dx. Deferred

four conditions exists, the NOS diagnosis may be the most appropriate designation of the disorder to use:

1. The person conforms to the general criteria of the disorder, but the symptoms do not meet the criteria for a specific disorder. The symptoms may be below the threshold for a disorder, but clinically significant, or the symptoms may be atypical or mixed.
2. The person does not meet the criteria for any DSM-IV disorder in the main classification, but is in clinically significant distress. The criteria for some symptom patterns of this nature are included in Appendix B: Criteria Sets and Axes Provided for Further Study (pp. 703-761). These disorders are being considered for inclusion in the main classification system, but are undergoing further research before a decision is made to give the disorders full status. These disorders can be diagnosed under the NOS category for specific disorders. For example:

   300.15 Dissociative Disorder NOS, **Dissociative Trance Disorder**

   Some disorders have the possible Appendix B disorder explained in the NOS category, whereas others do not. The diagnostician should remain alert to the possible use of the Appendix B disorders in unclear circumstances.

3. Etiology is uncertain. This can occur when it is unknown whether the disorder is due to a GMC, is substance induced, or is primary.

Tip: In the DSM-IV, primary mental disorder refers to a disorder that is not due to a general medical condition (GMC) or is not substance induced (see p. 165).

---

4. The diagnostician does not have time to complete data collection, data are inconsistent or contradictory, but the symptoms can be placed within a class of disorders.

Indication of Diagnostic Uncertainty

The DSM-IV provides several ways to indicate diagnostic uncertainty:

1. Use the V codes included in the section of the manual titled "Other Conditions That May Be a Focus of Clinical Attention." This section of the DSM-IV lists conditions that may or not be related to diagnosis of a mental disorder but are a focus of clinical attention. These conditions can be recorded on Axis I. The name of the condition is preceded by a numeric code that begins with the letter *V.* These conditions are often referred to as the "V codes."

Tip: Most payers for mental health services will not reimburse for V-code conditions.

---

2. Use 799.9 Diagnosis or Condition Deferred on Axis I or 799.9 Diagnosis Deferred on Axis II. These codes are used when the diagnostician does not have enough information to make a diagnosis and is unable to even make a tentative diagnosis (provisional diagnosis).
3. Use 300.9 Unspecified Mental Disorder (nonpsychotic). This code is used when the mental disorder present is not covered in the DSM-IV, when no NOS category is appropriate, or when a nonpsychotic disorder is apparent but not enough information is available to diagnose a DSM-IV disorder.
4. The Not Otherwise Specified category (NOS) for a disorder can be used. This category was explained previously.
5. A specific diagnosis is given with the "(Provisional)" designation. This designation was explained earlier.

Frequently Used Criteria

The Frequently Used Criteria section explains four types of common criteria. The first criteria are used to exclude certain diagnoses and to suggest others. The DSM-IV classification uses criteria sets in making determinations about what conditions must be met to diagnose a specific disorder. The criteria for each disorder are listed with alphabetic characters in the "diagnostic dialogue boxes" that summarize the disorder. These criteria are of two types—inclusion and exclusion. Inclusion criteria are conditions, behaviors, and symptoms that a person must have to be diagnosed with the disorder, and when certain conditions, behaviors, or symptoms do or do not exist, the person does not have that disorder. Exclusion criteria are generally used to assist with differential diagnosis. Certain phrases are used with exclusion criteria, such as the following:

- **"Criteria have never been met for . . . "** Used to establish a lifetime hierarchy among disorders. For example, the diagnosis Major Depressive Disorder cannot be given after a Manic Episode has occurred, and the diagnosis must be changed to Bipolar Disorder.
- **"Criteria are not met for . . . "** Used to define the relationship between disorders or subtypes. This is explained as the specifier With Melancholic Features takes precedence over With Atypical Features in a Major Depressive Episode.
- **"does not occur exclusively during the course of . . . "** Prevents diagnosing a disorder when the symptoms occur only in the course of another disorder. For example, Bulimia Nervosa is not diagnosed separately if it occurs only during occurrences of Anorexia Nervosa.
- **"not due to the direct physiological effects of a substance (e.g., a drug of abuse, a medication) or a general medical condition."** Used to indicate that substance-induced and general medical conditions are ruled out as causative factors before the disorder is diagnosed.
- **"not better accounted for by . . . "** Used to indicate that disorders mentioned in the criterion must be considered in the differential diagnosis. Clinical judgment is used when boundaries between disorders cannot be established.

The second common criteria set is for substance-induced disorders. It is often difficult to determine if symptoms are substance induced, and two criteria have been added to the substance-induced disorders to aid the diagnostician in making this distinction. These criteria provide general guidelines, but clinical judgment remains the determinant of whether the symptoms are a result of the physiological effects of a substance. The criteria are as follows:

- There is evidence from the history, physical examination, or laboratory findings that either the symptoms developed during or within a month of Substance Intoxication or Withdrawal, or medication use caused the disorder.
- The disturbance is not better accounted for by a disorder that is not substance induced. Indicators of this are (1) the symptoms preceded the onset of substance use; (2) the symptoms persist for approximately one month after acute withdrawal or intoxication has stopped; (3) symptoms are in excess of what would be expected given the type, duration, or amount of the substance used; or (4) other evidence exists suggesting an independent, non-substance-induced disorder. See page 193 for further information about these criteria.

The third criteria set is for a Mental Disorder Due to a General Medical Condition. The following criterion is applied to every mental disorder that is attributed to a GMC: There is evidence from the history, physical examination, or laboratory findings that the disturbance is the direct physiological result of a general medical condition. See page 166 for further discussion of this criterion.

The fourth criteria set is the criteria for clinical significance. This is a brief, but important, discussion. The mental disorder definition used by the DSM-IV requires the person to have clinically significant impairment or distress to be diagnosed with a disorder. To remind the diagnostician of this, most disorders include a clinical significance criterion stating "causes clinically significant distress or impairment in social, occupational, or other important areas of functioning" (p. 7). This statement establishes a threshold of degree of impaired functioning in deciding whether a person has a mental disorder. Clinical judgment is crucial in determining clinical significance and in making a diagnosis. These skills can be developed through experience in evaluating many clients, familiarity with all criteria for the different disorders, as well as reading practice guidelines and attending continuing education seminars for specific disorders.

Types of Information in the DSM-IV Text

The diagnostic classification for each disorder is organized according to a standard set of headings that is slightly different from the DSM-III-R version. The following are the headings used in the DSM-IV (some are not used if information is unavailable in that area).

- *Diagnostic Features:* States the diagnostic criteria and sometimes provides illustrations.

Tip: The Diagnostic Features section begins with a key summarization of the disorder and is critical for beginning diagnosticians to read.

- *Subtypes/Specifiers:* Defines and explains subtypes and specifiers if they are used with the disorder. Not included with all disorders.
- *Recording Procedures:* Provides guidelines for reporting the name of the disorder and for selecting an ICD-9 diagnostic code. Can include instructions for using subtypes/specifiers. Not included with all disorders.
- *Associated Features and Disorders:* Usually contains three parts:

  1. associated descriptive features and mental disorders,
  2. associated laboratory findings, and
  3. associated physical examination findings and general medical conditions.

- *Specific Culture, Age, and Gender Features:* Provides guidance for taking into consideration cultural, developmental, or gender factors.
- *Prevalence*: Contains information on occurrence and lifetime prevalence, incidence, and lifetime risk. Data are reported for different settings when information exists.
- *Course:* Provides information on lifetime patterns and the usual evolution of the disorder.
- *Familiar Pattern:* Describes frequency of the disorder for first-degree biological relatives of the person compared with its frequency in the general population.
- *Differential Diagnosis:* Identifies how to differentiate the disorder from similar disorders.

These sections are followed by what I refer to as "diagnostic dialogue boxes" which are double-border boxes similar to this one:

■ Diagnostic Criteria

The DSM-IV system refers to these boxes as "diagnostic criteria." The tendency is to turn to the "diagnostic dialogue boxes" immediately when considering a disorder because the boxes appear to be a quick and easy way to apply a diagnosis, since the information in the boxes summarizes the disorder and outlines its criteria and symptoms. I do not recommend this strategy until one is thoroughly familiar with a disorder. When learning a disorder, one should carefully read the text sections for the disorder before moving to the diagnostic dialogue box. Crucial information about the disorder is explained in the text sections and may not be apparent in the box summary. Even experienced clinicians are often required to go to the text section to clarify the nature of a disorder. Also, the text section can be quite helpful in creating client confidence in the clinician. When the clinician has read about associated disorders, cultural features, or familial patterns, he or she can ask the client pertinent questions: "Have you ever had a problem with . . . ?" or "Has anyone in your family had . . . ?" This demonstrates that the clinician is familiar with the symptoms and behaviors that constitute the functional problems the client is experiencing. Such familiarity can be reassuring to the client.

Tip: The diagnostic criteria "boxes" feature two different symbols that precede the name of the disorder printed in bold at the top of the box. One symbol is a black square ■, and the other symbol is a white square □ . The black square is printed in the box where the criteria begin; if the criteria set continues on another page, the white square is used on the second page to indicate that previous material relates to that disorder. Continued criteria sets are also indicated by *(continued)* printed after the heading.

Tip: If you do not understand any item in the diagnostic dialogue box, return to the text section to find the answer. Never record a diagnosis when you do not understand all the information in the diagnostic dialogue box!

DSM-IV Organizational Plan

This discussion gives an overview of the sections of the manual that deal with classification of disorders. Simply stated, the classification system has two major divisions. The first division, which is the bulk of the manual, contains sixteen diagnostic classes with over 300 disorders; the second division is a brief one titled "Other Conditions That May Be a Focus of Clinical Attention." The sixteen classes of disorders are explained in Visual 3.4, and Visual 3.5 details the categories of the second division.

VISUAL 3.4. Classes of DSM-IV Disorders

- **Disorders Usually First Diagnosed in Infancy, Childhood, or Adolescence**

1. While *usually* diagnosed in infancy, childhood, and adolescence, the disorders in this section can be diagnosed in adults if it can be determined they meet the criteria for the disorders.

2. Infants, children, and adolescents can be diagnosed with disorders in other sections of the manual if they meet the criteria for the disorder.

- **Delirium, Dementia, and Amnestic and Cognitive Disorders**
- **Mental Disorders Due to a General Medical Condition Not Elsewhere Classified**
- **Substance-Related Disorders**

In DSM-III-R these disorders were grouped together under the heading of *Organic Mental Syndromes and Disorders.* The terminology "organic mental disorder" is not used in the DSM-IV.

These disorders are presented before the other disorders because of their importance in differential diagnosis.

- **Schizophrenia and Other Psychotic Disorders**
- **Mood Disorders**
- **Anxiety Disorders**
- **Somatoform Disorders**
- **Factitious Disorders**
- **Dissociative Disorders**
- **Sexual and Gender Identity Disorders**
- **Eating Disorders**
- **Sleep Disorders**
- **Impulse-Control Disorders Not Elsewhere Classified**
- **Adjustment Disorders**
- **Personality Disorders**

Classes grouped on the basis of shared features, except for Adjustment Disorders, which are based on common etiology.

Other Conditions That May Be a Focus of Clinical Attention

Psychological Factors Affecting Medical Condition
Medication-Induced Movement Disorders
Other Medication-Induced Disorders
Relational Problems
Problems Related to Abuse or Neglect
Additional Conditions That May Be a Focus of Clinical Attention
Condition is focus of treatment and person does not have mental disorder.
Person has mental disorder but it is unrelated to the problem.
Person has mental disorder related to the problem, but the condition is severe enough to need independent clinical attention.

Recorded on Axis I

VISUAL 3.5. Summary of "Other Conditions That May Be a Focus of Clinical Attention" Section of the DSM-IV

Problem is focus of diagnosis or treatment and person has no mental disorder, has a coexisting, unrelated mental disorder, or has problem related to mental disorder.

Psychological Factors Affecting Medical Condition

316	Psychological Factor Affecting Medical Condition

Medication-Induced Movement Disorders

332.1	Neuroleptic-Induced Parkinsonism
333.92	Neuroleptic Malignant Syndrome
333.7	Neuroleptic-Induced Acute Dystonia
333.99	Neuroleptic-Induced Acute Akathisia
333.82	Neuroleptic-Induced Tardive Dyskinesia
333.1	Medication-Induced Postural Tremor
333.90	Medication-Induced Movement Disorder NOS

Other Medication-Induced Disorder

995.2	Adverse Effects of Medication NOS

Relational Problems

V61.9	Relational Problem Related to a MD or GMC
V61.20	Parent-Child Relational Problem
V61.10	Partner Relational Problem
V61.8	Sibling Relational Problem
V62.81	Relational Problem NOS

Problems Related to Abuse or Neglect

V61.21	Physical Abuse of Child (*Note:* Coded as 995.54 if victim clinical focus)
V61.21	Sexual Abuse of Child (*Note:* Coded as 995.53 if victim clinical focus)
V61.21	Neglect of Child (*Note:* Coded as 995.52 if victim clinical focus)
V61.1	Physical Abuse of Adult (*Note:* Coded as V61.12 if focus of clinical attention is perpetrator and abuse is by partner, V62.83 if focus of clinical attention is perpetrator and abuse is by person other than partner, 995.81 if victim clinical focus)

Additional Conditions That May Be a Focus of Clinical Attention

V15.81	Noncompliance With Treatment (e.g., discomfort, medication side-effects, cost, religion, culture, personality traits, PDs)
V65.2	Malingering (e.g., intentional production of symptoms motivated by external inducements, i.e., avoidance of military, work, or to gain financial compensation)
V71.01	Adult Antisocial Behavior (antisocial behavior not due to a MD)
V71.02	Child or Adolescent Antisocial Behavior (antisocial behavior not due to MD)
V62.89	Borderline Intellectual Functioning (IQ range 71-84); *Note:* Coded on Axis II.
780.9	Age-Related Cognitive Decline
V62.82	Bereavement
V62.3	Academic Problem
V62.2	Occupational Problem
313.82	Identity Problem
V62.89	Religious or Spiritual Problem
V62.4	Acculturation Problem
V62.89	Phase of Life Problem

Source: American Psychiatric Association, 1994, pp. 675-686. Reprinted with permission from the *Diagnostic and Statistical Manual of Mental Disorders,* Fourth Edition. Copyright 1994 American Psychiatric Association.

DSM-IV CLASSIFICATION

The disorders summarized in Visual 3.4 are presented in detail in the front of the DSM-IV as a "table of contents" titled "DSM-IV Classification," which appears from page 13 to page 24 of the manual. Diagnosticians should become familiar with this section, as it is the best way to learn the classes, their arrangement, and the disorders within each classification.

Tip: In the "DSM-IV Classification" from page 13 to page 24, the gray-shaded areas represent the sixteen classes. The disorders for each class are printed below the gray-shaded heading. The disorder numeric codes are printed to the left of the disorder, making this section of the manual a nice reference tool for finding codes. The page location of the disorder text is printed to the right in parentheses.

MULTIAXIAL ASSESSMENT

The "Multiaxial Assessment" section at the beginning of the DSM-IV (pp. 25-35) explains the multiaxial system that is the recommended format for recording and reporting a diagnosis. The multiaxial format, introduced in the DSM-III (1980), is used to promote a comprehensive evaluation of the person. The system uses the following five axes to record a diagnosis:

Axis I	Clinical Disorders
	Other Conditions That May Be a Focus of Clinical Attention
Axis II	Personality Disorders
	Mental Retardation
Axis III	General Medical Conditions (GMCs)
Axis IV	Psychosocial and Environmental Problems
Axis V	Global Assessment of Functioning (GAF)

This section of the DSM-IV explains each axis and gives a listing of the disorders that are recorded on each axis (see pp. 26-27). These pages are helpful references for remembering the distinction between Axis I and Axis II disorders. This section includes an explanation of the GAF scale, which is printed on page 32. The clinician should refer to this page when learning the elements of the GAF. The section concludes with an example of a multiaxial diagnosis, a multiaxial reporting form, and examples of how to record a diagnosis when the multiaxial format is not used.

Chapter 4 provides a detailed explanation of how to perform and record a multiaxial diagnosis based on this section of the DSM-IV.

DISORDERS CATEGORIES

The specific categories of disorders are not discussed in detail here. Each category is covered individually in its own chapter (see Chapters 5-21).

ADDITIONAL CODES

Another section of the DSM-IV that is important to discuss at this point is titled "Additional Codes" (p. 687). This simple, one-page section lists the codes to use when the case involves an unspecified mental disorder, one not included in the DSM-IV; no diagnosis is made on Axis I or Axis II; or the diagnosis is deferred. The codes listed in this section are as follows:

300.9 Unspecified Mental Disorder (nonpsychotic)
(Indicates a mental disorder not in the DSM-IV, no appropriate NOS category, or insufficient information to make a diagnosis.)

V71.09 No Diagnosis or Condition on Axis I
(Indicates no mental disorder or condition is found to be present on Axis I.)

799.9 Diagnosis or Condition Deferred on Axis I
(Indicates insufficient information to make an Axis I diagnosis.)

V71.09 No Diagnosis on Axis II
(Indicates no mental disorder or condition is found to be present on Axis II.)

799.9 Diagnosis Deferred on Axis II
(Indicates insufficient information to make an Axis II diagnosis.)

Tip: When recording a multiaxial diagnosis, never leave an axis blank even if no disorder is diagnosed on the axis. Enter the appropriate "V code" from the additional codes section. If an axis is left blank, anyone reading the multiaxial diagnosis cannot determine if the diagnostician simply forgot to enter the diagnosis or there is no diagnosis on the axis. For example, entering the code V71.09 No Diagnosis on Axis I indicates that the diagnostician reviewed the person and found no disorder or condition on that axis.

APPENDIXES

The DSM-IV has ten appendixes, which are summarized on pages 10 and 11. Visual 3.6 provides a visual summary of the appendixes. Diagnosticians should become familiar with the appendixes. They contain important information that can be helpful in doing effective diagnosis, such as Appendix A, which contains decision trees for differential diagnosis, and information that is essential to diagnosis under certain conditions, such as Appendix I, which contains an outline for a cultural formulation and a glossary of culture-bound syndromes.

Visual 3.7 illustrates the criteria for the diagnosis of Dysthymic Disorder, found on page 349 in the DSM-IV. This illustration identifies many of the factors described in this chapter. This visual is also to be used with Visuals 4.5 and 4.6 in Chapter 4 that illustrate a diagnosis and treatment plan based on Dysthymic Disorder.

INDEX

A section of the DSM-IV that cannot be overlooked is the index. The index can be a quick way to find many disorders, conditions, and symptoms. Some index items have two-page references. The first page number is the page on which the discussion of the disorder begins. The second page reference is in parentheses and refers to the page where the diagnostic criteria "box" for that disorder begins. For example, the listing for Antisocial Personality Disorder appears as:

Antisocial personality disorder, 645 (649)

Page 645 is where the descriptive material for Antisocial Personality Disorder begins, and page 649 is where the diagnostic criteria for Antisocial Personality Disorder begin.

RECOMMENDED READING

A number of books are available to aid in learning how to diagnose and record the classes of disorders in the DSM-IV. Videotapes and audiotapes are also available for learning proposes. The following are the most commonly used DSM-IV resource materials.

The Internet is a good resource for information about specific disorders. One limitation of the Internet as a resource is that some well-known

VISUAL 3.6. DSM-IV Appendixes Overview

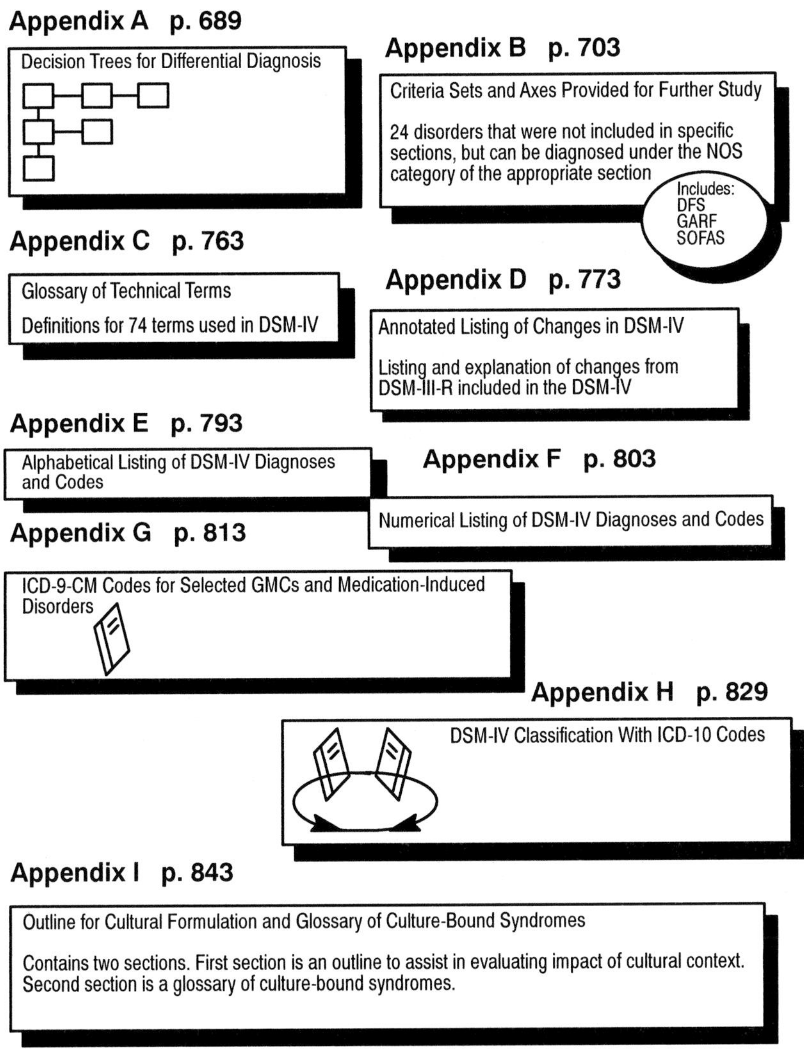

Source: American Psychiatric Association, 1994, DSM-IV, pp. 689-873.

VISUAL 3.7. Illustration of Diagnostic Criteria for 300.4 Dysthymic Disorder

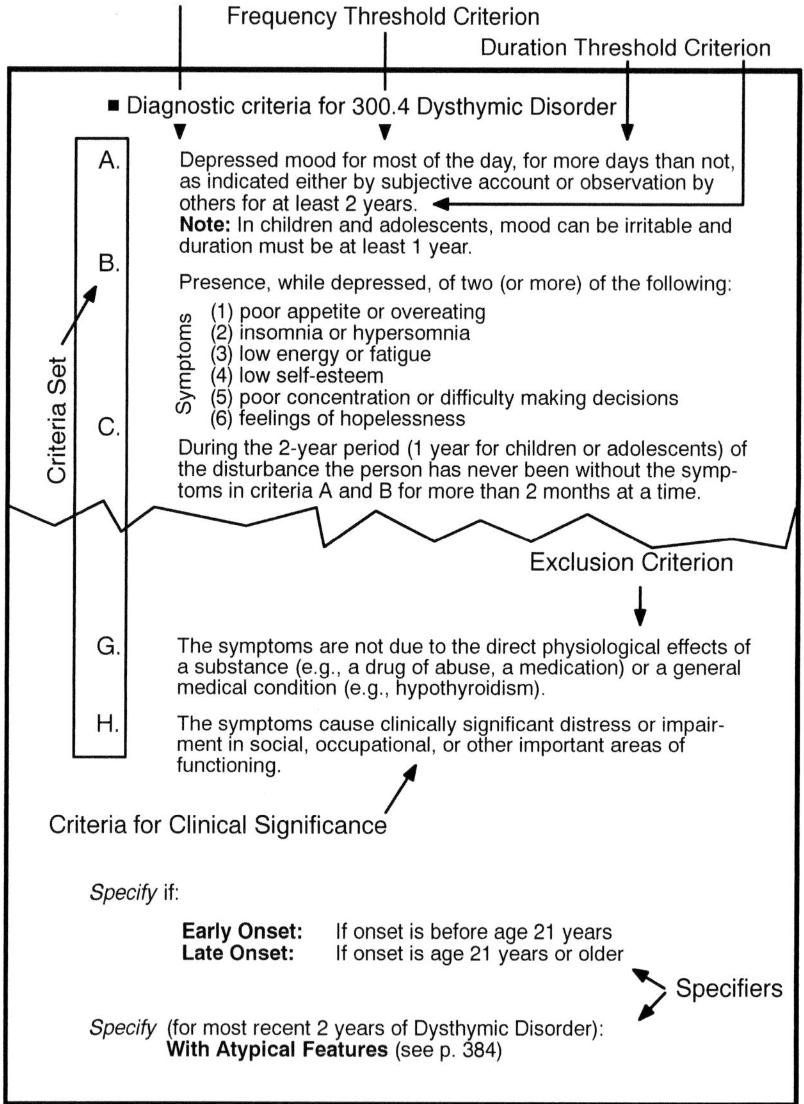

Source: American Psychiatric Association, 1994, pp. 345-349. Reprinted with permission from the *Diagnostic and Statistical Manual of Mental Disorders,* Fourth Edition. Copyright 1994 American Psychiatric Association.

disorders (e.g., Autistic Disorder, Obsessive-Compulsive Disorder, and Bipolar Disorder) have so many Web sites that searching for the most helpful ones can be very time-consuming. I have found that it is better to purchase books that aid in finding good Web sites containing DSM-IV disorders information rather than performing a search myself. The best Internet-related resource to date for the DSM-IV disorders is Morrison and Stamps's book *DSM-IV Internet Companion.*

American Psychiatric Association (1994). *Diagnostic and Statistical Manual of Mental Disorders,* Fourth Edition. Washington, DC: American Psychiatric Association.

American Psychiatric Association (1994). *DSM-IV Sourcebook,* Volume 1. Washington, DC: American Psychiatric Association.

Edgerton, J. and Campbell, R. J. (1994). *American Psychiatry Glossary.* Washington, DC: American Psychiatric Association.

Fauman, M. A. (1994). *Study Guide to DSM-IV.* Washington, DC: American Psychiatric Association.

First, M. B., Frances, A., and Pincus, H. N. (1995). *DSM-IV Handbook of Differential Diagnosis.* Washington, DC: American Psychiatric Association.

First, M. B., Gibbon, M., Spitzer, R. L., Williams, J. B. W., and Benjamin, L. (1997). *Structured Clinical Interview for DSM-IV Axis II Disorders (SCID-II).* Washington, DC: American Psychiatric Association.

First, M. B., Spitzer, R. L., Gibbon, M., and Williams, J. B. W. (1997). *Structured Clinical Interview for DSM-IV Axis I Disorders (SCID-I), Clinical Version.* Washington, DC: American Psychiatric Association.

Frances, A. (1995). *DSM-IV Audio Review.* Washington, DC: American Psychiatric Press.

Frances, A. and First, M. B. (1998). *Your Mental Health: A Layman's Guide to the Psychiatrist's Bible.* New York: Scribner.

Frances, A., First, M. B., and Pincus, H. N. (1995). *DSM-IV Guidebook: The Essential Companion to the* Diagnostic and Statistical Manual of Mental Disorders. Washington, DC: American Psychiatric Association.

Frances, A. and Ross, R. (1996). *DSM-IV Case Studies: A Guide to Differential Diagnosis.* Washington, DC: American Psychiatric Press.

House, A. E. (1999). *DSM-IV Diagnosis in the Schools.* New York: Guilford.

Kaplan, H. I. and Sadock, B. J. (1998). *Synopsis of Psychiatry: Behavioral Sciences/Clinical Psychiatry,* Eighth Edition. Baltimore, MD: Williams and Wilkins.

Kennedy, J. A. (1992). *Fundamentals of Psychiatric Treatment Planning.* Washington, DC: American Psychiatric Press.

Morrision, J. (1994). *The First Interview: Revised for DSM-IV.* New York: Guilford.

Morrison, J. (1995). *DSM-IV Made Easy: The Clinicians' Guide to Diagnosis.* New York: Guilford.

Morrison, M. R. and Stamps, R. E. (1998). *DSM-IV Internet Companion.* New York: Norton.

Othmer, E. and Othmer, S. C. (1994). *The Clinical Interview Using DSM-IV, Volume 1: Fundamentals.* Washington, DC: American Psychiatric Association.

Othmer, E. and Othmer, S. C. (1994). *The Clinical Interview Using DSM-IV, Volume 2: The Difficult Patient.* Washington, DC: American Psychiatric Association.

Pliszka, S. R., Carlson, C. L., and Swanson, J. M. (1999). *ADHD with Comorbid Disorders.* New York: Guilford.

Rapoport, J. L. and Ismond, D. R. (1996). *DSM-IV Training Guide for Diagnosis of Childhood Disorders.* New York: Brunner/Mazel.

Samuels, S. K. and Sikorsky, S. A. (1998). *Clinical Evaluations of School-Aged Children,* Second Edition. Sarasota, FL: Professional Resource Press.

Spitzer, R. L., Gibbon, M., Skodol, A. E., Williams, J. B. W., and First, M. B. (1995). *DSM-IV Casebook.* Washington, DC: American Psychiatric Association.

Video/Audio/Electronic Resources

Diagnosis According to the DSM-IV (1994). New York: Newbridge Communications.

DSM-IV Audio Review (1995). Washington, DC: American Psychiatric Association.

DSM-IV Video Case Reviews (1995). Washington, DC: American Psychiatric Association.

DSM-IV Videotaped Clinical Vignettes (1995). New York: Brunner/Mazel.

Electronic DSM-IV Plus, Version 3.0 (1999). Washington, DC: American Psychiatric Association.

Highlights of the DSM-IV (1996). Washington, DC: American Psychological Association.

Video Review of Psychiatry (1999). New York: Specialty Preparation Inc.

REFERENCE

American Psychiatric Association (1994). *Diagnostic and Statistical Manual of Mental Disorders,* Fourth Edition. Washington, DC: American Psychiatric Association.

Chapter 4

The Multiaxial System

INTRODUCTION

The heart of the DSM-IV system is the multiaxial format that uses five levels or areas to perform a thorough diagnosis. This system, introduced in the DSM-III, recognizes the complexity of diagnosis and the interrelatedness of the many factors that are components of a mental disorder diagnosis. The multiaxial system generally takes into account psychological, physical, internal, external, developmental, and social factors. The five axes that make up the system are as follows:

Axis I: Clinical Disorders
Other Conditions That May Be a Focus of Clinical Attention

Axis II: Personality Disorders
Mental Retardation

Axis III: General Medical Conditions

Axis IV: Psychosocial and Environmental Problems

Axis V: Global Assessment of Functioning

Visual 4.1 summarizes the five axes.

AXIS I: CLINICAL DISORDERS AND AXIS II: PERSONALITY DISORDERS AND MENTAL RETARDATION

Axis I and Axis II are the key components of the multiaxial system and are used to record the 340 disorders in the classification system. The distinction between the two axes has a somewhat historical basis. Axis I is

VISUAL 4.1. DSM-IV Multiaxial System Overview

Axis I Clinical Disorders

ICA Disorders (excluding Mental Retardation)
Delirium, Dementia, Amnesia, Other Cognitive Disorders
Mental Disorders Due to General Medical Condition
Substance-Related Disorders
Schizophrenia and Other Psychotic Disorders
Mood Disorders
Anxiety Disorders
Somatoform Disorders
Factitious Disorders
Dissociative Disorders
Sexual and Gender Identity Disorders
Eating Disorders
Sleep Disorders
Impulse-Control Disorders NEC
Adjustment Disorders
Other Conditions That May Be Focus of Clinical Attention

Axis II Personality Disorders and Mental Retardation

Paranoid Personality Disorder
Schizoid Personality Disorder
Schizotypal Personality Disorder
Antisocial Personality Disorder
Borderline Personality Disorder
Histrionic Personality Disorder
Narcissistic Personality Disorder
Avoidant Personality Disorder
Dependent Personality Disorder
Obsessive-Compulsive Personality Disorder
Personality Disorder NOS
Mental Retardation

Axis III General Medical Conditions

Infectious and Parasitic Diseases
Neoplasms
Endocrine, Nutritional, Metabolic, Immunity Disorders
Diseases of the Blood and Blood-Forming Organs
Diseases of the Nervous System and Sense Organs
Diseases of the Circulatory System
Diseases of the Respiratory System
Diseases of the Digestive System
Diseases of the Genitourinary System
Complications of Pregnancy, Childbirth, and the Puerperium
Diseases of the Skin and Subcutaneous Tissues
Diseases of the Musculoskeletal System and Connective Tissue
Congenital Anomalies
Certain Conditions Originating in the Perinatal Period
Symptoms, Signs, and Ill-Defined Conditions
Injury and Poisoning

Axis IV Psychosocial/ Environmental Problems

Problems with primary support group
Problems related to the social environment
Educational problems
Occupational problems
Housing problems
Economic problems
Problems with access to health care services
Problems related to the legal system/crime
Other psychosocial and environmental problems

Axis V Global Assessment of Functioning

100 / 91
90 / 81
80 / 71
70 / 61
60 / 51
50 / 41
40 / 31
30 / 21
20 / 11
10 / 1
0

Source: American Psychiatric Association, 1994, pp. 25-35. Reprinted with permission from the *Diagnostic and Statistical Manual of Mental Disorders,* Fourth Edition. Copyright 1994 American Psychiatric Association.

used to record what in the past were viewed as neuroses and psychoses, and Axis II is used to record what were referred to as character disorders. Neuroses were considered deficiencies and limitations that could impair, but not chronically alter, almost all areas of functioning and could be effectively relieved with intervention. Character disorders were viewed as long-standing defects ingrained in the developmental process of childhood that caused major, lifelong dysfunction in most aspects of life and were not generally amenable to treatment. This is most likely why payers consistently reimburse clinicians for Axis I disorders and not Axis II disorders, since Axis I disorders can be changed through intervention, whereas Axis II disorders are unalterable, and paying for treatment of intractable disorders is an inefficient use of funds.

In the current system, Axis I is used to record clinical disorders in the main section of the DSM-IV (pp. 37-673), as well as other conditions that may be a focus of clinical attention, which are found in a separate section near the end of the manual (pp. 675-686). Axis II is used for reporting personality disorders and mental retardation. A separate axis is included for personality disorders and mental retardation to ensure that they are not overlooked, since Axis I disorders are more evident during an assessment. Axis II can also be used to record maladaptive personality features and defense mechanisms. The habitual maladaptive defense mechanisms are listed in Appendix B of the DSM-IV (pp. 751-757). Personality features and defense mechanisms are recorded without codes. Examples of how to record these factors are on page 33 of the DSM-IV.

Tip: Remember from Chapter 3 that the principal diagnosis is recorded as the first diagnosis on Axis I. If Axis I and Axis II diagnoses are made, and the principal diagnosis is on Axis II, the phrase "(Principal Diagnosis)" is entered after the diagnosis is recorded. The phrase "(Reason for Visit)" can also be used. If no diagnosis is on Axis I or Axis II, enter V71.09 No Diagnosis on Axis I/II. If diagnosis is deferred on Axis I or Axis II, enter 799.9 Diagnosis Deferred on Axis I/II. If the diagnosis is provisional, enter the word "(Provisional)" after the diagnosis.

AXIS III: GENERAL MEDICAL CONDITIONS

Axis III is used to record coexisting physical disorders that may be associated with a mental disorder or may be independent of the mental disorder but related to its treatment. Disorders recorded on Axis III are found in the ICD-9-CM *(International Classification of Diseases,* Ninth

Revision, Clinical Modification). Appendix G of the DSM-IV has a summary listing of the medical conditions that are to be listed on Axis III. The GMCs listed in Appendix G are only some of the many ICD-9 disorders that can be recorded on Axis III. The ICD-9-CM code and name of the disorder should be written in the same format as Axis I and Axis II disorders.

Tip: Any disorder listed on Axis III by a mental health professional who is not a physician should be followed by "As Reported By . . . " and the person who reported the Axis III disorder to the diagnostician. Some examples of how to list this person are "Identified Patient," "Primary Care Physician," "Mother," "Father," "Foster mother," or the person's name can be entered.

When a mental disorder is believed to be the direct result of a general medical condition, a Mental Disorder Due to a General Medical Condition should be recorded on Axis I, and the general medical condition should be recorded on Axis I and Axis III. Details of this type of diagnosis are explained in the "Mental Disorders Due to a General Medical Condition" section of the DSM-IV, which begins on page 165. This diagnosis should be made by a physician or in consultation with a physician. It is usually difficult to distinguish primary mental disorder and mental disorders due to GMCs. This difficulty is compounded because GMCs can exacerbate the symptoms of a mental disorder without causing the mental disorder. The two disorders can be connected through nonphysiological means, or the coexistence of the physical and mental disorders can be coincidental. For example, anxiety disorder symptoms can be precipitated by a psychosocial stressor rather than resulting directly from the physiological effects of a GMC. An example of how to record a mental disorder directly due to a general medical condition is shown below:

Axis I: 293.83 Mood Disorder Due to Hypertensive Heart Disease With Congestive Heart Failure, Severe

Axis II: V71.09 No Dx. on Axis II

Axis III: 402.91 Hypertensive heart disease with congestive heart failure as reported by primary care physician, Dr. John Smith

---

Tip: When dealing with the etiology connection between mental disorders and GMCs, read carefully the section "Mental Disorders Due to a General Medical Condition" (pp. 165-174). Three of these disorders are included in the section, but criteria for eight of these disorders are within other classes of disorders in the manual.

AXIS IV: PSYCHOSOCIAL AND ENVIRONMENTAL PROBLEMS (PEPs)

Axis IV is used to report psychosocial and environmental problems (PEPs) that may influence diagnosis, treatment, and prognosis of mental disorders. This section was overhauled for the DSM-IV. In DSM-III-R, the section was titled "Severity of Psychosocial Stressors" and contained eleven categories, each of which was assessed on a scale from 0 to 6 based on the severity of the stressor. For the DSM-IV, the title of the section was changed, the categories were reduced to nine, the specific factors for children and adolescents were eliminated, and the rating scale was eliminated. In the DSM-IV, psychosocial and environmental problems are listed in each category and are not rated.

A PEP can represent a range of events: a negative life event or experience; an environmental difficulty, deficiency, or impediment; a family dysfunction or distress; an interpersonal conflict or stress; absence of social supports; lack of resources; or any other problem that exists within the context of the person's mental disorder. PEPs can also develop as a consequence of the person's mental disorder.

The list of PEPs can be quite long for some people. The diagnostician must make a clinical judgment regarding which PEPs are the most significant in relation to the person's mental disorder. While all relevant PEPs should be listed, very long lists of PEPs should be avoided. If the list becomes too long, the practitioner may have to prioritize the PEPs and include only the most significant ones.

To control the number of PEPs listed, only PEPs evident during the year preceding the evaluation are listed. PEPs existing for more than one year can be listed if they continue to contribute to the mental disorder or are a focus of intervention. An example of this would be a prior rape that contributes to a diagnosis of dysthymic disorder and continues to be a focus in the treatment to address the dysthymia.

PEPs that become a primary focus of clinical attention can be recorded on Axis I using a code from the section titled "Other Conditions That May Be a Focus of Clinical Attention" (pp. 675-686).

Nine categories of PEPs are described on pages 29 and 30 of the DSM-IV. The categories are as follows:

1. Problems with primary support group
2. Problems related to the social environment
3. Educational problems
4. Occupational problems
5. Housing problems
6. Economic problems
7. Problems with access to health care services
8. Problems related to interaction with the legal system/crime
9. Other psychosocial and environmental problems

PEPs should be recorded in very brief phrases, and narrative statements should be avoided. At the same time, the phrase should include enough detail to convey understanding of the problem in a general sense. For example, instead of "poor academic performance" record "poor grades in science, math, and art." Instead of "loss of job" record "loss of job due to absenteeism."

AXIS V: GLOBAL ASSESSMENT OF FUNCTIONING (GAF)

Axis V provides a scale that gives a crude estimate of the person's current overall level of functioning. This information can be useful in establishing degree of impairment, planning treatment, and estimating outcome. The scale ranges from 0 to 100, with 100 representing superior functioning and 1 representing severe impairment and potential to harm self and others. A 0 is entered if inadequate information is available to assign a score. The GAF numeric scale is accompanied by text indicators used in assigning a score. Visual 4.2 summarizes the GAF. The actual GAF scale is on page 32 of the DSM-IV. The GAF scale applies only to psychological, social, and occupational functioning. Impairment due to physical or environmental functioning is excluded from the criteria for this scale. The rating assigned to the person should be based on the level of functioning at the time of the evaluation. This is done by listing the time frame in parentheses after recording the score. Multiple ratings at different times can be listed when appropriate, such as when the person has had a psychiatric hospital admission. The admission and discharge GAF scores can be indicative of the course of hospitalization. For example:

Axis V: GAF = 55 (at admission)
GAF = 70 (at discharge)

VISUAL 4.2. DSM-IV Global Assessment of Functioning (GAF) Scale

SUPERIOR FUNCTION	100–91	Superior functioning in wide range of activities; no symptoms.
ABSENT MINIMAL	90–81	Absent or minimal symptoms; good functioning in all areas; no more than everyday problems.
TRANSIENT	80–71	Symptoms are transient and expectable reactions to psychosocial stressors; no more than slight impairment in SOS functioning.
MILD	70–61	Some mild symptoms; some difficulty in SOS functioning; some meaningful interpersonal relationships.
MODERATE	60–51	Moderate symptoms; moderate difficulty in SOS functioning.
SERIOUS	50–41	Serious symptoms; serious impairment in SOS functioning.
IMPAIRED REALITY TESTING	40–31	Some impairment in reality testing or communication, or SOS functioning; serious impairment in family relations, judgment, thinking, or mood.
SERIOUS IMPAIRMENT	30–21	Behavior is considerably influenced by delusions or hallucinations or serious impairment of communication or judgment.
DANGER TO SELF, OTHERS	20–11	Some danger of hurting self or others, or occasionally fails to maintain minimal personal hygiene, or gross impairment in communication.
PERSISTENT DANGER	10–01	Persistent danger of severely hurting self or others, or persistent inability to maintain personal hygiene, or serious suicidal act with clear expectation of death.
INADEQUATE INFORMATION	0	Inadequate information.

Source: American Psychiatric Association, 1994, pp. 30-32. Reprinted with permission from the *Diagnostic and Statistical Manual of Mental Disorders,* Fourth Edition. Copyright 1994 American Psychiatric Association.

Note: SOS = Social, Occupational, School

ADDITIONAL FUNCTIONING ASSESSMENT SCALES

Social and Occupational Functioning Assessment Scale (SOFAS)

In settings in which it is appropriate to assess social and occupational functioning or disability impairment independent of psychological functioning, practitioners can use the Social and Occupational Functioning Assessment Scale (SOFAS), which is included in Appendix B: Criteria Sets and Axes Provided for Further Study of the DSM-IV (pp. 760-761). This scale may be integrated as a full feature of future DSM manuals if research on the scale proves it to be a reliable and useful measure. The SOFAS scale is based on the same numerical rating scale (0-100) as the GAF but uses slightly different criteria than the GAF.

Global Assessment of Relational Functioning (GARF) Scale

A related scale for assessing relationship functioning that has been included in Appendix B is the Global Assessment of Relational Functioning (GARF) Scale. Practitioners who do marriage, couples, and family therapy will find this scale helpful. The GARF scale uses the same numerical ratings (0-100) as the GAF, with detailed measurement criteria. Yingling and colleagues (1998) wrote a book titled *GARF Assessment Sourcebook,* which is a guide to using the GARF scale. Visual 4.3 summarizes the GARF scale.

Defensive Functioning Scale (DFS)

The Defensive Functioning Scale (DFS) (pp. 751-753) is included in Appendix B and is under consideration for inclusion as a scale in future versions of the DSM. Some have argued that this scale is one of the few remaining elements of the DSM-IV based on the work of psychoanalytically oriented theoreticians such as Adolph Meyer (see Chapter 2). Some psychodynamic practitioners believe that the DSM-IV lacks useful guidelines for their form of clinical practice (Frances, First, and Pincus, 1995). The DFS is based on defense mechanisms or coping styles that protect the person against anxiety, awareness of danger, or effects of stressors. The defense mechanisms are categorized in groups referred to as *Defense Levels.* To use the DFS, the clinician identifies up to seven defense mechanisms, in order of prominence, that are evident during the evaluation. The DFS is recorded in two parts:

1. *Current defenses or coping styles:* the clinician records up to seven defenses or coping strategies.
2. *Predominant current defense level:* the clinician records one of seven levels of functioning listed in the DSM-IV.

The DFS is further described and illustrated in Visual 22.2 in Chapter 22.

VISUAL 4.3. DSM-IV Global Assessment of Relational Functioning (GARF) Scale Summary

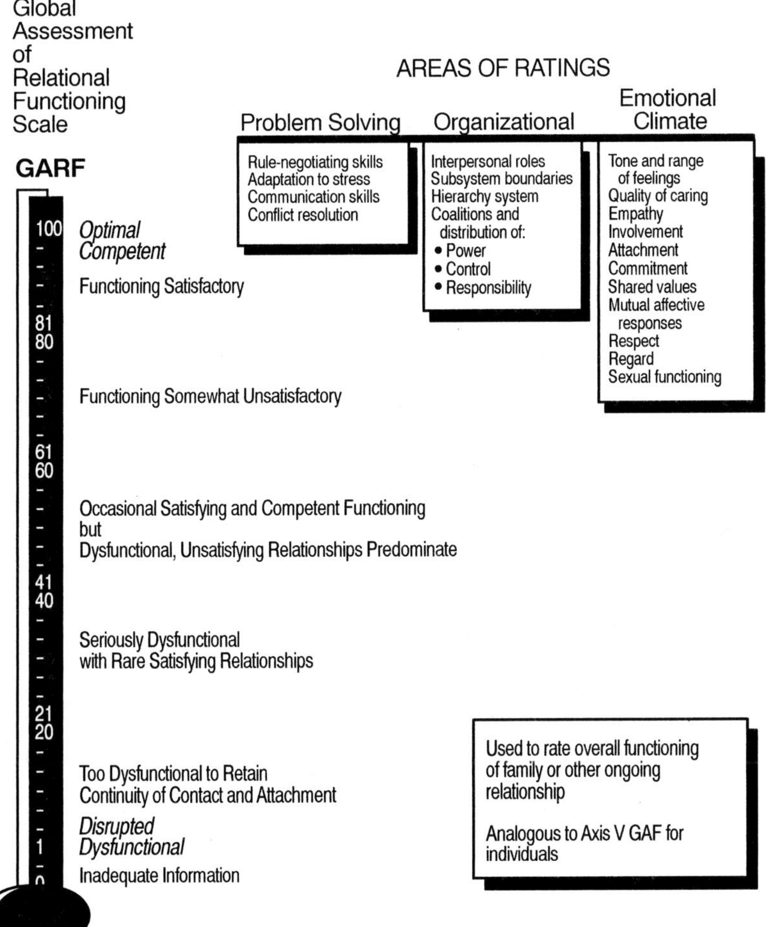

Source: American Psychiatric Association, 1994, pp. 758-759.

Tip: A caution about GAF scores is worth noting. GAF scores assigned by clinicians are being used by others to make decisions. For example, some managed care organizations use "GAF cutoff scores" to determine qualification for treatment or admission to psychiatric facilities. Other organizations use GAF scores to make decisions not necessarily related to the person's mental status. For example, the author is aware of one city housing authority that uses GAF scores of people discharged from state mental hospitals to determine eligibility for public housing. Clinicians can do little about these practices except raise concerns regarding such uses of GAF scores. These misapplications of GAF scores are pointed out here to alert practitioners to the importance of making GAF assessment as accurate as possible. It is also important to enter the time of the GAF score, which is required by the DSM-IV guidelines, to alert users that these scores can change significantly in a short period of time, depending on the person's circumstances.

Tip: The Social and Occupational Functioning Assessment Scale (SOFAS), Global Assessment of Relational Functioning (GARF) Scale, and Defensive Functioning Scale (DFS) are discussed in more detail in Chapter 23.

RULE OUT

The phrase "rule out" is not used in the DSM-IV as it was in previous editions of the manual. Rule out's most probable replacement is "(Provisional Diagnosis)." Rule out is appropriate in certain situations, such as when the possibility of a disorder may exist or be developing, in which you would not use the diagnosis-deferred designation; for example, with a child with possible symptoms of bipolar disorder whose father has bipolar disorder. The decision to use diagnosis deferred or rule out is a clinical judgment. The term rule out is no longer used as a multiaxial system term. However, the diagnostician should use a conceptual rule-out process in each case. Most disorders in the DSM-IV have rule-out-oriented diagnostic criteria referred to as exclusion criteria. The two most common exclusion criteria are related to ruling out substances or general medical conditions as a cause of the disorder. Other factors or disorders that must be commonly ruled out in the assessment process are malingering or factitious disorder, cultural influences, age-appropriate behaviors, and other conditions that may be a focus of clinical attention, such as physical abuse, sexual abuse, and neglect in children. Visual 4.4 illustrates the rule-out process the diagnostician should use in making each diagnosis.

VISUAL 4.4. Rule-Out Process and Differential Diagnosis

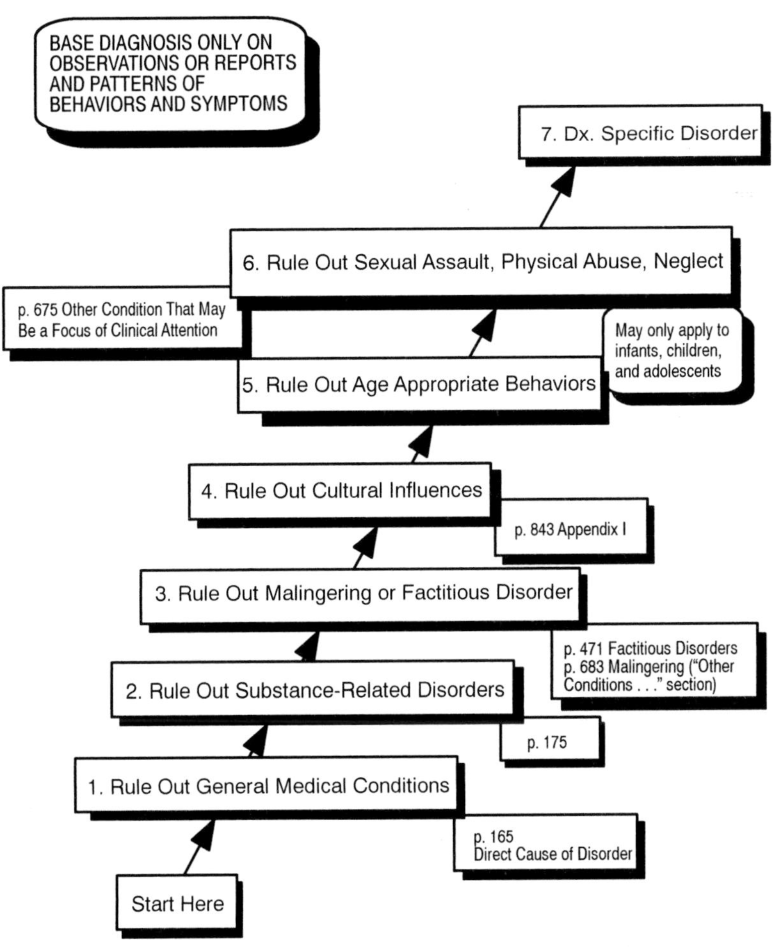

DIAGNOSTIC ILLUSTRATION

Visual 4.5 is an illustration of most of the information explained in this chapter. It features the diagnosis of a sixteen-year-old high school student named Mary, who was sexually assaulted by an uncle when she was six

VISUAL 4.5. Multiaxial Diagnosis Illustration

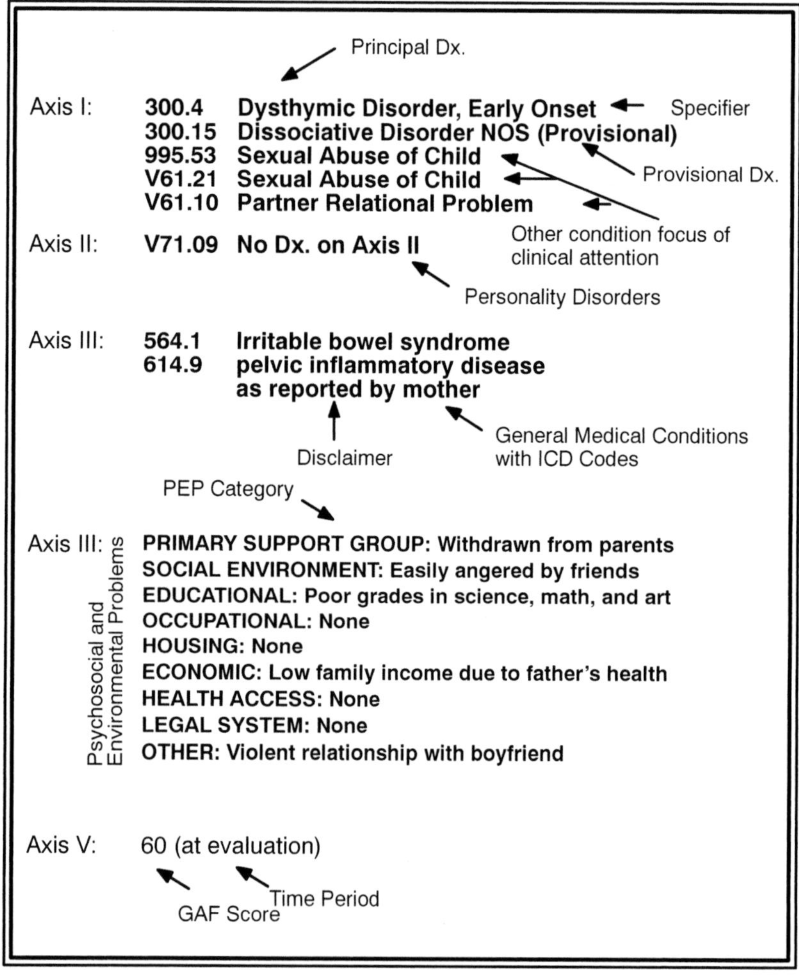

Source: American Psychiatric Association, 1994, pp. 25-31.

years old and twelve years old. The uncle lived in another state, visited the family twice, and lived with the young woman's parents during the two visits. On both of these visits he sexually assaulted Mary when her parents were not at home. She did not reveal the sexual assaults until she entered therapy at age sixteen. Mary entered therapy after appearing in court for fondling a six-year-old boy she was baby-sitting for a family that lived in Mary's neighborhood. At the time of the intake evaluation at a mental health center, Mary and her parents described to the therapist symptoms of dysthymia. She was moody, at times refused to eat, was described as "lazy," and "wanted to sleep all the time." The parents had difficulty getting her to engage in family activities, and she believed she "could not do anything right." The parents became upset because Mary repeatedly would not make even the smallest decision about her life or daily events. Mary had the symptoms of dysthymia for many years, and for the last three years, she had been functioning poorly at school, at home, and in social relationships. She was considering dropping out of school. Mary had an older boyfriend with whom she argued frequently, and he had been emotionally and physically abusive of Mary. Mary would complain to her parents that she wanted to break off the relationship with this boy, but she could not bring herself to do it. Mary was sometimes forgetful, unresponsive, and seemingly unable to hear what her parents and others would say to her. She was treated by her family physician for irritable bowel syndrome three years ago, and one year ago she was diagnosed with pelvic inflammatory disease.

On Axis I, Mary received several diagnoses and other conditions that may be a focus of clinical attention. Mary was diagnosed as having Dysthymic Disorder, Early Onset, most likely associated with the childhood sexual abuse. She also had symptoms of dissociation, but the diagnostician gave Mary the diagnosis on a provisional basis because, although she was fairly certain Mary would meet the criteria for this disorder, she wanted to interview the parents further about the symptoms of this disorder. The practitioner wanted to give Mary a standardized dissociative measure before fully assigning the disorder. The sexual abuse of this young woman is recorded as 995.53 because she was a victim of sexual abuse, and she also received the "other condition" of V61.21 Sexual Abuse of Child because she had fondled a child she was baby-sitting. The DSM-IV has separate codes for a person who is abused and for one who is an abuser. This differential coding applies to physical abuse, sexual abuse, and neglect (p. 682). Mary received the additional "other condition" of V61.10 Partner Relational Problem because of her violent relationship with her boyfriend.

On Axis II, Mary received no diagnosis, so the code and description V71.09 No Dx. on Axis II was recorded.

On Axis III, the mother reported that Mary had been diagnosed by the family primary care physician as having irritable bowel syndrome and pelvic inflammatory disease. These disorders are common in childhood sexual abuse cases.

On Axis IV, Mary and her parents reported she had become withdrawn from her family, and was easily angered by her friends, which cut her off from social supports. She was receiving poor grades in school in the subjects of science, math, and art. Economic problems existed in the form of low family income because of the father's inability to work due to his health. No occupational, housing, health access, or legal system problems were noted. In the area of the open-ended "other" category, the practitioner listed the violent relationship with the boyfriend to give more specificity to the V61.10 Partner Relational Problem identified on Axis I.

Mary's GAF score was 60 at the time of the evaluation. This means that Mary was having moderate problems in family, social, and school functioning.

TREATMENT PLANNING

Practitioners are increasingly required to formulate treatment plans that are clearly stated and based on sound criteria and standardized practice guidelines. Treatment plans must be stated in behavioral terms and be measurable. Goals, problems, and outcomes must be clearly identified. Another frequent expectation is that the treatment plan will be linked to the diagnosis. This expectation is another reason why a person should do a thorough multiaxial diagnosis. Axis I and Axis II relate to the symptoms and behaviors that can be targeted in a treatment plan, and Axis IV is critical to psychosocial and environmental factors that are basic to a treatment plan. The diagnostic criteria in the diagnostic dialogue boxes can be directly linked to treatment goals and outcome statements.

To assist practitioners in developing treatment plan items, an example is provided in Visual 4.6. This visual illustrates how treatment planning can be linked with any disorder in the DSM-IV. For consistency, this treatment planning example is based on the diagnosis for Mary presented in Visual 4.5. The diagnostic criteria for Dysthymic Disorder are listed in the box at the top of the visual. The second box includes problem statements generated from the diagnostic criteria. The third box lists the target behaviors and goals of intervention. The numbers in each box correspond and are linked, and this is indicated by the arrows that point to item one in each box. The reader can follow each set of symptoms, problems, and goals through each box by number. Where more than one goal is linked to a problem and symptom, subsets of "a" and "b" have been used.

VISUAL 4.6. Integration of DSM-IV Diagnosis and Treatment Planning

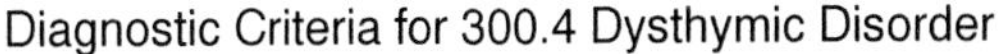

Diagnostic Criteria for 300.4 Dysthymic Disorder

A. Depressed mood for most of the day, for more days than not, as indicated either by subjective account or observation by others, for at least two years. *Note:* In children and adolescents, mood can be irritable and duration must be at least one year.
B. Presence, while depressed, of two (or more) of the following:
   1. Poor appetite or overeating
   2. Insomnia or hypersomnia
   3. Low energy or fatigue
   4. Low self-esteem
   5. Poor concentration or difficulty making decisions
   6. Feelings of hopelessness

Problem Statements
(As Identified by Therapist, IP, and Spouse)

1. Overeating at lunch and dinner most days
2. Difficulty getting to sleep three to four nights per week
3. Feeling of low energy and fatigue four to five days per week
4. Sense of low self-worth 90 percent of the time
5. Indecision regarding a change of jobs
6. Indecision regarding care and discipline of children
7. Statements reflecting feelings of dread and hopelessness three to five times per week

Target Behaviors and Goals
(As Defined by Therapist and IP)

1. Reduce overeating at lunch and dinner by 75 percent (ST).
2. Develop conscious dreaming activities to reduce sleeplessness by 80 percent (ST).
3a. Increase physical activity by 60 percent to reduce fatigue (ST).
3b. Develop cognitive strategies to reduce low energy by 75 percent (LT).
4a. Develop cognitive strategies to increase positive self-statements to counter and eliminate negative self-statements (LT).
4b. Identify and eliminate statements that distort comments by others regarding I.P. self-worth (LT).
5. Explore pros and cons of job change (LT).
6a. Identify strategies that are effective in increasing comforting touch of children by 60 percent (LT).
6b. Identify and eliminate marital conflicts regarding discipline of children (LT).
6c. Identify and eliminate marital conflicts regarding discipline of children (LT).
6c. Refer to parenting skills course offered by school (ST).
7. Develop cognitive awareness of hopeful situations three to five times per week (LT).

Note:
IP = Identified Patient
ST = Short Term
LT = Long Term

Source: American Psychiatric Association, 1994, pp. 345-349. Diagnostic criteria reprinted with permission from the *Diagnostic and Statistical Manual of Mental Disorders,* Fourth Edition. Copyright 1994 American Psychiatric Association.

Treatment planning should be a joint effort of the practitioner, the client, and family members, if relevant, and this has been indicated in the visual. Treatment plans do not need to follow the format presented in this illustration. The visual has been organized in this manner to highlight how diagnosis and treatment planning should be linked. Treatment plans can be formatted in many ways, but the content suggested in the visual should be included in any treatment plan.

A second illustration of the diagnosis-treatment planning link is provided in Visual 4.7 to give additional guidelines for practitioners. The case associated with this treatment plan involved a twelve-year-old child who was placed in a group home because the father was in jail and the mother was dying of AIDS. The child was having many relational problems with staff and residents.

NONAXIAL FORMAT

The DSM-IV does not require a multiaxial format for reporting mental disorders, and the police will not come and put you in jail for failure to follow the guidelines presented in this book. However, I would recommend strongly that all mental health professionals use the multiaxial format to make a thorough diagnosis in every case. When practitioners do not follow the DSM-IV guidelines for formatting diagnosis, they are open to criticism about not knowing how to perform diagnosis in general. In addition, using the multiaxial format helps to ensure that the diagnostician has not missed any major aspect of the person's functioning.

HOW TO STUDY

Having gained an understanding of the organization of the manual and the conceptualization of the multiaxial system, the reader can move to a more detailed study of the manual. Visual 4.8 summarizes a strategy for studying the DSM-IV based on the information presented in Chapters 3 and 4.

RECOMMENDED READING

First, M. B., Spitzer, R. L., Gibbon, M., and Williams, J. B. W. (1997). *Structured Clinical Interview for DSM-IV Axis I Disorders (SCID-I), Clinical Version*. Washington, DC: American Psychiatric Association.

First, M. B., Gibbon, M., Spitzer, R. L., Williams, J. B. W., and Benjamin, L. (1997). *Structured Clinical Interview for DSM-IV Axis II Disorders (SCID-II)*. Washington, DC: American Psychiatric Association.

VISUAL 4.7. Integration of DSM-IV Diagnosis and Treatment Planning

Diagnostic Criteria for 313.81 Oppositional Defiant Disorder

A. Pattern of negativistic, hostile, and defiant behavior lasting at least six months, during which four (or more) of the following are present:
   1. Loses temper
   2. Argues with adults
   3. Defies or refuses to comply with adult requests or rules
   4. Deliberately annoys people
   5. Blames others for his/her mistakes or misbehavior
   6. Touchy or easily annoyed by others
   7. Angry and resentful
   8. Spiteful or vindictive

B. The disturbance in behavior causes clinically significant impairment in social, academic, or occupational functioning.

C. The behavior does not occur exclusively during the course of a Psychotic or Mood Disorder.

D. Criteria are not met for Conduct Disorder, and if the individual is age eighteen years or older, criteria are not met for Antisocial Personality Disorder.

Problem Statements
(As Identified by Therapist, Resident, Caseworker, and Parents)

1. Loses temper and shouts at three to four staff members three to six times per week.
2. Daily argues with Program Director about rules and other management issues.
3. Stays out after curfew two to three nights per week during home visits.
4. Taunts other residents three to five times daily (especially Tina J.).
5. Daily blames other resident noisiness for failure to complete homework.
6. Argues with other residents about trivial matters three to six times per week.
7. Daily verbalizes anger at parents for placing her at Happy Hills Center.
8. Lies to staff about other residents' activities three to five times per week (especially about Mary K., Tanya H., and Nancy B.).

Target Behaviors and Goals
(As Defined by Therapist, Staff, Resident, Caseworker, and Parents)

1. Reduce shouting at staff by 75 percent (ST).
2. Reduce arguing with Program Director by 80 percent (ST).
3a. Eliminate curfew violation through incentive plan (ST).
3b. Structure activities to eliminate curfew violations (LT).
4a. Eliminate taunting by suggesting alternative verbalizations (ST).
4b. Identify and eliminate statements that distort comments by others and lead to taunts (LT).
5. Decrease blaming of others by 75 percent through cognitive restructuring (LT).
6. Decrease arguing with other residents by 60 percent (ST).
7. Decrease anger at parents through cognitive restructuring (LT).
8a. Increase self-esteem statements by 75 percent (ST).
8b. Extinguish lying to staff through ignoring reports about other residents (ST).

Source: American Psychiatric Association, 1994, pp. 345-349.

VISUAL 4.8. How to Study the DSM-IV and What to Code

HOW TO STUDY

1. Read "Introduction" (includes history, research, ICD-10 relationship, mental disorder definition, limitations, clinical judgment, forensics, culture, treatment planning, GMCs, and organization). pp. xv-xxv
2. Read "Use of the Manual" (includes coding, specifiers, recurrence, principal/provisional Dx., NOS, clinical significance criteria, types of information in DSM-IV, and organization). pp. 1-11
3. Review "DSM-IV Classification" (includes 18 categories of disorders (headings shaded gray, pp. 13-24); pay special attention to sections "Additional Conditions that May Be a Focus of Clinical Attention" (pp. 675-686) and "Additional Codes" (p. 687).
4. Read "Multiaxial Format" (Includes 5 axes explanations, examples, and nonaxial format). pp. 25-35
5. Review "Appendixes A through J (especially focus on "Defensive Functioning Scale," "GARF Scale," and "SOFAS," pp. 751-761). pp. 689-873
6. Review "Index" (Note 2 numbers—disorder discussion page and criteria "boxes" in parentheses). pp. 875-886.

USABLE SCALES

100/91, 90/81, 80/71, 70/61, 60/51, 50/41, 40/31, 30/21, 20/11, 10/1, 0

GAF GARF SOFAS use this scale

GAF (psychological, social, and occupational functioning; exclude physical or environmental limitations) p. 32

GARF (functioning of family or ongoing relationship; covers problem-solving, organization, and emotional climate) p. 758

SOFAS (focus on social and occupational functioning; includes consideration of GMCs in making assessment/variable time measurements) p. 760

Defensive Functioning Scale (DFS) (evaluation of defenses or coping styles based on 7 measures of defense levels/current and past times) p. 751

Recording Form: DFS
A. Current defenses or coping styles: list in order, beginning with most prominent defenses or coping styles
1.
2.
3.
4.
5.
6.
7.
B. Predominant current defense level:

High adaptive level
Mental inhibitions level
Minor-image distorting level
Disavowal level
Major-image distorting level
Action level
Level of defensive dysregulation

WHAT TO CODE

Clinical Disorders (Axis 1) (pp. 37-627)
Other Conditions That May Be a Focus of Clinical Attention (Axis 1) (pp. 675-686)
Personality Disorders (Axis 2) (pp. 629-673)
Mental Retardation (Axis 2) (pp. 39-46)
Additional Codes (Axis 1) (p. 687)
GMCs (Axis 3) (Appendix G)

DO NOT CODE

Major Depressive, Manic, Mixed, Hypomanic episodes (pp. 317-338)
Panic Attack or Agoraphobia (pp. 394-397)

REFERENCES

American Psychiatric Association (1994). *Diagnostic and Statistical Manual of Mental Disorders,* Fourth Edition, Washington, DC: American Psychiatric Association.

Frances, A., First, M. B., and Pincus, H. A. (1995). *DSM-IV Guidebook: The Essential Companion to the* Diagnostic and Statistical Manual of Mental Disorders. Washington, DC: American Psychiatric Press.

Yingling, L. C., Miller, W. E., McDonald, A. L., and Galewaler, S. T. (1998). *GARF Assessment Sourcebook: Using the DSM-IV Global Assessment of Relational Functioning*. New York: Brunner/Mazel.

Chapter 5

Disorders Usually First Diagnosed in Infancy, Childhood, or Adolescence (ICA Disorders)

DISORDERS

Mental Retardation

317	Mild Mental Retardation
318.0	Moderate Mental Retardation
318.1	Severe Mental Retardation
318.2	Profound Mental Retardation
319	Mental Retardation, Severity Unspecified
V62.89	Borderline Intellectual Functioning (in section, "Other Conditions That May Be a Focus of Clinical Attention." *Note:* Recorded on Axis II)

Learning Disorders (Formerly Academic Skills Disorders)

315.00	Reading Disorder
315.1	Mathematics Disorder
315.2	Disorder of Written Expression
315.9	Learning Disorder NOS
V62.3	Academic Problem (in section "Other Conditions That May Be a Focus of Clinical Attention")

Motor Skills Disorder

315.4	Developmental Coordination Disorder

Communication Disorders

315.31	Expressive Language Disorder
315.32	Mixed Receptive-Expressive Language Disorder
315.39	Phonological Disorder (formerly Developmental Articulation Disorder)
307.0	Stuttering
307.9	Communication Disorder NOS

Pervasive Developmental Disorders

299.00	Autistic Disorder
299.80	Rett's Disorder
299.10	Childhood Disintegrative Disorder
299.80	Asperger's Disorder
299.80	Pervasive Developmental Disorder NOS (including Atypical Autism)

Attention-Deficit and Disruptive Behavior Disorders

314.xx	Attention-Deficit/Hyperactivity Disorder
	.01 Combined Type
	.00 Predominantly Inattentive Type
	.01 Predominantly Hyperactive-Impulsive Type
314.9	Attention-Deficit/Hyperactivity Disorder NOS
312.xx	Conduct Disorder
	.81 Childhood-Onset Type
	.82 Adolescent-Onset Type
	.89 Unspecified Onset
313.81	Oppositional Defiant Disorder
312.9	Disruptive Behavior Disorder NOS
V71.02	Child or Adolescent Antisocial Behavior (in section "Other Conditions That May Be a Focus of Clinical Attention")

Feeding and Eating Disorders of Infancy or Early Childhood

307.52	Pica
307.53	Rumination Disorder
307.59	Feeding Disorder of Infancy or Early Childhood

Tic Disorders

307.23 Tourette's Disorder
307.22 Chronic Motor or Vocal Tic Disorder
307.21 Transient Tic Disorder
307.20 Tic Disorder NOS

Elimination Disorders

___._ Encopresis
787.6 With Constipation and Overflow Incontinence
307.7 Without Constipation and Overflow Incontinence
307.6 Enuresis (not due to a GMC)

Other Disorders of Infancy, Childhood, or Adolescence

309.21 Separation Anxiety Disorder
313.23 Selective Mutism (formerly Elective Mutism)
313.89 Reactive Attachment Disorder of Infancy or Early Childhood
307.3 Stereotypic Movement Disorder (formerly Stereotypy/Habit Disorder)
313.9 Disorder of Infancy, Childhood, or Adolescence NOS
V61.20 Parent-Child Relational Problem (in section, "Other Conditions That May Be a Focus of Clinical Attention")
V61.8 Sibling Relational Problem (in section, "Other Conditions That May Be a Focus of Clinical Attention")
V61.21 Physical Abuse of Child (in section, "Other Conditions That May Be a Focus of Clinical Attention")
995.54 Physical Abuse of Child (in section, "Other Conditions That May Be a Focus of Clinical Attention")
V61.21 Sexual Abuse of Child (in section, "Other Conditions That May Be a Focus of Clinical Attention")
995.53 Sexual Abuse of Child (in section, "Other Conditions That May Be a Focus of Clinical Attention")
V61.21 Neglect of Child (in section, "Other Conditions That May Be a Focus of Clinical Attention")
995.52 Neglect of Child (in section, "Other Conditions That May Be a Focus of Clinical Attention")

FUNDAMENTAL FEATURES

Ten categories of disorders including forty-four coded disorders make up this section. Visual 5.1 provides a summary of the disorders in this section.

VISUAL 5.1. Summary of DSM-IV Disorders Usually First Diagnosed in Infancy, Childhood, or Adolescence

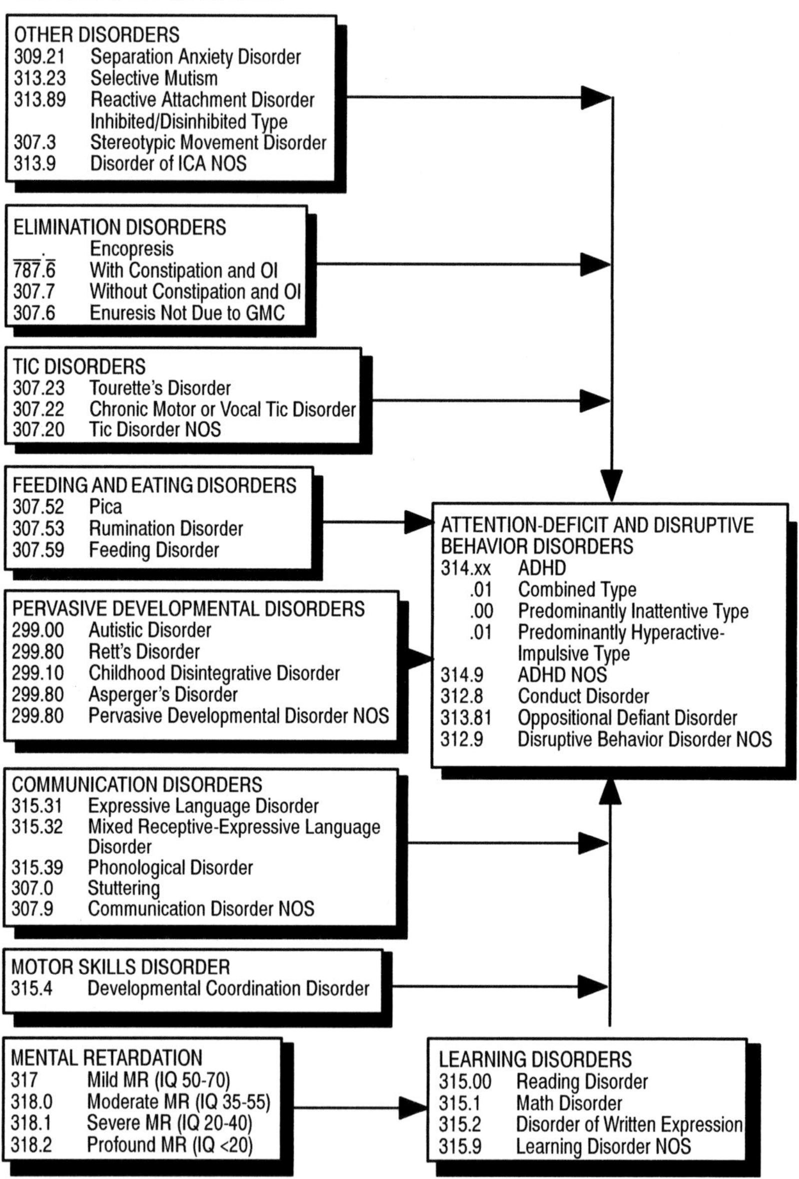

Source: American Psychiatric Association, 1994, pp. 37-121.

The arrows in the visual indicate possible connections for diagnosticians to be alert to when evaluating children. The Attention-Deficit and Disruptive Behavior Disorder section accounts for the majority of diagnoses given in this class of disorders, and other disorders can often be overlooked.

Note that the terminology of this class of disorders uses the word *usually.* Disorders of infancy, childhood, or adolescence can be diagnosed in adults if the diagnostician is able to trace the symptoms sufficiently far back in the person's history to ensure the person, as a child or adolescent, met the criteria for the disorder. For example, if an adult male, age twenty-four, is believed to have Attention-Deficit/Hyperactivity Disorder (ADHD), the diagnostician must be able to determine that the man experienced onset of the symptoms before age seven because that is one of the inclusion criteria for the disorder. If the age of onset criterion and other criteria of the disorder are met, the man can be diagnosed with the disorder. The same pattern of establishing for adults whether the criteria are met holds for all other ICA Disorders.

If an adult does not meet the full symptoms and criteria for the disorder, but did as an infant, a child, or an adolescent (ICA), then the disorder can be diagnosed with the specifier **In Partial Remission**. If the person met the criteria for a disorder as a child, but has no symptoms as an adult, then the diagnosis can be listed with the designation **Prior History**.

Diagnoses of disorders in other sections of the DSM-IV can be given to ICAs if they meet the criteria for the disorder. Some disorders in other sections of the manual have criteria notations that make duration, frequency, or inclusion criteria exceptions for children. For example, in Dysthymic Disorder, the symptoms in Criterion A must be present for two years, but a notation indicates that for children the duration criterion is one year (p. 349). This is illustrative of the importance of reading criteria carefully and fully when making a diagnosis.

Factors associated with age of onset of ICA disorders are described in the text section of each individual disorder titled Specific Culture, Age and Gender Features.

Personality Disorders are diagnosed in persons under eighteen years of age only when the features of the disorder have persisted for at least one year.

Antisocial Personality Disorder cannot be diagnosed in a person under age eighteen years (see p. 645). Under age eighteen, the symptoms and behavior associated with Antisocial Personality Disorder are included in the diagnosis of Conduct Disorder or the condition Child or Adolescent Antisocial Behavior.

In addition to the forty-four disorders in this section, a series of conditions that can be listed on Axis I are included in the section "Other Conditions That May Be a Focus of Clinical Attention." The following conditions are most relevant to ICAs:

- Relational Problems
- Problems Related to Abuse or Neglect
- Child or Adolescent Antisocial Behavior
- Borderline Intellectual Functioning
- Bereavement
- Academic Problem
- Identity Problem

INFANT AND CHILD GAF

The DSM-IV has only a generalized GAF form that is more usable with adults and does not relate to the symptoms and behaviors of very small children. Visual 5.2 contains an alternative infant and toddler GAF and a child and adolescent GAF.

SUBTYPES AND SPECIFIERS

The major DSM-IV Child Disorders Subtypes and Specifiers follow. As mentioned in Chapter 3, subtypes and specifiers do not follow a specific pattern. Some subtypes have individual coding numbers (see ADHD), and others do not (see Conduct Disorder). Specifiers are often tied to the individual disorder.

Attention-Deficit/Hyperactivity Disorder
Subtypes: 314.01 AD/HD Disorder, Combined Type
314.00 AD/HD Disorder, Predominantly Inattentive Type
314.01 AD/HD Disorder, Predominantly Hyperactive-Impulsive Type

Conduct Disorder
Subtypes: 312.81 Conduct Disorder, Childhood-Onset Type
312.82 Conduct Disorder, Adolescent-Onset Type
312.89 Conduct Disorder, Unspecified Onset
Specifiers: Mild, Moderate, Severe

307.21 Transient Tic Disorder
Specifiers: Single Episode, Recurrent

VISUAL 5.2. Infant and Toddler and Child and Adolescent GAF Scale

Infant and Toddler GAF Scale

100-91	Normal functioning in all developmental areas. Appropriate reflexes are within normal limits. Infant/toddler has met all developmental milestones related to physical development, self-help skills, communication skills, cognitive skills, language skills, and emotional development.
90-81	Minimal developmental delays in one or two areas of the physical development, self-help skills, communication skills, cognitive skills, language skills, and emotional development that are not due to a general medical condition. Infant/toddler may have "fussy" or uneasy temperament. Development delays are transient and episodic.
80-71	Developmental delays in one or two areas of physical development, self-help skills, communication skills, cognitive skills, language skills, and emotional development as well as feeding or eating problems of short duration (less than four weeks). Other developmental delays appear to be emerging, but infant/toddler is responding to professional or caregiver intervention.
70-61	Prolonged periods of language, cognitive, and intellectual developmental delays are present, and infant/toddler is not responding to professional or caregiver intervention.
60-51	Physical and self-help developmental milestones are attained with assistance from a caregiver, but language, communication, and social deficits are significant, and infant/toddler is not responsive to professional or caregiver intervention.
50-41	Physical and self-help developmental milestones are not met. Language, communication, and social deficits are significant, and infant/toddler is not responsive to professional or caregiver intervention. Infant/toddler has significant impairment in communicating needs to caregiver.
40-31	Significantly impaired language, communication, and cognitive developmental deficits. Infant/toddler is not responsive to caregiver interaction, commands, or directives. Periods of fixed gaze.
30-21	Physical and self-help skills absent and interaction is minimal. Infants exhibit persistent crying, and toddlers, frequent aggression or complete withdrawal. Self-injurious behavior may be present.
20-11	Significant delays in all areas of development. Withdrawal and nonresponsivenses to human contact. Cries when touched. Self-injurious behavior may be present.
10-1	Profound failure to meet any developmental milestones, and infant/toddler is not responsive to caregivers. Infant/toddler meets the criteria for nonorganic failure to thrive syndrome.
0	Inadequate information
NOTE:	Assignment of the infant/toddler GAF score should be based on use of standardized instruments that measure development, infant observation/clinical observation, and a clinical interview/play session when appropriate.

VISUAL 5.2 *(continued)*

Child and Adolescent GAF Scale

100-91	Superior functioning in most activities. Life's problems are easily managed and understood with caregiver support. Is generally a well-liked child. No symptoms.
90-81	Minimal symptoms (e.g., mild anxiety about complex school assignments). Good functioning and adjustment in most areas. Interested in a wide range of family, school, and social activities. Feels fundamentally secure at home and at school.
80-71	If symptoms present, they are temporary and expectable reactions to psychosocial stressors. Slight impairment in home, school, and social functioning, but child rebounds after brief crisis period.
70-61	Some mild symptoms. Some difficulty in home, school, or peer functioning (e.g., occasional truancy or small thefts from family members or peers). Some symptoms arising from normal developmental crises (e.g., nail-biting, nightmares, slight change in school performance, anxiety over loss of boyfriend/girlfriend, or some drug use that creates family tension).
60-51	Moderate symptoms (e.g., flat affect, minimal speech, occasional anxiety reactions). Difficulty functioning at home, in school, and in relation to peers (e.g., frequent fights with peers, withdrawal, temper tantrums, bullying others, no friends or small circle of friends, frequent drug use, frequent inattention to schoolwork, required to repeat grade, frequent school suspensions, and serious self-doubts and low self-esteem).
50-41	Serious symptoms (e.g., suicidal ideation, severe obsessional rituals, frequent stealing). Severe disruption of relationships with caregivers, school officials, or peers (e.g., serious substance abuse, serious attacks on others, permanent suspension from school, fired from several jobs).
40-31	Some poor reality testing. Major impairment of judgment and thinking. Many conflicts with caregivers, school, and peers (e.g., destructive behavior, self-harming behavior, severe psychosomatic complaints, compulsive behavior, obsessions, anxiety, somatic delusions, major developmental delays, refusal to attend school, withdrawal and isolation, hallucinations).
30-21	Unable to function in most areas. Serious disruption of relationships with caregivers and peers. School functioning requires permanent suspension. Serious impairment of communication and judgment.
20-11	Needs constant supervision to prevent hurting self or others. Gross impairment of reality testing, cognition, communication, affect, or personal hygiene (e.g., suicide attempts, age-inappropriate smearing of feces, incoherent or unable to communicate).
10-1	Needs constant supervision (twenty-four hour care). Constant threat to self and/or others. Autistic, symbiotic, psychotic, or borderline children/adolescents can appear from 1 to 30 on this scale based on ability to function.
0	Inadequate information

Encopresis
Subtypes: 787.6 With Constipation and Overflow Incontinence
307.7 Without Constipation and Overflow Incontinence

307.6 Enuresis
Subtypes: Nocturnal Only
Diurnal Only
Nocturnal and Diurnal

309.21 Separation Anxiety Disorder
Specifier: Early Onset

313.89 Reactive Attachment Disorder of Infancy or Early Childhood
Subtypes: Inhibited Type
Disinhibited Type

307.3 Stereotypic Movement Disorder
Specifier: With Self-Injurious Behavior

CHANGES IN ICA DISORDERS FROM DSM-III-R TO DSM-IV

A number of changes were made in the ICA Disorders in the DSM-IV. A summary of the changes are presented in Visual 5.3. The details of the changes are contained in Appendix D of the DSM-IV.

AGE OF ONSET

The ages of onset for ICA Disorders are presented in Visual 5.4. This visual can aid in ensuring that the child meets the age criteria for a given disorder while keeping in mind other disorders in this section. It is designed to limit searching through the DSM-IV manual section by section to determine ages of onset. The reader should note, however, that some disorders have an approximate age of onset while others have a specific age of onset for diagnosing the disorder.

DIFFERENTIAL DIAGNOSIS

Visual 5.4 graphically presents the differential diagnosis of DSM-IV ICA Disorders. Suggestions for differential diagnosis can be determined

VISUAL 5.3. DSM-IV Changes from DSM-III-R Related to Childhood and Adolescence

Note: A summary of all DSM-IV changes from DSM-III-R have been included in this Visual since many of the adult disorders apply to children.

Details of the following summary items are provided in Appendix D of the DSM-IV.

Axis Changes

Axis II: Pervasive Developmental Disorders, Learning Disorders, Motor Skills Disorder, and Communication Disorders moved to Axis I

Axis III: Appendix G added listing of selected GMCs and ICD-9 codes that are listed on Axis III.

Axis IV: Used to report psychosocial and environmental problems rather than intensity of set stressors.

Axis V: GAF changed from 1-90 to 0-100. Appendix B contains GAF for social, occupational, and relational (GARF) functioning.

New Disorders Introduced into DSM-IV

Rett's Disorder
Childhood Disintegrative Disorder
Asperger's Disorder
Feeding Disorder of Infancy or Early Childhood
Bipolar II Disorder
Acute Stress Disorder
Substance-Induced Sexual Dysfunction
Narcolepsy
Breathing-Related Sleep Disorder

DSM-III-R Disorders Deleted from DSM-IV or Subsumed into Other Categories

Cluttering
Overanxious Disorder of Childhood
Avoidant Personality Disorder
Undifferentiated Attention-Deficit Disorder
Passive-Aggressive Personality Disorder

Appendixes

Appendix A:	Decision Trees for Differential Dx.	Expansion based on GMCs.
Appendix B:	Criteria Sets and Axes for Further Study	Expanded to include new proposals.
Appendix C:	Glossary of Technical Terms	New terms added and old ones refined.
Appendix D:	Listing of Changes in DSM-IV	New format.
Appendix E:	Alphabetical Listing of Codes	Revised to update.
Appendix F:	Numerical Listing of Codes	Revised to update.
Appendix G:	ICD-9 Codes for GMCs	New.
Appendix H:	DSM-IV Classification with ICD-10	DSM codes with ICD-10 system.
Appendix I:	Outline for Cultural Formulation . . .	Aids in multicultural use of DSM.
Appendix J:	DSM-IV Contributors	Updated list of contributors.

VISUAL 5.3 *(continued)*

Disorders Usually First Diagnosed in Infancy, Childhood, or Adolescence	
Mental Retardation	Modified to conform to AAMR definition.
Learning Disorders	Change from Academic Skills Disorders.
Communication Disorders	Consolidates speech and language disorders.
Expressive Language Disorder	Moved to Axis I.
Mixed Receptive-Expressive Language Disorder	Replaces Developmental Repetitive Language Disorder.
Phonological Disorder	Changed from Developmental Articulation Disorder.
Stuttering	Expanded criteria.
Pervasive Developmental Disorder	Moved to Axis I.
Autistic Disorder	Reduced inclusion items from sixteen to twelve.
Rett's Disorder	Added.
Childhood Disintegrative Disorder	Added.
Asperger's Disorder	Added.
ADHD	Reduced to one category.
Conduct Disorder	Added 2 symptoms (staying out all night and intimidating others).
Oppositional Defiant Disorder	"Uses absence language" deleted and impairment criterion added.
Feeding and Eating Disorders Infancy and Early Childhood	Changed to allow placement of Anorexia Nervosa and Bulimia in separate section.
Pica	Changed to allow use with other disorders.
Rumination Disorder	Weight criteria eliminated.
Feeding Disorders of Infancy or Early Childhood	Added.
Tic Disorders	Upper age of Dx. reduced from twenty-one to eighteen.
Encopresis	Duration requirement reduced from six to three months.
Enuresis (not due to GMC)	Frequency and duration threshold raised.
Separation Anxiety Disorder	Two symptom categories combined and duration requirement increased to four weeks.
Selective Mutism	Name changed from Elective Mutism and symptoms added.
Reactive Attachment Disorder of Infancy or Early Childhood	Subtypes added.
Stereotypic Movement Disorder	Changed from Stereotype/Habit Disorder.
Delirium, Dementia, and Other Cognitive Disorders	Replaces Organic Mental Disorders category.
Delirium	Added one category and deleted one category.
Dementia	Reorganized and simplified.
Amnestic Disorders	Simplified and refined.
Substance-Related Disorders	Combined in one category.
Substance Dependence	Symptoms reduced from nine to seven. Duration criterion deleted.
Substance Abuse	Symptoms expanded from two to four.
Substance Intoxication	Substance list refined.
Substance Withdrawal	Substance list refined.
Table of Substance-Induced Disorders	Expanded.
Schizophrenia/Psychotic Disorders	Combines Schizophrenia, Delusional Disorder, and Psychotic Disorder NOS.
Substance-Induced Psychotic Disorder	Added.

VISUAL 5.3 *(continued)*

Mood Disorders	
Major Depressive Disorder	Two criterion added.
Manic Episode	Duration criterion of one week reinstated.
Mixed Episode	Elevated from subtype to full set of criteria.
Hypomanic Episode	Elevated from subtype to full set of criteria.
Dysthymic Disorder	Refined criteria.
Bipolar Disorders	Divided into BPD 1and 2.
Substance-Induced Mood Disorder	Changed from Organic Mood Disorder.
Anxiety Disorders	
Specific Phobia	Changed from Simple Phobia.
Social Phobia	Subsumes Avoidant Disorder of Childhood.
Obsessive-Compulsive Disorder	Distinguishes obsessions and compulsions.
Posttraumatic Stress Disorder	Refinement of criteria.
Acute Stress Disorder	Added.
Generalized Anxiety Disorder	Subsumes Overanxious Disorder of Childhood.
Substance-Induced Anxiety Disorder	Changed from Organic Anxiety Disorder.
Somatoform Disorders	
Somatization Disorder	Thirty-five symptoms refined to four groupings.
Conversion Disorder	Refined criteria.
Hypochondriasis	New specifier.
Body Dysmorphic Disorder	Refined criteria.
Dissociative Disorders	
Dissociative Amnesia	Changed from Psychogenic Amnesia.
Dissociative Fugue	Changed from Psychogenic Fugue.
Dissociative Identity Disorder	Changed from Multiple Personality Disorder.
Sexual and Gender Identity Disorders	
Gender Identity Disorder	Subsumes Gender Identity Disorders of Childhood/ Adolescence.
Eating Disorders	
Anorexia Nervosa	Refined and moved from childhood disorders.
Bulimia Nervosa	Refined and moved from childhood disorders.
Sleep Disorders	Reorganized in four sections.
Circadian Rhythm Sleep Disorder	Changed from Sleep-Wake Schedule Disorder.
Nightmare Disorder	Changed from Dream Anxiety Disorder.
Insomnia Related to Another MD	Added.
Sleep Disorder Due to a GMC	Added.
Substance-Induced Sleep Disorder	Added.
Impulse-Control Disorders	
Intermittent Explosive Disorder	Some criteria deleted.
Adjustment Disorders	Duration criteria extended six months after stressor. Acute and chronic stressors added.
Other Conditions That May Be a Focus of Clinical Attention	Changed from Conditions Not Attributable to a Mental Disorder. Several conditions added.
Relational Problems	Refined.
Problems Related to Abuse/ Neglect	Added.

VISUAL 5.4. Summary Guide for Differential Diagnosis of DSM-IV ICA Disorders

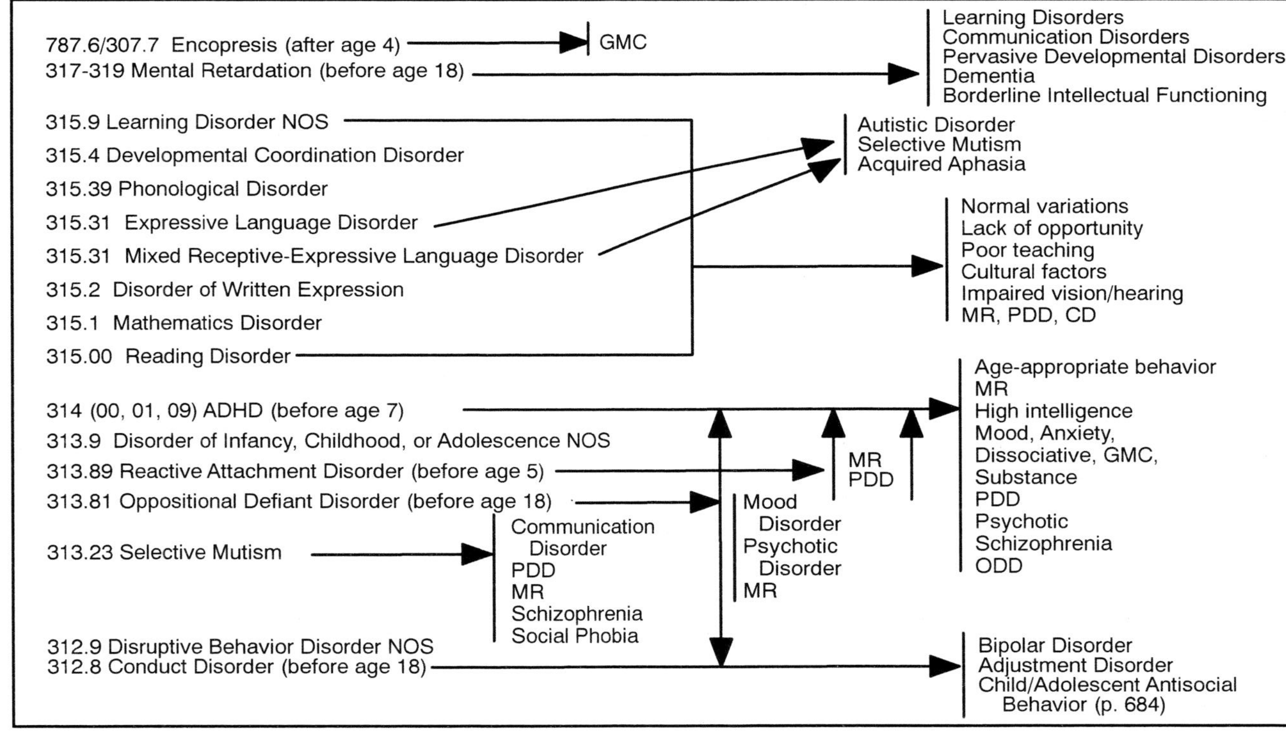

VISUAL 5.4 *(continued)*

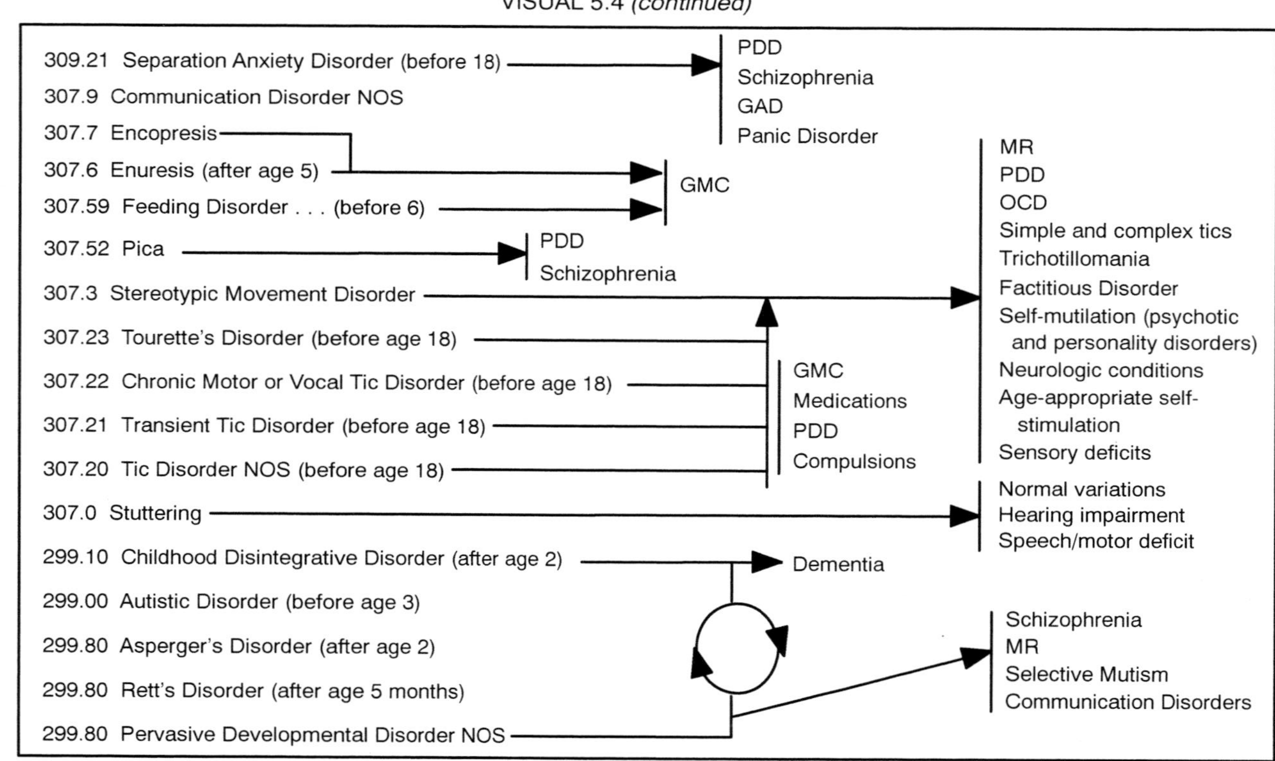

by following the arrows from left to right. Further information regarding differential diagnosis is provided in the explanations of the individual ICA disorders, following Recommended Reading.

RECOMMENDED READING

House, A. E. (1999). *DSM-IV Diagnosis in the Schools.* New York: Guilford.

Kamphaus, R. W. and Frick, P. J. (1996). *Clinical Assessment of Child and Adolescent Personality and Behavior.* Boston: Allyn and Bacon.

Lewis, M. and Volkmar, F. (1990). *Clinical Aspects of Child and Adolescent Development,* Third Edition. Philadelphia, PA: Lea and Febiger.

Mash, E. J. and Terdal, L. G. (1997). *Assessment of Childhood Disorders,* Third Edition. New York: Guilford.

Olin, J. T. and Keatinge, C. (1998). *Rapid Psychological Assessment.* New York: Wiley.

Rapoport, J. L. and Ismond, D. R. (1996). *DSM-IV Training Guide for Diagnosis of Childhood Disorders.* New York: Brunner/Mazel.

Samuels, S. K. and Sikorsky, S. (1998). *Clinical Evaluations of School-Aged Children,* Second Edition. Sarasota, FL: Professional Resource Press.

Vance, H. B. (1998). *Psychological Assessment of Children: Basic Practices for School and Clinical Settings.* New York: Wiley.

Wicks-Nelson, R. and Israel, A. C. (1997). *Behavior Disorders of Childhood,* Third Edition. Upper Saddle River, NJ: Prentice-Hall.

Wodrich, D. L. (1997). *Children's Psychological Testing: A Guide for Nonpsychologists,* Third Edition. Baltimore, MD: Brooks.

MENTAL RETARDATION

317	Mild Mental Retardation
318.0	Moderate Mental Retardation
318.1	Severe Mental Retardation
318.2	Profound Mental Retardation
319	Mental Retardation, Severity Unspecified

Fundamental Features

- Significantly subaverage general intellectual functioning accompanied by significant limitations in adaptive functioning in life skills.

- To make this diagnosis, the person must have an IQ below 70 to meet the threshold criteria, as measured by standardized intelligence tests, and the person must have identifiable impaired functioning related to adaptive skills, as reported by several reliable sources and, if possible, through standardized measures of adaptive functioning. The criteria are illustrated in Visual 5.5.
- Onset of symptoms must be before age eighteen.
- When IQ scores of 71 to 84 are achieved on standardized intelligence tests, the person should be given the condition V62.89 Borderline Intellectual Functioning. This condition is recorded on Axis II (see p. 684).
- Mental Retardation is recorded on Axis II.

Recommended Standardized Measures

- AAMR Adaptive Behavior Scales, Second Edition
- Adaptive Behavior Inventory (ABI)
- Kauffman Assessment Battery for Children (K-ABC)
- Kaufman Brief Intelligence Test (K-BIT)
- Stanford-Binet
- Vineland Adaptive Behavior Scales
- Wechsler Intelligence Scales for Children

LEARNING DISORDERS

315.00 Reading Disorder
315.1 Mathematics Disorder
315.2 Disorder of Written Expression
315.9 Learning Disorder NOS

Fundamental Features

- Formerly Academic Skills Disorders.
- The Learning Disorders are straightforward in their presentation and have precise criteria.
- Diagnosed on the basis of scores achieved on individually administered standardized tests of reading, mathematics, or written expression substantially below expected age, education, and level of intelligence.
- The learning problems significantly impair academic performance and achievement or activities of daily living that require reading, math, and writing skills.

VISUAL 5.5. Mental Retardation Criteria Summary

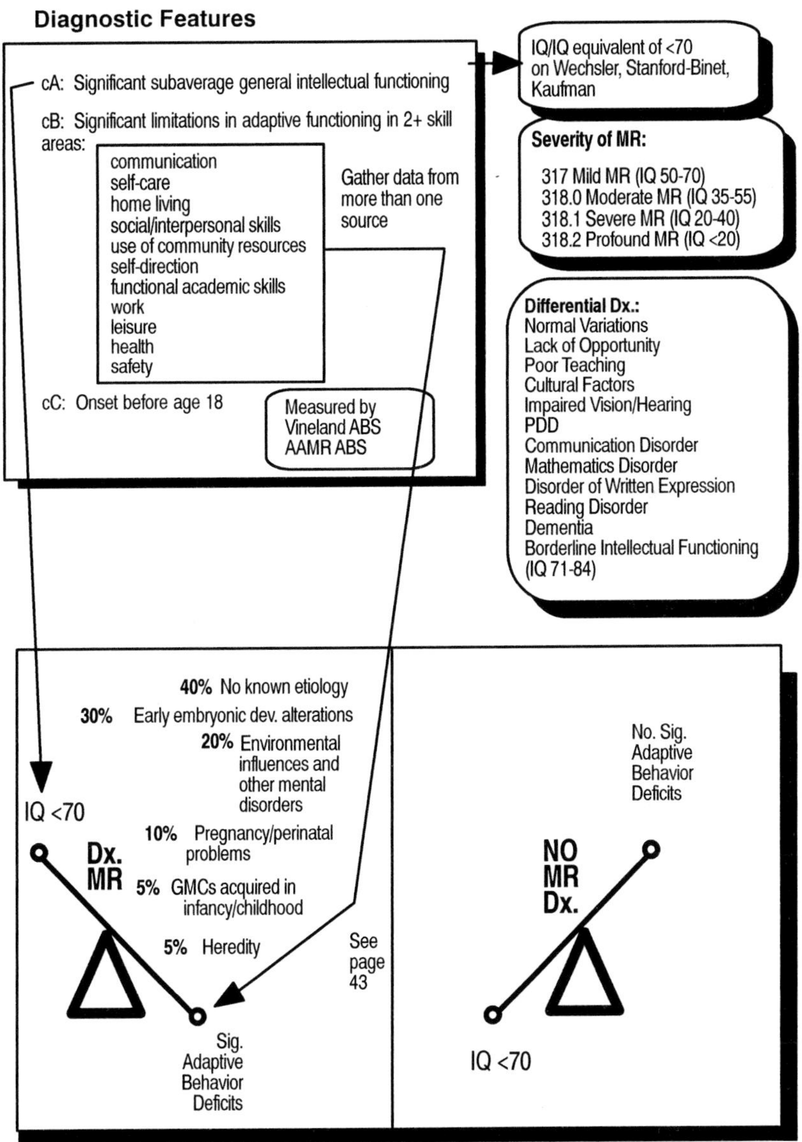

Source: American Psychiatric Association, 1994, pp. 39-46. Reprinted with permission from the *Diagnostic and Statistical Manual of Mental Disorders,* Fourth Edition. Copyright 1994 American Psychiatric Association.

- Can be accompanied by discouragement, low self-concept, and poor social skills.
- Person can be at risk for dropping out of school.
- Screen for coexisting Conduct Disorder, Oppositional Defiant Disorder, ADHD, Major Depressive Disorder, Dysthymic Disorder, Communication Disorder, and Developmental Coordination Disorder.

Differential Diagnosis

Differential diagnosis should include screening for Mental Retardation Pervasive Developmental Disorder and Communication Disorders. When any disorder is diagnosed in one of these categories, disorders in the other two categories should be ruled out to ensure a thorough and accurate diagnosis.

Recommended Standardized Measures

- Test of Written Language, Third Edition (TOWL-3)
- Gray Oral Reading Tests, Third Edition (GORT-3)
- Wide Range Achievement Test 3 (WRAT3)

MOTOR SKILLS DISORDER

Fundamental Features

- This category includes only one disorder, 315.4 Developmental Coordination Disorder.
- The fundamental feature is noticeable impairment of developmental motor coordination, as reflected in walking, crawling, sitting, standing, handwriting, etc.
- These developmental delays must cause problems in academic performance and activities of daily living.
- Differential diagnosis includes reviewing for mental retardation, neurological disorders, pervasive developmental disorders, and ADHD.
- Assessment should include thorough review of family history.

COMMUNICATION DISORDERS

315.31 Expressive Language Disorder
315.32 Mixed Receptive-Expressive Language Disorder
315.39 Phonological Disorder (formerly Developmental Articulation Disorder)
307.0 Stuttering
307.9 Communication Disorder NOS

- Expressive Language Disorder and Mixed Receptive-Expressive Language Disorder are diagnosed through administration of standardized tests of language development and skills. The person must score substantially below norms for age and grade level.
- The communication delays impair academic, occupational, or social functioning.
- Language Disorders can be acquired (due to neurological or other GMCs) or developmental (not associated with any known neurological condition) in origin. Visual 5.6 provides an overview of the conceptualizations that form the basis of the receptive/expressive language disorders.
- Language comprehension is not as easily diagnosed as delays or problems in language production.

Tip: It is important to note that receptive language disorders cannot be diagnosed within the DSM system as a specific disorder in the absence of an expressive language delay or problem. Some children have receptive language deficits without expressive language problems, as illogical as this may seem. In some preliminary research, children with above-average intelligence who experienced traumatic events were found to have receptive language delays without expressive language deficits. Children with receptive language delays or problems and normal or above-average expressive language skills can be diagnosed as Communication Disorder NOS.

- When an acquired receptive and expressive language disorder occurs between ages three to nine years and is accompanied by seizures, it is referred to as Landau-Kleffner syndrome.

Differential Diagnosis

- Differential diagnosis should include Autistic Disorder, Mental Retardation, hearing impairment, severe environmental deprivation, or psychological trauma.

- Communication disorders due to deprivation or trauma usually remit when the deprivation or trauma ceases.

Tip: Early diagnosis is important. Estimates are that language deficits are present in 20 percent of younger school-age children and 65 percent of children who experience deprivation or trauma. Language delays can improve significantly with six to eight weeks of intensive school-based intervention programs.

- Because of the extent of receptive and expressive language disorders and the apparent underdiagnosis of these disorders, a summary of the full criteria are printed in Visuals 5.6 and 5.7.
- Diagnosticians need to be alert to cultural factors in language disorders, especially when the person is in a bilingual environment.
- Phonological Disorder is related to the failure to use speech sounds appropriate to developmental milestones. Types of problems are errors in sound production, use, representation, or organization.
- Stuttering is a deficit in normal fluency and time patterning of speech that is not age appropriate.

Visual 5.8 illustrates the process of receptive and expressive language. Language disorders are widespread. Approximately 20 percent of school-age children have some form of language disorder, and approximately 65 percent of children who have been abused have receptive-expressive language disorders. Language-processing skills can be assessed as early as the first year of life, and diagnosis is important because there is a window of opportunity for addressing developmental language problems. This window of opportunity is roughly the first five years of life. If language disorders are diagnosed at later ages, they are resistant to treatment. Fortunately, if this form of language disorder is diagnosed early, it can be effectively treated with brief intervention.

Recommended Standardized Measures

- Comprehensive Receptive and Expressive Vocabulary Test (CREVT)
- Comprehensive Receptive and Expressive Vocabulary Test Adult (CREVT-A)

VISUAL 5.6. 315.31 Expressive Language Disorder (ELD)

Diagnostic Features

- The fundamental feature of Expressive Language Disorder is an impairment in expressive language development, as demonstrated by scores on standardized, individually administered measures of expressive language that are substantially below those obtained from standardized measures of both nonverbal intellectual capacity and receptive language development (Criterion A).
- Interferes with academic or occupational achievement or social communication (Criterion B).
- Symptoms do not meet criteria for Mixed Receptive-Expressive Language Disorder or Pervasive Developmental Disorder (Criterion C).
- If mental retardation, speech-motor sensory deficit, or environmental deprivation present, language difficulties are in excess of those associated with these disorders (Criterion D).
- If speech-motor or sensory deficit or neurological condition present, coded on Axis III.
- Linguistic features vary and include limited amount of speech, limited range of vocabulary, difficulty acquiring new words, word finding, or vocabulary errors, shortened sentences, simplified grammatical structures, limited varieties of grammatical structures, limited varieties of sentence structure and types, omission of critical parts of sentences, use of unusual word order, slow rate of language development.
- Nonlinguistic functioning (measured by performance intelligence tests) and language comprehension skills are usually within normal limits.
- ELD is acquired or developmental.

Associated Features and Disorders

- Phonological Disorder in younger children.
- Disturbance in fluency and language formulation involving rapid rate and erratic rhythm of speech.
- Disturbance in language structuring ("Cluttering," e.g., erratic and dysrhythmic speech with rapid and jerky spurts).
- When acquired, may also include acquired motor articulation problems, phonological errors, slow speech, syllable repetitions, and monotonous intonation and stress patterns.
- School problems (e.g., writing to dictation, copying sentences, and spelling).
- Mild impairment in receptive language skills.
- History of motor developmental milestone delay.
- Developmental Coordination Disorder often present.
- Enuresis common.
- Social withdrawal.

VISUAL 5.6 *(continued)*

- ADHD.
- EEG abnormalities.
- Abnormal neuroimaging.
- Dysarthric behaviors (imperfect articulation of speech due to disturbance of muscle control).
- Apraxic behavior (poor coordination w/o impairment of muscles or senses).
- Other neurological signs.

Specific Culture and Gender Features

- Culture: must consider bilingual effects.
- Developmental ELD more common in males.

Prevalence

- 3 to 5 percent of children estimated to have developmental ELD.
- Acquired ELD less common.

Course

- Developmental recognized by age three (milder forms detected in adolescence).
- Acquired ELD occurs at any age and onset is sudden.
- Developmental ELD outcome is variable (50 percent outgrow).
- Acquired ELD course depends on the severity of the neural pathology.

Familial Pattern

- Developmental ELD associated with a family history of communication or learning disorders.
- Acquired ELD not associated with family history.

Differential Diagnosis

- Distinguish from MR-ELD.
- ELD not diagnosed if criteria for Autistic Disorder or PDD are met.
- Symptoms of ELD present in mental retardation, hearing impairment, other sensory deficits, speech motor deficits, severe environmental deprivation (ELD clears rapidly when environmental deprivation eliminated). Dx. ELD if symptoms in excess of those associated with these disorders.
- Distinguish from Disorder of Written Expression, Selective Mutism (do careful history to detect normal language in some situations), and Acquired Aphasia.

Source: American Psychiatric Association, 1994, pp. 55-58. Reprinted with permission from the *Diagnostic and Statistical Manual of Mental Disorders,* Fourth Edition.

VISUAL 5.7. 315.32 Mixed Receptive-Expressive Language Disorder (MRELD)

Diagnostic Features

- The essential feature of Mixed Receptive-Expressive Language Disorder is an impairment in both receptive and expressive language development, as demonstrated by scores on standardized, individually administered measures of both receptive and expressive language development substantially below those obtained from standardized measures of both nonverbal intellectual capacity and receptive language development (Criterion A).
- Interferes with academic or occupational achievement or social communication (Criterion B).
- Symptoms do not meet criteria for Pervasive Developmental Disorder (Criterion C).
- If mental retardation, speech-motor sensory deficit, or environmental deprivation present, language difficulties are in excess of those associated with these disorders (Criterion D).
- If speech-motor or sensory deficit or neurological condition present, coded on Axis III.
- Linguistic features vary and include limited amount of speech, limited range of vocabulary, difficulty acquiring new words, word finding, or vocabulary errors, shortened sentences, simplified grammatical structures, limited varieties of grammatical structures, limited varieties of sentence structure and types, omission of critical parts of sentences, use of unusual word order, slow rate of language development, and impairment in receptive language development (e.g., difficulty understanding words, sentences, or specific types of words).
- Since development of expressive language depends on receptive skills, a pure receptive language disorder (analogous to Wernicke's aphasia in adults) is very rare.
- MRELD is acquired or developmental.

Associated Features and Disorders

- Similar to ELD disorder.
- Symptoms less obvious than expressive language symptoms.
- Child may intermittently appear not to hear, to be confused, or not to be paying attention when spoken to.
- Child may follow commands incorrectly, give inappropriate responses to questions.
- Exceptionally quiet or excessively talkative.
- Conversation skills poor or inappropriate.
- Deficits in sensory information processing are common.
- Phonological Disorder, Learning Disorders, ADHD, Developmental Coordination Disorder, and Enuresis often present.
- EEG abnormalities.
- Abnormal neuroimaging.
- A form of acquired MRELD is Landau-Kleffner syndrome, which has onset at about three to nine years and is accompanied by seizures.

VISUAL 5.7 *(continued)*

Specific Culture and Gender Features

- Culture: must consider bilingual effects.
- Developmental ELD more common in males.

Prevalence

- 3 percent of children estimated to have developmental MRELD.
- MRELD less common than ELD.

Course

- Developmental type can often be recognized by age four (milder forms detected upon entering school).
- Acquired ELD occurs at any age and onset is sudden.
- Developmental MRELD outcome is variable, but less positive than ELD.
- Acquired ELD course depends on the severity of the neural pathology.

Familial Pattern

- Developmental MRELD associated with a family history of communication or learning disorders.
- Acquired MRELD not associated with family history.

Differential Diagnosis

- Distinguish from ELD.
- MRELD not diagnosed if criteria for Autistic Disorder or PDD are met.
- Symptoms of MRELD present in mental retardation, hearing impairment, other sensory deficits, speech-motor deficits, severe environmental deprivation (MRELD clears rapidly when environmental deprivation eliminated). Dx. MRELD if symptoms in excess of those associated with these disorders.
- Distinguish from Disorder of Written Expression, Selective Mutism (do careful history to detect normal language in some situations), and Acquired Aphasia.

Source: American Psychiatric Association, 1994, pp. 58-61. Reprinted with permission from the *Diagnostic and Statistical Manual of Mental Disorders,* Fourth Edition. Copyright 1994 American Psychiatric Association.

Recommended Reading

Czerniewska, P. (1992). *Learning About Writing: The Early Years*. Malden, MA: Blackwell.

Fletcher, P. and MacWhinney, B. (1996). *The Handbook of Child Language*. Malden, MA: Blackwell.

Underwood, G. and Batt, W. (1996). *Reading and Understanding: An Introduction to the Psychology of Reading*. Malden, MA: Blackwell.

VISUAL 5.8. Conceptualization of Receptive and Expressive Language Disorders

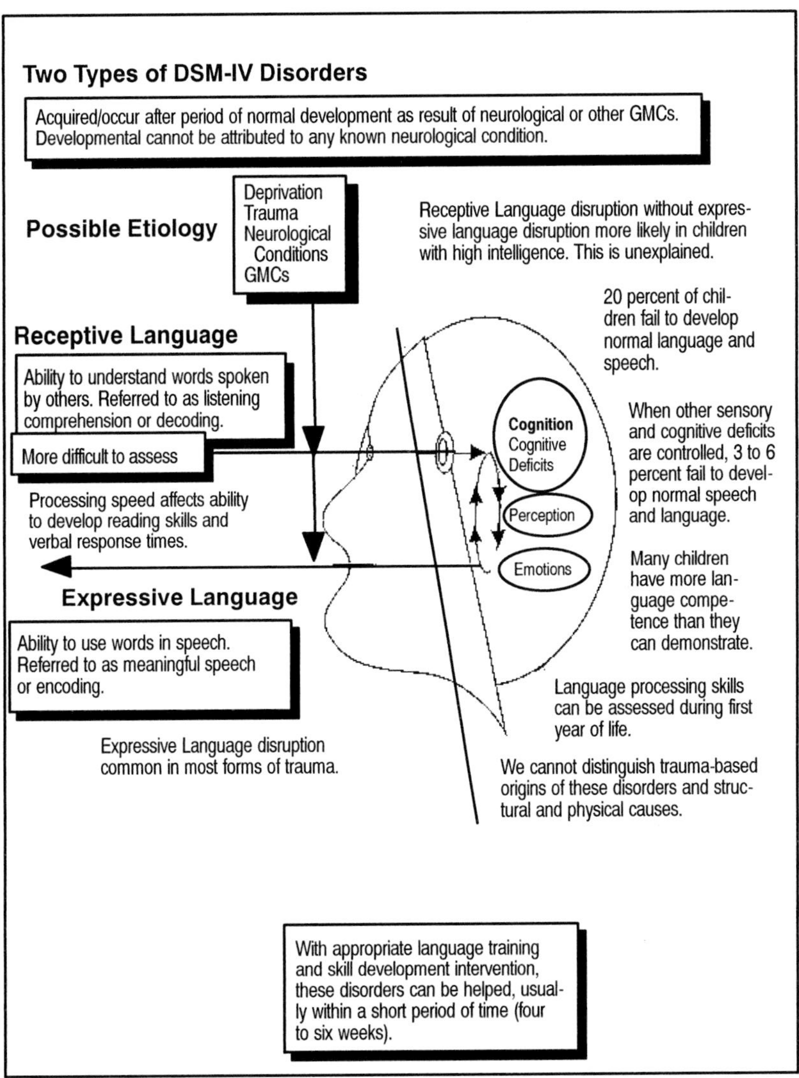

Source: American Psychiatric Association, 1994, pp. 55-61.

PERVASIVE DEVELOPMENTAL DISORDERS (PDDs)

299.00 Autistic Disorder
299.80 Rett's Disorder
299.10 Childhood Disintegrative Disorder
299.80 Asperger's Disorder
299.80 Pervasive Developmental Disorder NOS (including Atypical Autism)

Fundamental Features

- The essential feature of these disorders is a severe and pervasive impairment in social interaction skills, communication skills, or stereotyped behavior, interests, and skills.
- Usually detected during the early years of life.
- Usually coexists with Mental Retardation (code on Axis II).
- Often associated with coexisting GMCs (code on Axis III).
- These disorders are not necessarily associated with later development of schizophrenia.

Tip: Always do a thorough family assessment in the PDDs to rule out any familial disorders that may have contributed to the onset of PDDs.

- In late onset of these disorders some research evidence suggests that environmental teratogens (agents that can cause disruptions in biological and developmental processes) may be involved in etiology.
- A unique feature of Asperger's Disorder is the lack of clinically significant language delays. This can be a key factor in differential diagnosis.
- Some refer to this set of disorders as a "spectrum" disorder, in that a pervasive developmental disorder is a single disorder that manifests in degrees, and each disorder represents a level of intensity and extent of the symptoms of the disorder. Within the DSM-IV system, the focus is more on the age of onset of the disorder and nature of the symptoms in drawing the distinction between the different disorders. Visual 5.9 summarizes the age of onset factors in these disorders as well as the criteria and key features.

Recommended Standardized Measures

- Bayley Scales of Infant Development, Second Edition (BSID-II)
- Developmental Profile II (DP-II)
- Gilliam Autism Rating Scale (GARS)

Recommended Reading

Attwood, T. (1998). *Asperger's Syndrome: A Guide for Parents and Professionals*. London: Jessica Kingsley.

Cohen, S. (1998). *Targeting Autism: What We Know, Don't Know, and Can Do to Help Young Children with Autism and Related Disorders*. Berkeley, CA: University of California Press.

Kozloff, M. A. (1998). *Reaching the Autistic Child: A Parent Training Program*. Cambridge, MA: Brookline Books.

Rapoport, J. L. and Ismond, D. R. (1996). *DSM-IV Training Guide for Diagnosis of Childhood Disorders*. New York: Brunner/Mazel.

ATTENTION-DEFICIT AND DISRUPTIVE BEHAVIOR DISORDERS

314.01	ADHD, Combined Type
314.00	ADHD, Predominantly Inattentive
314.01	ADHD, Predominantly Hyperactive-Impulsive Type
314.9	ADHD NOS
312.81	Conduct Disorder, Childhood-Onset Type
312.82	Conduct Disorder, Adolescent-Onset Type
312.89	Conduct Disorder, Unspecified Onset
313.81	Oppositional Defiant Disorder
312.9	Disruptive Behavior Disorder NOS

Attention-Deficit/Hyperactivity Disorder

Fundamental Features

- This disorder is one of the most widely known disorders in the DSM system. The disorder consists of a pattern of inattention and/or hyperactivity or impulsivity. Its criteria are illustrated in Visual 5.10.

VISUAL 5.9. Pervasive Developmental Disorders Criteria (Also Referred to As "Pervasive Developmental Spectrum Disorders")

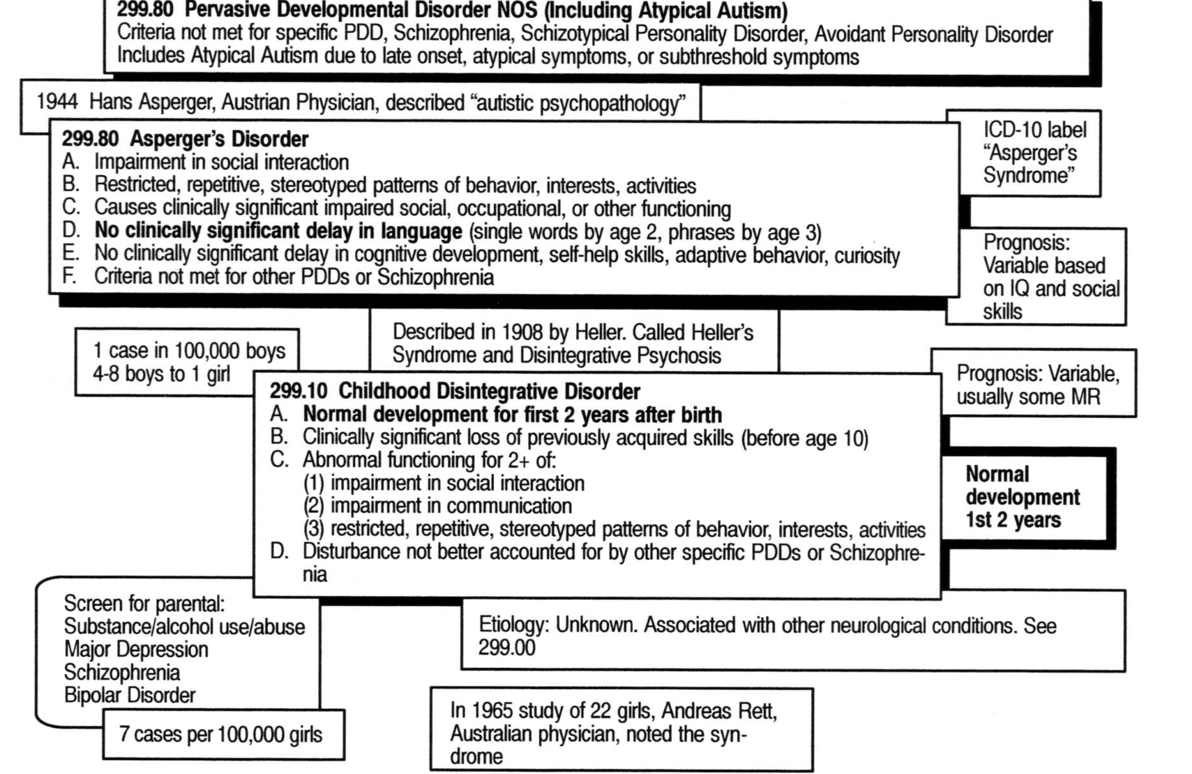

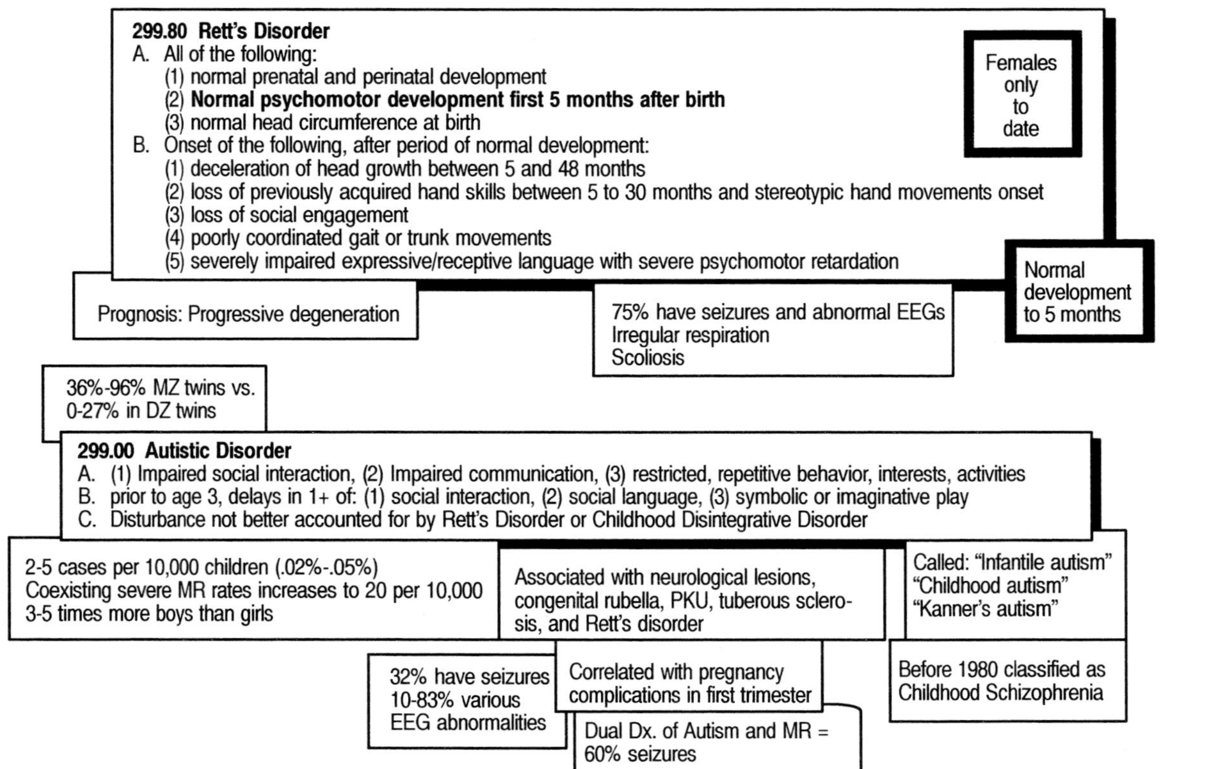

Source: American Psychiatric Association, 1994, pp. 65-78. Reprinted with permission from the *Diagnostic and Statistical Manual of Mental Disorders,* Fourth Edition. Copyright 1994 American Psychiatric Association.

VISUAL 5.10. Attention-Deficit/Hyperactivity Disorder Criteria

A. Either 1 or 2:
1. Six or more maladaptive and developmentally inconsistent symptoms of *inattention* for at least six months.

Inattention

a. fails at close attention to details or makes careless mistakes
b. difficulty sustaining attention often
c. does not seem to listen when spoken to
d. does not follow through on instructions and fails to finish tasks
e. difficulty organizing tasks and activities
f. avoids, dislikes tasks that require sustained mental effort
g. loses things necessary for tasks and activities
h. easily distracted by external stimuli
i. forgetful in daily activities

INATTENTION

2. Six or more of the following maladaptive and developmentally inconsistent symptoms of *hyperactivity-impulsivity* for at least six months.

Hyperactivity

a. fidgets with hands or feet or squirms in seat
b. leaves seat in class or other situations where remaining seated is expected
c. runs or climbs excessively in situations where it is inappropriate
d. difficulty playing quietly
e. "on the go" or acts as if "driven by a motor"
f. talks excessively

HYPERACTIVITY

Impulsivity

g. blurts out answers before questions are completed
h. difficulty awaiting turn
i. interrupts or intrudes on others

IMPULSIVITY

B. Some AD/HD symptoms that caused impairment were present before age 7.

C. Impairment from symptoms present in two or more settings (school, work, home).

D. Evidence of clinically significant impairment in social, academic, or occupational functioning.

E. Symptoms do not occur exclusively during a PDD, Schizophrenia, or other Psychotic Disorder and are not better accounted for by another MD (Mood Disorder, Anxiety Disorder, Dissociative Disorder, or PD).

Coding based on Type:

314.01 AD/HD, Combined Type: If both Criteria A1 and A2 met for past six months

314.00 AD/HD, Predominantly Inattentive Type: If Criterion A1 met but Criterion A2 not met for past six months.

314.01 AD/HD, Predominantly Hyperactive-Impulsive Type: If Criterion A2 met but Criterion A1 not met for past six months.

Coding note: For persons (especially adolescents and adults) currently having symptoms that no longer meet full criteria, specify "In Partial Remission."

Source: American Psychiatric Association, 1994, pp. 83-85. Reprinted with permission from the *Diagnostic and Statistical Manual of Mental Disorders*, Fourth Edition. Copyright 1994 American Psychiatric Association.

- The onset of symptoms of this disorder must occur before age seven. This disorder can be diagnosed in adults if the onset of the symptoms can be established to have first occurred by age seven.
- The criteria symptoms must be present in at least two settings (school, home, or work).
- The core features of this disorder are three sets of symptoms relating to inattention, hyperactivity, and impulsivity. The criteria for the disorder require that the person have at least six of nine symptoms of inattention and a total of six symptoms from the hyperactivity-impulsivity symptom groups.
- The three subtypes of this disorder are Predominantly Inattentive Type, Predominantly Hyperactive-Impulsive Type, and Combined Type, in which the person has inattention and hyperactivity-impulsivity.
- Some children who develop this disorder are later diagnosed with Oppositional Defiant Disorder, Conduct Disorder, and Antisocial Personality Disorder.
- Usually first diagnosed after entering school.

Differential Diagnosis

- Differential diagnosis should take into account age-appropriate activity level in active children, parents with low tolerance for child activity, Mental Retardation, oppositional behavior, understimulating environment, and PDD.

Recommended Standardized Measures

- Conners' Rating Scales-Revised (CRS-R)
- Connors' Adult ADHD Rating Scales (CAARS)
- ADHD Rating Scale-IV (ADHDRS-IV)

Recommended Reading

Barkley, R. A. (1990). *Attention Deficit Hyperactivity Disorder: A Handbook for Diagnosis and Treatment,* Second Edition. New York: Guilford.

Greenberg, G. S. and Horn, W. F. (1991). *Attention Deficit Hyperactivity Disorder: Questions and Answers for Parents.* Champaign, IL: Research Press.

Ingersoll, B. (1988). *Your Hyperactive Child: A Parent's Guide to Coping with Attention Deficit Disorder.* New York: Doubleday.

Pliszka, S. R., Carlson, C. L., and Swanson, J. M. (1999). *ADHD with Comorbid Disorders*. New York: Guilford.

Triolo, S. J. (1998). *Attention Deficit Hyperactivity Disorder in Adults*. Philadelphia, PA: Accelerated Development.

Conduct Disorder

Fundamental Features

- This single disorder is focused on a pattern of behavior in which the rights of others or age-appropriate societal norms are violated. These behaviors are assessed in four groups: (1) aggression that causes or threatens harm to people or animals, (2) acts that cause property harm or damage, (3) deceit or theft, and (4) serious violations of rules. The criteria specify levels of these behaviors during the past year and past six months.
- Conduct Disorder is one of the most frequently diagnosed disorders in childhood.
- Conduct Disorder can be diagnosed in persons over eighteen years of age if they do not meet the criteria for Antisocial Personality Disorder. Persons under age eighteen cannot be diagnosed with Antisocial Personality Disorder.
- Deviant behavior is present in multiple settings, such as home, school, and community.
- The three subtypes are Childhood Onset (onset of symptoms prior to age ten), Adolescent Onset (onset of symptoms after age ten), and Unspecified Onset (age of onset is unknown). Recent research suggests that onset for serious, internally driven Conduct Disorder is at a very early age (prior to age five), whereas late onset of the disorder (after age ten) is more likely peer group motivated and more amenable to treatment. Visual 5.11 provides a model for assessing the onset of Conduct Disorder and the most appropriate intervention methods.
- This disorder requires the diagnostician to enter a severity specifier of Mild, Moderate, or Severe as part of the diagnosis.

Differential Diagnosis

- For Conduct Disorder, the typical differential diagnosis would include Oppositional Defiant Disorder, ADHD, Manic Episode, and Child or Adolescent Antisocial Behavior.

VISUAL 5.11. Conduct Disorder Diagnosis Summary

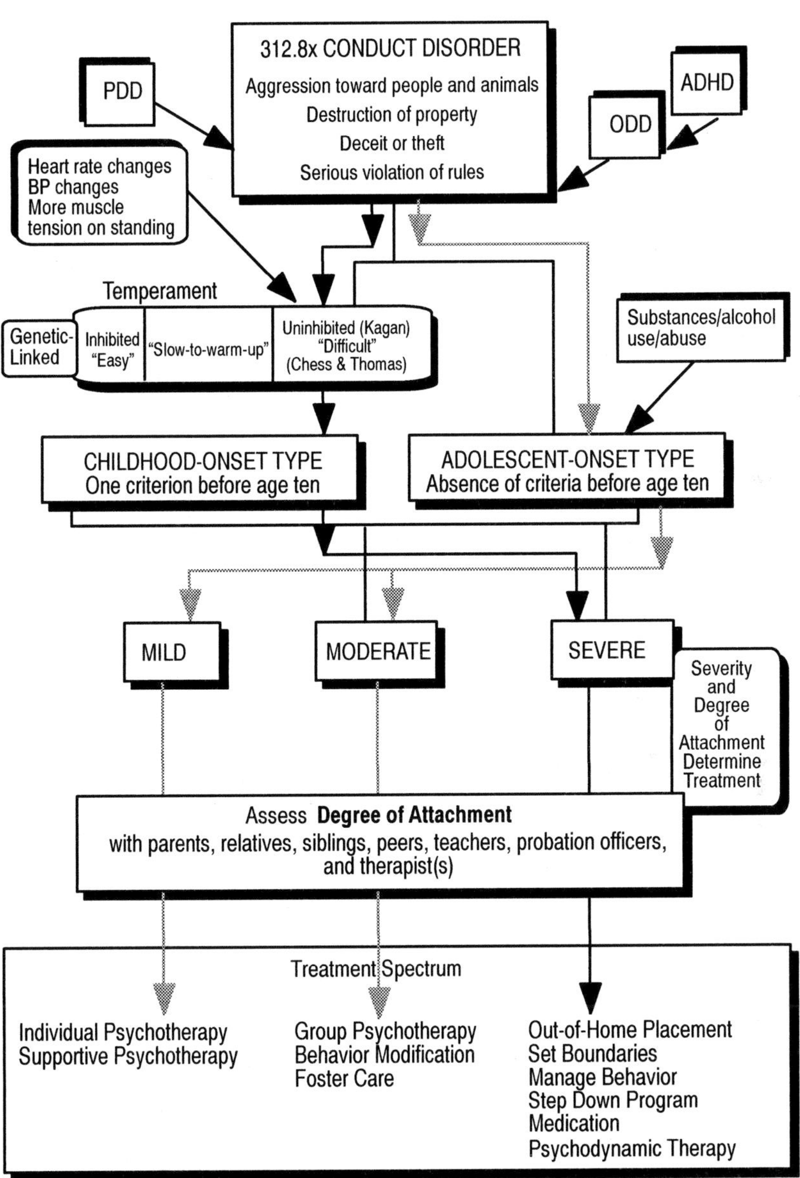

Source: American Psychiatric Association, 1994, pp. 85-91.

Recommended Standardized Measures

- Children's Inventory of Anger (CHIA)
- Devereux Scales of Mental Disorders (DSMD)
- Louisville Behavior Checklist (LBC)
- Burks' Behavior Rating Scales (BBRS)
- See also the scales for Oppositional Defiant Disorder

Recommended Reading

Chess, S. and Thomas, A. (1996). *Temperament: Theory and Practice.* New York: Brunner/Mazel.

Flannery, D. J. and Huff, C. R. (1998). *Youth Violence: Prevention, Intervention, and Social Policy.* Washington, DC: American Psychiatric Press.

Henggeler, S. W., Schoenwald, S. K., Borduin, C. M., Roland, M. D., and Cunningham, P. B. (1998). *Multisystemic Treatment of Antisocial Behavior in Children and Adolescents.* New York: Guilford.

Kagan, J. (1984). *The Nature of the Child.* New York: Basic Books.

Oppositional Defiant Disorder

Fundamental Features

- This disorder can be viewed as a less intense version of the Conduct Disorder diagnosis. The key features are negative, disobedient, and hostile behavior toward authority figures that persists for at least six months.
- To meet the criteria for the disorder, the behavior, in the diagnostician's judgment, must be beyond the bounds of age-appropriate childhood opposition or adolescent adjustment.
- Aggression can occur toward adults and peers, but it is not as severe as that seen in Conduct Disorder.

Differential Diagnosis

- The key disorders in differential Diagnosis of Oppositional Defiant Disorder are Conduct Disorder, Mood Disorders, Psychotic Disorders, Communication Disorders, or age-appropriate behaviors.

Recommended Standardized Measures

- Devereux Scales of Mental Disorders (DSMD)
- Social Behavioral Assessment Inventory (SBAI)
- See also the scales for Conduct Disorder

Recommended Reading

Barkley, R. A. and Benton, C. M. (1998). *Your Defiant Child: Eight Steps to Better Behavior.* New York: Guilford.

Barkley, R. A., Edwards, G. H., and Robin, A. L. (1999). *Defiant Teens: A Clinician's Manual for Assessment and Family Intervention.* New York: Guilford.

Disruptive Behavior Disorder NOS

This diagnosis is used for conduct or oppositional behavior that does not meet the full criteria for Conduct Disorder or Oppositional Defiant Disorder, but symptoms or behavioral problems exist that are clinically significant.

FEEDING AND EATING DISORDERS OF INFANCY OR EARLY CHILDHOOD

307.52 Pica
307.53 Rumination Disorder
307.59 Feeding Disorder of Infancy or Early Childhood

Pica

Fundamental Features

- Pica is a rare disorder that occurs mostly in young children, the elderly, and people with mental retardation. The fundamental feature of this disorder is repeated eating of substances that are not nutritional for a period of at least one month.
- The type of substances eaten usually vary with age. Younger children eat plaster, paint, string, hair, or cloth. Older children eat animal feces, sand, insects, leaves, and pebbles. Adolescents and adults eat clay, soil, or wood.

- The disorder is not diagnosed if the eating of substances is part of a culturally sanctioned ritual or practice.
- If the eating behavior is part of another mental disorder, such as Mental Retardation, Pervasive Developmental Disorder, or Schizophrenia, it must be so severe that it warrants independent clinical attention.

Differential Diagnosis

Differential diagnosis includes Mental Retardation, Pervasive Developmental Disorder, Schizophrenia, Kleine-Levin syndrome, Rumination Disorder, Feeding and Eating Disorder of Infancy or Early Childhood, Anorexia Nervosa, and Bulimia.

Rumination Disorder

Fundamental Features

- The singular feature of this disorder is regurgitation and rechewing of food that develops in early childhood after a period of normal development and lasts for at least one month.

Differential Diagnosis

- The clinician should consider the following disorders when doing differential diagnosis for this disorder: GMCs, normal vomiting of childhood, Anorexia Nervosa, or Bulimia Nervosa.

Feeding Disorder of Infancy or Early Childhood

Fundamental Features

- The singular feature of this disorder is the failure to eat adequately and is indicated by failure to gain weight or significant weight loss during a one-month period.

Differential Diagnosis

- The essential feature of differential diagnosis for this disorder is to review for GMCs.

TIC DISORDERS

307.23 Tourette's Disorder
307.22 Chronic Motor or Vocal Tic Disorder
307.21 Transient Tic Disorder
307.20 Tic Disorder NOS

Fundamental Features

- Tics are sudden, recurring, nonrhythmic, stereotyped motor movements or vocalizations.
- Tics can be made worse by stress.
- Tics can decrease when the person is engaged in focused activities.
- Tics usually diminish significantly during sleep.
- Tics are typed as simple or complex.
- Examples of simple motor tics are eye blinking, neck jerking, shoulder shrugging, facial grimaces, and coughing. Simple vocal tics include throat clearing, grunting, sniffing, snorting, and barking. Complex motor tics can be facial gestures, grooming behaviors, jumping, touching, stamping, and smelling objects. Common complex vocal tics are repeating words and phrases out of context, coprolalia (use of socially unacceptable or obscene words), palilalia (repeating one's own sounds or words), and echolalia (repeating the sound, word, or phrase last heard).
- Tourette's Disorder involves multiple motor and one or more vocal tics that have occurred many times each day for more than one year. Chronic Motor or Vocal Tic Disorder involves single or multiple motor or vocal tics that have occurred many times almost daily for at least one year. Transient Tic Disorder involves single or multiple motor and/or vocal tics that occur many times a day, almost every day, for at least four weeks, but no longer than twelve months.

Differential Diagnosis

- Abnormal movements that accompany GMCs, Medication-Induced Movement Disorder NOS, Stereotypic Movement Disorder, PDDs, or compulsions should be considered as part of differential diagnosis.

ELIMINATION DISORDERS

___._ Encopresis (two subtypes)
787.6 With Constipation and Overflow Incontinence
307.7 Without Constipation and Overflow Incontinence
307.6 Enuresis (not due to a GMC)

Fundamental Features

Tip: When encountering the symptoms of enuresis and encopresis, the diagnostician should inquire whether the child has had a medical examination within the past thirty days that included evaluation of these symptoms, since, in many cases, the symptoms can be caused by a medical condition.

- The essential feature of Encopresis is repeated passage of feces in inappropriate places, such as in clothing or on floors. Most often this is an involuntary act, but it can be intentional. These incidents must occur at least once a month for at least three months. The child must be at least four years of age. If the child has developmental delays, he/she must have attained a mental age of at least four years.
- The main feature of Enuresis is frequent voiding of urine during the day or night in bedding or clothes. This is usually involuntary, but can be intentional. The voiding must occur at least twice a week for at least three months or cause clinically significant distress or impairment in social, academic, or other areas of functioning. The child must be at least five years of age. If the child has developmental delays, he/she must have a mental age of at least five years. The diagnostician must specify Nocturnal (night) Only, Diurnal (day) Only, or Nocturnal and Diurnal.

Differential Diagnosis

- GMCs should be considered when evaluating for Encopresis. According to the DSM-IV Differential Diagnosis section for this disorder, Encopresis is diagnosed only when constipation is present during a GMC, and fecal incontinence related to other GMCs, such as chronic diarrhea, would not justify a DSM-IV diagnosis.
- The basic differential diagnosis for Enuresis is to review for GMCs. According to the DSM-IV Differential Diagnosis section for this disorder, Enuresis can be diagnosed if the condition existed before the onset of the GMC and persists after treatment of the GMC.

OTHER DISORDERS OF INFANCY, CHILDHOOD, OR ADOLESCENCE

309.21 Separation Anxiety Disorder
313.23 Selective Mutism

313.89 Reactive Attachment Disorder of Infancy or Early Childhood
307.3 Stereotypic Movement Disorder
313.9 Disorder of Infancy, Childhood, or Adolescence NOS

Separation Anxiety Disorder

Fundamental Features

- This disorder consists of excessive anxiety regarding separation from the home or the caregivers. The anxiety must be clinically judged to be in excess of age-appropriate fears, and its duration must be at least four weeks.
- Visual 5.12, which summaries this disorder, has been included because of the increase in violence outside the home in places such as schools and day care centers. The visual can aid diagnosticians when faced with children who have realistic fears based on a threatening incident versus children who have separation anxiety for no apparent reason. The visual may aid in performing differential diagnosis based on Generalized Anxiety Disorder, Acute Stress Disorder, or PTSD.

Differential Diagnosis

- Differential diagnosis includes PDDs, Schizophrenia, Generalized Anxiety Disorder, Panic Disorder With Agoraphobia, Agoraphobia Without History of Panic Disorder, or Conduct Disorder.

Selective Mutism

Fundamental Features

- Selective Mutism is the failure to speak in specific social situations (such as in school, day care, when with playmates or relatives) in which speaking is expected. The person usually speaks in other situations.
- The mutism must be present for at least one month and not limited to the first month of school.
- This disorder is excluded if the person does not speak because of a lack of knowledge of a situation or because of embarrassment due to a communication disorder.

VISUAL 5.12. 309.21 Separation Anxiety Disorder Criteria Summary

FUNDAMENTAL FEATURE

Excessive anxiety concerning separation from the home or from those to whom the person is attached

DIAGNOSTIC CRITERIA

A. Developmentally inappropriate excessive anxiety about separation from home/person with 3+ of:
   1. Recurrently excessive distress upon separation
   2. Persistent/excessive worry about losing or harm to major attachment figure
   3. Persistent/excessive worry events will cause separation
   4. Reluctance or refusal to go to school or elsewhere because of separation fear
   5. Fearful or reluctance to be alone or without attachment person
   6. Refusal to go to sleep without nearness of attachment figure
   7. Repeated nightmares with separation theme
   8. Repeated complaints of physical symptoms when separation occurs/anticipated

B. Duration of four weeks plus

C. Onset before age eighteen

D. Causes clinically significant distress/impairment in social, academic, or other areas

E. Does not occur during course of PDD, Schizophrenia, other Psychotic Disorder, or Panic Disorder

ASSOCIATED FEATURES

Usually:
- Close-knit families
- On separation, shows social withdrawal, apathy, sadness, poor concentration
- Fear of animals, monsters, darkness, muggers/burglars, kidnappers, car accidents, plane travel
- Concerns about death
- Becomes angry when facing separation
- When alone reports unusual perceptions (seeing things)
- Leads to family conflict and frustration
- Compliant and eager to please
- Depressed mood

PREVALENCE, COURSE, FAMILIAL PATTERN

- Present in 4 percent of children/young adolescents
- Develops after life stress
- Onset before preschool age to eighteen
- Periods of intensity and remission
- More common in first degree relatives
- More frequent in mothers with panic disorder

DIFFERENTIAL DIAGNOSIS

- PDD
- Schizophrenia
- Generalized Anxiety Disorder
- Panic Disorder With Agoraphobia
- Agoraphobia Without History of Panic Disorder
- Conduct Disorder

Source: American Psychiatric Association, 1994, pp. 110-113. Reprinted with permission from the *Diagnostic and Statistical Manual of Mental Disorders,* Fourth Edition.

- Persons with mutism will sometimes communicate by gestures, nodding the head, or short utterances.

Differential Diagnosis

- Differential Diagnosis must consider Communication Disorder, Lack of knowledge of language, PDD, Schizophrenia, other Psychotic Disorder, severe Mental Retardation, or Social Phobia.

Tips: Often children with Selective Mutism will not talk in the clinical interview. Sometimes the child can be asked to communicate with the clinician by whispering to the caregiver who then relays the information to the clinician. I have even administered standardized tests in this manner.

If the caregiver/family member of the person has a camcorder, the therapist should ask the caregiver to provide a videotape of the person talking in the home for review to assess the accuracy of the degree of mutism and to assess for other communication disorders.

If the person is reported not to speak in any situations, the person should be referred for medical evaluation.

For diagnostic guidelines for this disorder, see a special section on Selective Mutism in *Developmental and Behavioral Pediatrics* (Stein, Rapin, and Yapko, 1999).

Reactive Attachment Disorder

Fundamental Features

- Reactive Attachment Disorder consists of disturbed and developmentally inappropriate social relatedness that begins before age five and is associated with grossly pathological care.
- The two types of this disorder are Inhibited Type and Disinhibited Type. The Inhibited Type child fails to initiate and respond in developmentally appropriate ways in social interactions. The Disinhibited Type child selects attachment figures and engages in socialization in an indiscriminate manner.
- With this disorder, the presumption is that pathological care of the child has occurred in the form of failure to meet the child's emotional and physical needs, and primary caregivers have changed frequently.

Tip: Before making this diagnosis, the clinician should ensure that pathological care has been documented. This would usually involve a finding of neglect and/or abuse by an agency that has completed a formal evaluation of the child and the caregivers.

Differential Diagnosis

- Differential Diagnosis should include Mental Retardation, PDD, and ADHD.

Recommended Reading

Ainsworth, M. D., Blehar, M. C., Waters, E., and Wall, S. (1978). *Patterns of Attachment: A Psychological Study of the Stranger Situation*. Hillsdale, NJ: Lawrence Erlbaum Associates.

Cassidy, J. and Shaver, P. R. (1999). *Handbook of Attachment: Theory, Research, and Clinical Applications*. New York: Guilford.

Stereotypic Movement Disorder

Fundamental Features

- This disorder is characterized by motor behavior that is repetitive, appears uncontrollable, and is not functional. The behavior significantly interferes with activities of daily living and can result in injury that requires medical intervention.
- The one specifier for this disorder is With Self-Injurious Behavior.

Differential Diagnosis

- Differential diagnosis should include a review for Mental Retardation, PDD, OCD, Tic Disorder, Trichotillomania, Factitious Disorder, self-mutilation associated with certain Psychotic and Personality Disorders, Involuntary Movements, and GMCs.

Disorder of Infancy, Childhood, or Adolescence NOS

This final category of the ICA disorders is designed to capture symptoms and behaviors judged by the clinician to constitute a mental disorder, but do not precisely meet the criteria of a specific DSM-IV disorder.

CONCLUSION

Visuals 5.13 and 5.14 provide a summary of the childhood and adult disorders that are commonly diagnosed in children. These visuals are based on general trends and do not reflect precise statistical findings. Visual 5.15 summarizes the ages of onset for ICA disorders. Not all disorders specify an age of onset, but the visual offers a crude measure of the developmental progression of the onset of some ICA disorders.

REFERENCES

American Psychiatric Association (1994). *Diagnostic and Statistical Manual of Mental Disorders,* Fourth Edition. Washington, DC: American Psychiatric Association.

Stein, M. T., Rapin, I., and Yapko, D. (1999). Challenging Case: Selective Mutism. *Developmental and Behavioral Pediatrics,* 20(1): 38-41.

VISUAL 5.13. Frequently Used DSM-IV ICA Disorders

312.8x Conduct Disorder
Repeated violation of age-appropriate societal norms

313.81 Oppositional Defiant Disorder
Negative, defiant, and hostile behavior toward authority figures for at least six months

ATTENTION-DEFICIT/HYPERACTIVITY DISORDER
314.9 AD/HD NOS
314.01 AD/HD, Combined Type
314.00 AD/HD, Predominantly Inattentive Type
314.01 AD/HD, Predominantly Hyperactive-Impulse Type
Inattention and/or hyperactivity-impulsivity outside normal range

PERVASIVE DEVELOPMENTAL DISORDERS

299.80 Pervasive Developmental Disorder NOS (including Atypical Autism)
299.80 Asperger's Disorder. Severe, sustained impairment of social interaction and restricted, repetitive patterns of behavior — New
299.80 Rett's Disorder. Multiple deficits after a period of normal functioning during first five months — New

Now coded on Axis I

299.10 Childhood Disintegrative Disorder. Regression of functioning after two years of normal development — New
299.00 Autistic Disorder. Impaired developmental social interaction and communication; restricted activities and interests

FEEDING AND EATING DISORDERS
307.52 Pica. Persistent eating of nonnutritive substances for one month plus
307.53 Rumination Disorder. Repeated regurgitation and rechewing food in infancy for one month plus after period of normal development
307.59 Feeding Disorder. Persistent failure to eat adequately (with no weight gain or weight loss) for one month plus

Screen for GMCs, stress, acute chronic depression, alcohol/drug abuse, personality disorder in mother.

35 percent of infants have feeding problems.
1 to 2 percent have serious eating problems.
Feeding problems persist into adulthood.
Pica associated with bulimia nervosa in adolescence.

VISUAL 5.14. Frequently Used Adult DSM-IV Disorders for ICA Diagnosis

300.4 Dysthymic Disorder
Chronic depression for two years

296.3x Major Depressive Disorder, Recurrent
At least two-week period of depressive mood and loss of interest in activities

296.2x Major Depressive Disorder, Single Episode
At least two-week period of depressive mood and loss of interest in activities

300.02 Generalized Anxiety Disorder
Excessive anxiety and worry for a number of events for six months or more

309.81 Posttraumatic Stress Disorder
Exposed to traumatic event with symptoms for more than one month in which:
1. experienced/witnessed event that threatened death or serious injury
2. person's response involved fear, helplessness, horror

Acute Symptoms < than three months

Chronic Symptoms > than three months

Delayed Onset Six months after stressor

308.3 Acute Stress Disorder
Exposed to traumatic event within one month in which:
1. experienced/witnessed event that threatened death or serious injury
2. person's response involved fear, helplessness, horror

Adjustment Disorders

309.0 With Depressed Mood. Depression, tearfulness, hopelessness
309.24 With Anxiety. Nervousness, worry, jitteriness, separation fear
309.28 With Mixed Anxiety and Depressed Mood. Combination of depression and anxiety
309.3 With Disturbance of Conduct. Violation of rights of others and societal norms, truancy, vandalism, reckless driving, fighting, legal default
309.4 With Mixed Disturbance of Emotions and Conduct. Combined depression and/or anxiety and conduct disturbance
309.9 Unspecified. Physical complaints, social withdrawal, work or academic inhibition in response to unusual stressor.

Acute. Symptoms present less than six months

Chronic. Stressor persists more than six months

VISUAL 5.15. Average Age of Onset for ICA Disorders Summary

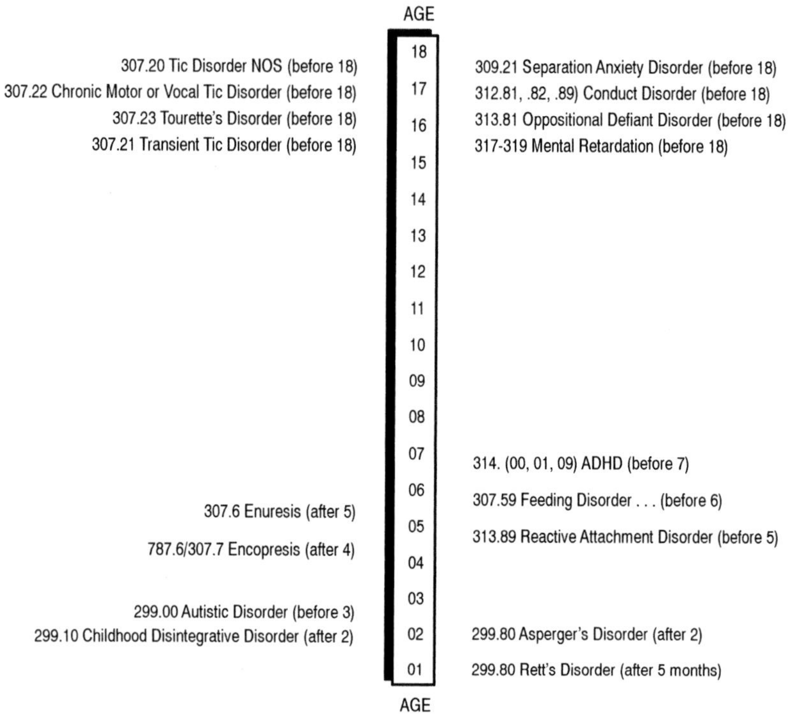

Disorders (left)	AGE	Disorders (right)
307.20 Tic Disorder NOS (before 18) 307.22 Chronic Motor or Vocal Tic Disorder (before 18) 307.23 Tourette's Disorder (before 18) 307.21 Transient Tic Disorder (before 18)	18	309.21 Separation Anxiety Disorder (before 18) 312.81, .82, .89) Conduct Disorder (before 18) 313.81 Oppositional Defiant Disorder (before 18) 317-319 Mental Retardation (before 18)
	17	
	16	
	15	
	14	
	13	
	12	
	11	
	10	
	09	
	08	
	07	314. (00, 01, 09) ADHD (before 7)
	06	307.59 Feeding Disorder . . . (before 6)
307.6 Enuresis (after 5)	05	313.89 Reactive Attachment Disorder (before 5)
787.6/307.7 Encopresis (after 4)	04	
299.00 Autistic Disorder (before 3)	03	
299.10 Childhood Disintegrative Disorder (after 2)	02	299.80 Asperger's Disorder (after 2)
	01	299.80 Rett's Disorder (after 5 months)
	AGE	

Disorders with no specific onset age or age appropriate onset

299.80	Pervasive Developmental Disorder NOS	315.00	Reading Disorder
307.3	Stereotypic Movement Disorder	315.1	Mathematics Disorder
307.0	Stuttering	315.2	Disorder of Written Expression
307.52	Pica	315.31	Expressive Language Disorder
307.9	Communication Disorder NOS	315.31	Mixed Receptive-Expressive Language Disorder
312.9	Disruptive Behavior Disorder NOS	315.39	Phonological Disorder
313.23	Selective Mutism	315.4	Developmental Coordination Disorder
313.9	Disorder of Infancy, Childhood, or Adolescence NOS	315.9	Learning Disorder NOS

Chapter 6

Delirium, Dementia, and Amnestic and Other Cognitive Disorders

DISORDERS

Delirium

293.0	Delirium Due to . . . (indicate GMC)
___._	Substance Intoxication Delirium (see p. 131 for substance-specific codes)
___._	Substance Withdrawal Delirium (see p. 132 for substance-specific codes)
___._	Delirium Due to Multiple Etiologies (code for each specific etiology)
780.09	Delirium NOS

Dementia

290.xx	Dementia of the Alzheimer's Type, With Early Onset (see pp. 140-141 for coding options)
290.xx	Dementia of the Alzheimer's Type, With Late Onset (see pp. 140-141 for coding options)
290.4x	Vascular Dementia (formerly Multi-Infarct Dementia) (see p. 144 for coding options)
294.1	Dementia Due to HIV Disease
294.1	Dementia Due to Head Trauma
294.1	Dementia Due to Parkinson's Disease
294.1	Dementia Due to Huntington's Disease
290.10	Dementia Due to Pick's Disease
290.10	Dementia Due to Creutzfeldt-Jakob Disease

294.1 Dementia Due to . . . (indicate GMC) (see pp. 146-152 for range of codes)
___._ Substance-Induced Persisting Dementia (see p. 154 for coding details)
___._ Dementia Due to Multiple Etiologies (see p. 155 for coding details)
294.8 Dementia NOS

Amnestic Disorders

294.0 Amnestic Disorder Due to . . . (indicate GMC)
___._ Substance-Induced Persisting Amnestic Disorder (see p. 162 for coding details)
294.8 Amnestic Disorder NOS

Other Cognitive Disorders

294.9 Cognitive Disorder NOS

FUNDAMENTAL FEATURES

- This class of disorders is divided into Delirium, Dementia, Amnestic Disorders, and Cognitive Disorders.
- In DSM-III-R these disorders were included in a section titled "Organic Mental Syndromes and Disorders." The term "organic mental disorder" is no longer used in the DSM system.
- A delirium is a disturbance of consciousness and change in cognition that develops in a brief period of time. Disorders in this set are listed according to suspected etiology.

Tip: Whenever there is a sudden onset of symptoms, as is the case in delirium, the clinician should always be alert to the possibility of a GMC or substance/alcohol use/abuse.

- Dementia is based on multiple cognitive deficits that include impairment in memory. Dementias are categorized according to the presumed etiology.
- An amnestic disorder reflects memory impairment while other significant cognitive impairments are absent.

- The category Cognitive Disorder NOS covers cognitive dysfunction believed to be due to a GMC or substance use that does not meet the criteria for disorders listed in this section.
- These disorders have unique coding features, and professionals who work with this class of disorders should refer to the specific disorders to establish accurate coding. The introductory listing of the disorders in this section refers to the disorders that have unique coding and includes the DSM-IV page numbers where the appropriate codes are provided.
- These disorders are more likely to be diagnosed by a physician. Visual 6.1 gives a summary conceptualization of these disorders.

REFERENCE

American Psychiatric Association (1994). *Diagnostic and Statistical Manual of Mental Disorders,* Fourth Edition. Washington, DC: American Psychiatric Association.

VISUAL 6.1. Delirium, Dementia, and Amnestic and Other Cognitive Disorders Criteria Summary

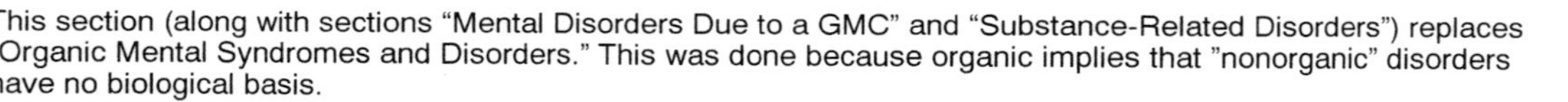

This section (along with sections "Mental Disorders Due to a GMC" and "Substance-Related Disorders") replaces "Organic Mental Syndromes and Disorders." This was done because organic implies that "nonorganic" disorders have no biological basis.

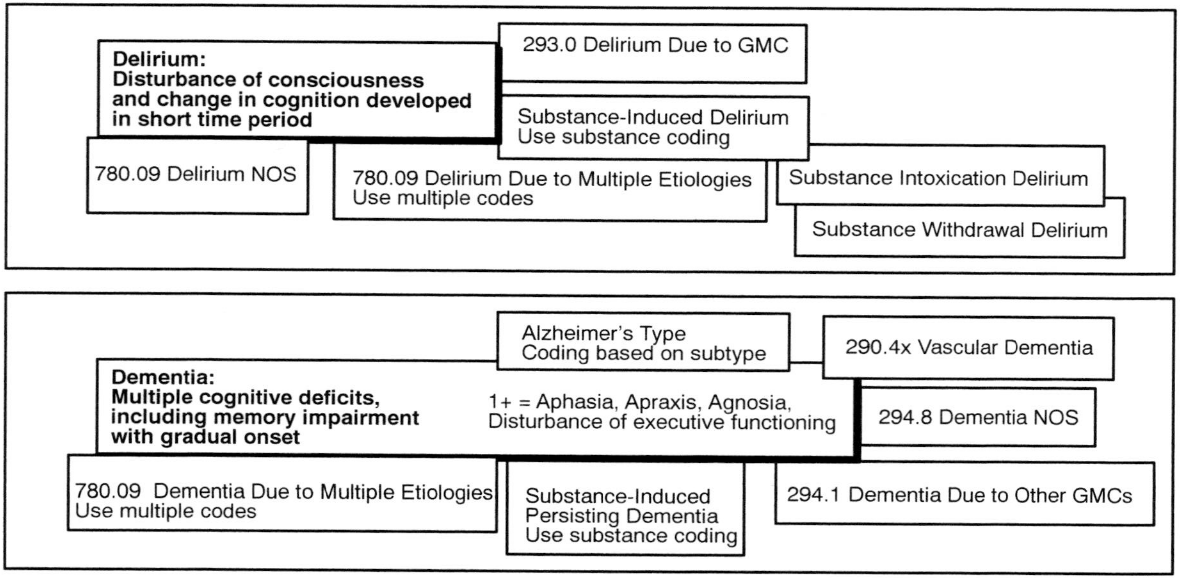

Delirium:
Disturbance of consciousness and change in cognition developed in short time period

293.0 Delirium Due to GMC

Substance-Induced Delirium
Use substance coding

Substance Intoxication Delirium

Substance Withdrawal Delirium

780.09 Delirium NOS

780.09 Delirium Due to Multiple Etiologies
Use multiple codes

Dementia:
Multiple cognitive deficits, including memory impairment with gradual onset

1+ = Aphasia, Apraxis, Agnosia, Disturbance of executive functioning

Alzheimer's Type
Coding based on subtype

290.4x Vascular Dementia

294.8 Dementia NOS

294.1 Dementia Due to Other GMCs

780.09 Dementia Due to Multiple Etiologies
Use multiple codes

Substance-Induced
Persisting Dementia
Use substance coding

VISUAL 6.1 *(continued)*

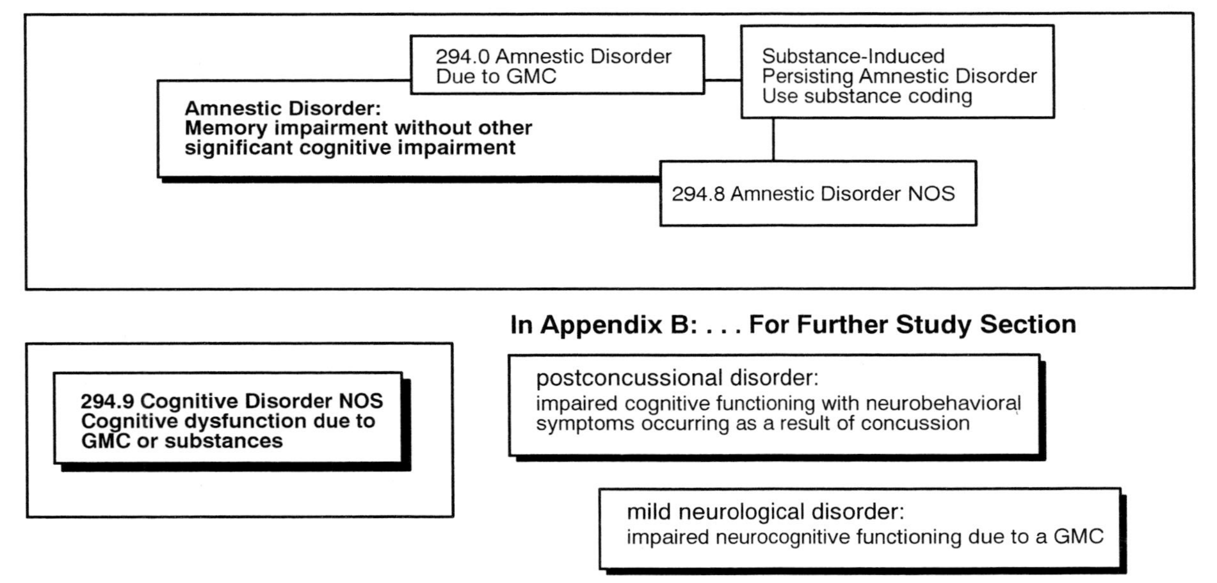

Source: American Psychiatric Association, 1994, pp. 123-174. Reprinted with permission from the *Diagnostic and Statistical Manual of Mental Disorders,* Fourth Edition. Copyright 1994 American Psychiatric Association.

Chapter 7

Mental Disorders Due to a General Medical Condition Not Elsewhere Classified

DISORDERS

293.89 Catatonic Disorder Due to a GMC
310.1 Personality Change Due to a GMC
293.9 Mental Disorder NOS Due to a GMC

FUNDAMENTAL FEATURES

- The essential feature of this set of disorders is that the person has mental symptoms that are determined by clinical judgment to be a direct physiological consequence of a general medical condition (GMC).
- This class of disorders would most likely be diagnosed by a physician or by a nonmedical mental health professional in close consultation with a physician.
- As with the previous section, "Delirium, Dementia, and Amnestic and Other Cognitive Disorders," disorders in this section were referred to as "organic" disorders in DSM-III-R. The term organic was retired for the DSM-IV.
- The term "general medical condition" refers to conditions that are recorded on Axis III of the DSM multiaxial system and, when listed on Axis III, are considered outside the mental disorders in the ICD. However, the reciprocal link between mental and physical disorders must be kept in mind.

- Some of the GMCs that produce mental symptoms are listed with disorders in the manual that share features with them. These disorders are listed in the lower left-hand corner of Visual 7.1.
- Three, out of 4, criteria are essential to the diagnosis of disorders in this section:

    1. Criterion B: evidence derived from history, physical examination, and laboratory findings shows that the symptoms are a direct physiological consequence of a GMC.
    2. Criterion C: the symptoms are not better accounted for by another mental disorder.
    3. Criterion D: the symptoms do not occur during an episode of a delirium.

- If the mental disorder is a direct physiological consequence of a physical disorder, code the mental condition and GMC disorder on Axis I and record the GMC on Axis III. If the mental disorder is not due to a GMC, record the mental disorder on Axis I or II and the GMC on Axis III. Appendix G of the DSM-IV lists summary ICD GMCs that can be used in recording Axis III diagnoses. Visual 7.2 illustrates diagnoses based on the explanation given here.

RECOMMENDED STANDARDIZED MEASURES

- Health Problems Checklist

RECOMMENDED READING

Morrison, J. (1997). *When Psychological Problems Mask Medical Disorders: A Guide for Psychotherapists.* New York: Guilford.

REFERENCE

American Psychiatric Association (1994). *Diagnostic and Statistical Manual of Mental Disorders,* Fourth Edition. Washington, DC: American Psychiatric Association.

VISUAL 7.1. Mental Disorders Due to a General Medical Condition (GMC) Criteria Summary

Fundamental Features

Presence of mental symptoms that are the direct physiological consequence of a GMC. Primary mental disorder refers to disorders that are not due to a GMC or substance induced.

If mental disorder a DIRECT PHYSIOLOGICAL CONSEQUENCE of the physical disorder, code physical disorder on Axis I and Axis III.

If mental disorder PSYCHOLOGICAL CONSEQUENCE of GMC, record mental disorder on Axis I and GMC on Axis III.

Use ICD-9 and ICD-10 codes in Appendix G.

Replaces section titled "Organic Mental Syndromes and Disorders."
Word organic eliminated, and disorders distributed in other sections.
Causative medical disorder coded on Axis III.
"Primary" mental disorder differentiated from that occurring "secondary" to a physical disorder.

293.89 Catatonic Disorder Due to a GMC
Catatonia due to direct physiological effects of a GMC

310.1 Personality Change Due to a GMC
Persistent personality disturbance as direct consequence of a GMC

TYPES:
Labile
Disinhibited
Aggressive
Apathetic
Paranoid
Other
Combined
Unspecified

293.9 Mental Disorder NOS Due to a GMC
Condition due to GMC but criteria not met for a specific mental disorder

MDs due to GMC in other sections

293.0 Delirium Due to GMC (p. 127)
___._ Dementia Due to GMC (p. 146)

294.0 Amnestic Disorder Due to GMC (p. 158)
293.8x Psychotic Disorder Due to GMC (p. 306)
293.83 Mood Disorder Due to GMC (p. 366)
293.89 Anxiety Disorder Due to GMC (p. 436)
___._ Sexual Dysfunction Due to GMC (p. 515)

780.5x Sleep Disorder Due to GMC (p. 597)

Source: American Psychiatric Association, 1994, pp. 165-174. Reprinted with permission from the *Diagnostic and Statistical Manual of Mental Disorders,* Fourth Edition.

VISUAL 7.2. Examples of Diagnosis for Mental Disorders Due to a General Medical Condition

DEPRESSION AS **DIRECT PHYSIOLOGICAL CONSEQUENCE** OF GMC

Axis I: 293.83 Mood Disorder Due to HIV Disease With Depressive Features

Axis II: V71.09 No Dx. on Axis II

Axis III: 042.2 AIDS, with specified malignant neoplasms as reported by Physician (Dr. R. U. Wright)

DEPRESSION AS **DIRECT PSYCHOLOGICAL CONSEQUENCE** OF GMC

Axis I: 309.28 Adjustment Disorder with Anxiety and Depressed Mood, Acute

Axis II: V71.09 No Dx. on Axis II

Axis III: 042.9 AIDS, unspecified as reported by IP and Physician (Dr. R. U. Wright)

DEPRESSION AS **DIRECT PSYCHOLOGICAL CONSEQUENCE** OF GMC

Axis I: 296.23 Major Depressive Disorder, Single Episode, Severe W/O Psychotic Features

Axis II: V71.09 No Dx. on Axis II

Axis III: 042.9 AIDS, unspecified as reported by IP and Physician (Dr. R. U. Wright)

Chapter 8

Substance-Related Disorders

DISORDERS

See Visual 8.1 and pages 16-19 in the DSM-IV.

FUNDAMENTAL FEATURES

- This section covers disorders related to taking a drug of abuse, including alcohol, the side effects of a medication, and toxin exposure. There are eleven classes of substances (see Visual 8.1) and polysubstances and other or unknown substances.
- Polysubstance Dependence refers to using at least three of the eleven substance classes in a twelve-month period.
- Prescription medications and over-the-counter medications can cause Substance-Related Disorders.
- Exposure to chemical substances (such as lead, some pesticides, and antifreeze) can cause Substance-Related Disorders.
- Substance Dependence refers to a cluster of cognitive, behavioral, and physiological symptoms indicating the person continues to use the substance despite substantial substance-related problems. A repeated pattern of self-administration usually results in tolerance, withdrawal, and compulsive drug use. Substance dependence diagnosis can be applied to every class of substances except caffeine.
- Substance Abuse is a pattern of substance use that results in recurrent and significant adverse consequences associated with frequent use of substances. This can result in significant impairment of activities of daily living.

Tip: The diagnosis of Substance Abuse is preempted by the diagnosis of Substance Dependence if the person's pattern of substance use has ever met the criteria for dependence for that class of substances.

VISUAL 8.1. Substance-Related Disorders Overview

Fundamental Features

Disorders related to taking a drug of abuse, medication side effects, and toxin exposure

Cluster of cognitive, behavioral, and physiological symptoms when continued use of substance despite significant substance-related problems

Differential Dx.

Non-substance-induced disorder if:
- Symptoms precede onset of substance use
- Symptoms persist 1 month after cessation
- Symptoms in excess of substance used
- Prior nonsubstance disorders
- Positive family history

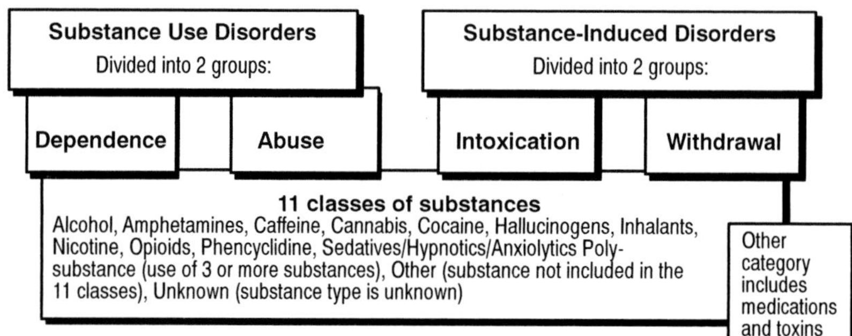

Substance-Induced Mental Disorders in Other Sections of the DSM-IV

Disorder	Section	Page
Substance-Induced:		
Delirium	Delirium, Dementia . . .	129
Persisting Dementia	Delirium, Dementia . . .	152
Persisting Amnestic Disorder	Delirium, Dementia . . .	161
Psychotic Disorder	Schizophrenia . . .	310
Mood Disorder	Mood Disorders	370
Anxiety Disorder	Anxiety Disorders	439
Sexual Dysfunction	Sexual and Gender . . .	519
Sleep Disorder	Sleep Disorders	601

For recording procedures for these disorders, see page 194 of the DSM-IV.

In Appendix B: . . . For Further Study Section

Caffeine Withdrawal:
Withdrawal syndrome due to abrupt cessation or reduction in use of caffeine-containing products after prolonged use

Source: American Psychiatric Association, 1994, pp. 175-272.

- Substance Intoxication is the occurrence of a reversible substance-specific syndrome due to recent ingestion or exposure to a substance. The maladaptive behavior or psychological effects associated with intoxication are the direct physiological result of the substance shortly after its use.
- Substance Withdrawal is manifested as a substance-specific maladaptive behavior change, with physiological and cognitive components that are due to cessation of, or reduction of, heavy and prolonged substance use. The substance syndrome causes clinically significant distress or impairment in multiple settings in which the person must function.
- Some Substance-Induced Disorders cause symptoms that are characteristic of other mental disorders, and these disorders are included in the specific class of disorders with which they share features. The disorders included in other sections are as follows:

Disorder	Section	Page
Substance-induced:		
Delirium	Delirium, Dementia . . .	129
Persisting Dementia	Delirium, Dementia . . .	152
Persisting Amnestic Disorder	Delirium, Dementia . . .	161
Psychotic Disorder	Schizophrenia . . .	310
Mood Disorder	Mood Disorders	370
Anxiety Disorder	Anxiety Disorders	439
Sexual Dysfunction	Sexual and Gender . . .	519
Sleep Disorder	Sleep Disorders	601

For recording procedures for these disorders, see page 194 of the DSM-IV.

ORGANIZATION

This section of the DSM-IV is structured somewhat differently from other sections and requires some study to master. Instead of having a discrete diagnosis for each class of substances, this section uses what Frances, First, and Pincus (1995) have called a "mix and match approach," in which the diagnosis starts with the name of the substance and then indicates the substance-related syndrome (dependence, intoxication, induced), and finally notes any specifiers that may apply. Visual 8.1 can help orient the reader to the organization of this section of the DSM-IV.

The Substance-Related Disorders are divided into two groups:

Substance-Use Disorders
Substance-Induced Disorders

Each of these groups is divided into two subgroups. Substance-Use Disorders are divided into:

Substance Dependence

1. For Substance Dependence the specifiers are
   - With Physiological Dependence
   - Without Physiological Dependence
2. The course specifiers for Substance Dependence are
   - Early Full Remission
   - Early Partial Remission
   - Sustained Full Remission
   - Sustained Partial Remission
   - On Agonist Therapy
   - In a Controlled Environment (These specifiers are defined on pages 179-180.)

Substance Abuse

Substance-Induced Disorders are quasi-divided into:

Substance Intoxication
Substance Withdrawal

For Substance-Induced Disorders the specifiers are

- With Onset During Intoxication
- With Onset During Withdrawal

Note: These specifiers are difficult to locate. See pages 177 and 191, and Appendix H.

Although these distinctions are made between the disorders, Substance-Induced Disorders are often an outcome of substance use. When this connection can be established, both disorders should be diagnosed (Frances, First, and Pincus, 1995).

Tip: Page 180 of the DSM-IV contains the only visual illustration that parallels the visuals used in this book! The visual gives a representation of the course specifiers for substance dependence.

Tip: Page 177 of the DSM-IV contains a table (Table 1) titled "Diagnoses Associated with Class of Substances." This table gives an overview of the organization of the Substance-Related Disorders section of the DSM-IV. If the reader is having trouble conceptualizing this section of the manual, I would strongly suggest studying this table.

Pages 195 to 270 of the DSM-IV provide the criteria for the diagnoses associated with the eleven classes of substances, which are as follows:

1. Alcohol
2. Amphetamines
3. Caffeine
4. Cannabis
5. Cocaine
6. Hallucinogens
7. Inhalants
8. Nicotine
9. Opioids
10. Phencyclidine
11. Sedatives/hypnotics/anxiolytics

Pages 270-272 give the criteria for Polysubstance-Related Disorder and Other (or Unknown) Substance-Related Disorders. The Polysubstance designation refers to the use of three or more substances; Other is used when the substance is not included in the previous eleven categories; Unknown indicates that the substance type is not known.

DIFFERENTIAL DIAGNOSIS

This section includes complex differential diagnoses for specific substances, since many substances have shared symptomology. General criteria for distinguishing Substance-Related Disorders from disorders that may have been masked by substances are as follows:

Non-substance-induced disorder if:

- symptoms precede onset of substance use;
- symptoms persistent one month after cessation of substance exposure;
- symptoms in excess of substance used;

- prior nonsubstance disorders exist; or
- positive family history for nonsubstance-related disorders.

RECOMMENDED STANDARDIZED MEASURES

- Addiction Severity Index (ASI)
- Brief Drinker Profile (BDP) (includes Michigan Alcoholism Screening Test [MAST])
- Maryland Addictions Questionnaire (MAQ)
- Substance Abuse Relapse Assessment (SARA)
- Substance Abuse Subtle Screening Inventory (SASSI)

RECOMMENDED READING

Frances, A., First, M. B., and Pincus, H. A. (1995). *DSM-IV Guidebook: The Essential Companion to the* Diagnostic and Statistical Manaul of Mental Disorders. Washington, DC: American Psychiatric Press.

Galanter, M. and Kleber, H. D. (1999). *Textbook of Substance Abuse Treatment*. Washington, DC: American Psychiatric Press.

Kaplan, H. I. and Sadock, B. J. (1998). *Synopsis of Psychiatry: Behavioral Sciences/Clinical Psychiatry,* Eighth Edition. Baltimore, MD: Williams and Wilkins.

Ray, O. (1995). *Drugs, Society, and Human Behavior.* New York: McGraw-Hill.

REFERENCES

American Psychiatric Association (1994). *Diagnostic and Statistical Manual of Mental Disorders,* Fourth Edition. Washington, DC: American Psychiatric Association.

Frances, A., First, M. B., and Pincus, H. A. (1995). *DSM-IV Guidebook: The Essential Companion to the* Diagnostic and Statistical Manual of Mental Disorders. Washington, DC: American Psychiatric Press.

Chapter 9

Schizophrenia and Other Psychotic Disorders

DISORDERS

295.xx Schizophrenia
  .30 Paranoid Type
  .10 Disorganized Type
  .20 Catatonic Type
  .90 Undifferentiated Type
  .60 Residual Type
295.40 Schizophreniform Disorder
295.70 Schizoaffective Disorder
297.1 Delusional Disorder
298.8 Brief Psychotic Disorder
297.3 Shared Psychotic Disorder (Folie à Deux)
293.xx Psychotic Disorder Due to . . . (indicate GMC)
  .81 With Delusions
  .82 With Hallucinations
___.__ Substance-Induced Psychotic Disorder (see p. 314 for substance-specific codes)
289.9 Psychotic Disorder NOS

FUNDAMENTAL FEATURES

In the DSM-III-R these disorders were divided into three sections: Schizophrenia, Delusional Disorder, and Psychotic Disorders Not Elsewhere Classified.

All disorders in this section of the DSM-IV have psychotic symptoms as a primary aspect of the disorder.

The terms psychosis and psychotic have been used in various ways throughout the history of classification (see Chapter 2). The most narrow definition of psychosis is a loss of reality-testing capability that is manifested by delusions and hallucinations about which the individual has no insight. A broader definition includes hallucinations even when the person has insight regarding their origin. The broadest definition includes hallucinations, delusions, as well as disorganized speech and grossly disorganized or catatonic behavior. Other definitions are quite broad and not based on specific symptoms, but instead use criteria of gross impairment that prevent the person meeting requirements of activities of daily living. Psychosis has also been defined as loss of ego boundaries or a gross impairment of reality testing. In the DSM-IV, different disorders emphasize different aspects of the definitions given here.

The DSM-IV uses the concept of positive and negative symptoms in defining Schizophrenia. Positive symptoms refer to an excess or distortion of normal functions, whereas negative symptoms refer to the loss or diminution of normal functions. In Schizophrenia Criterion A, the positive symptoms are distortions of inferential thinking (delusions), disturbance of perception (hallucinations), language and communication distortions (disorganized speech), and behavioral dysfunction (grossly disorganized or catatonic behavior). The negative symptoms include restriction in range and intensity of emotional expression (affect flattening), diminished production and fluency of thought and speech (alogia), and decline in the initiation of goal-directed behavior (avolition).

Delusions are erroneous beliefs that usually involve a misinterpretation of perceptions or experiences. Delusions are considered bizarre if they are clearly implausible, not understandable, and have no connection to ordinary life experiences.

Several of the disorders in this section are linked by the duration criterion to establish the diagnosis. Brief Psychotic Disorder, Schizophreniform Disorder, and Schizophrenia have essentially the same features and are distinguished by the duration of symptoms. The disorders are illustrated in Visual 9.1 and briefly summarized in the following pages.

Schizophrenia

Schizophrenia is characterized by positive and negative symptoms that have been present for at least one month, but some symptoms have persisted for at least six months and cause significant social or occupational dysfunction. The subtypes of Schizophrenia are as follows:

295.30 Schizophrenia, Paranoid Type

The person has prominent delusions or auditory hallucinations in the context of a relative preservation of cognitive functioning and affect. The delusions are usually persecutory and/or grandiose. Delusions of jealousy, religiosity, or somatization can be present.

VISUAL 9.1. Schizophrenia and Other Psychotic Disorders

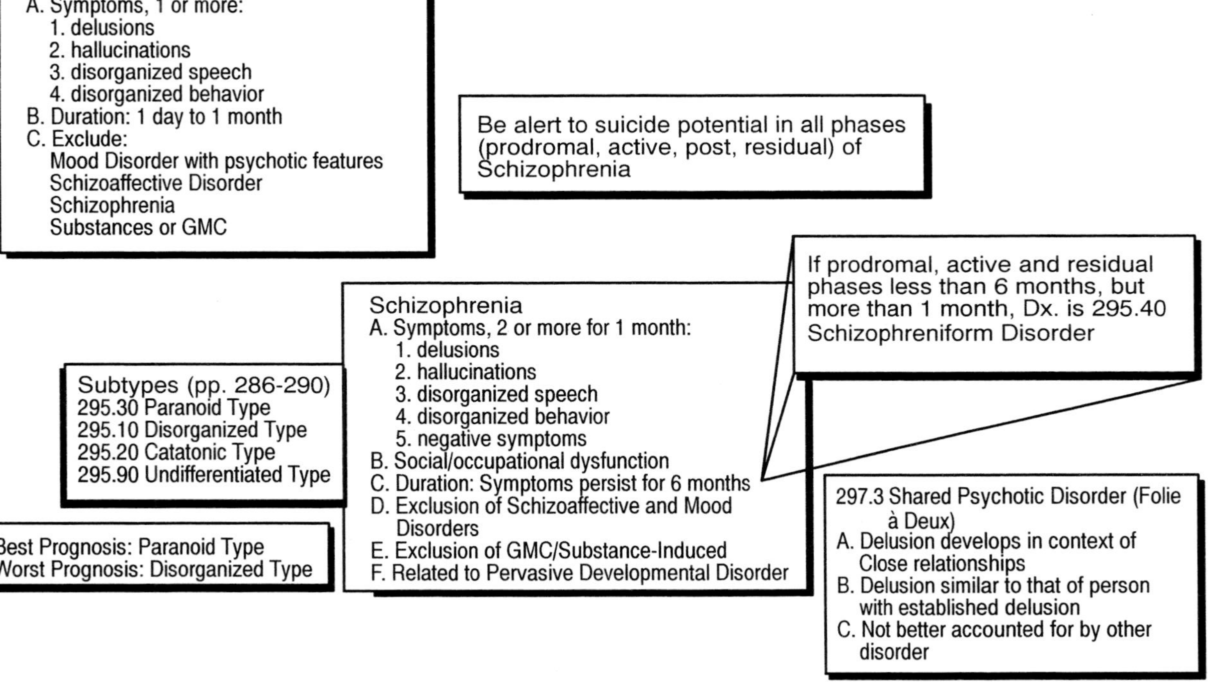

VISUAL 9.1 *(continued)*

295.70 Schizoaffective Disorder
A. Major depressive manic, or mixed episode concurrent with Criterion A for Schizophrenia
B. Delusions or hallucinations for at least 2 weeks in absence of mood symptoms
C. Mood episode present during active and residual phases
D. Exclude substances or GMC

297.1 Delusional Disorder
A. Nonbizarre delusions for 1 month
B. Schizophrenia Criterion A never met
C. Aside from delusions, functioning not markedly impaired
D. If mood episodes present, they are brief
E. Exclusion of substances or GMC

293.xx Psychotic Disorder Due to GMC
A. Prominent hallucinations or delusions
B. Disturbance direct physiological consequence of GMC
C. Exclude other mental disorder
D. Exclude course of delirium, xx coding .81 with delusions; .82 with hallucinations

Substance-Induced Psychotic Disorder
(Use code for specific substance)
A. Prominent hallucinations or delusions
B. Criterion A symptoms develop within 1 month of substance intoxication or withdrawal
C. Exclude other mental disorders
D. Excluse course of delirium

298.9 Psychotic Disorder NOS
Delusions, hallucinations, disorganized speech, disorganized behavior without specific information to make Dx.

In Appendix B . . . For Further Study Section

Alternative Dimensional Descriptors for Schizophrenia

Psychotic
Disorganized
Negative

postpsychotic depressive disorder of Schizophrenia

simple deteriorative disorder (simple Schizophrenia)

Source: American Psychiatric Association, 1994, pp. 273-315. Reprinted with permission from the *Diagnostic and Statistical Manual of Mental Disorders,* Fourth Edition.

295.10 Schizophrenia, Disorganized Type

Presence of disorganized speech and disorganized behavior and flat or inappropriate affect. These symptoms may be accompanied by inappropriate silliness and laughter.

295.20 Schizophrenia, Catatonic Type

Presence of marked psychomotor disturbance that can involve motor immobility, excessive motor activity, extreme negativism, mutism, peculiar involuntary movements, echolalia (senseless repetition of another person's speech), or echopraxia (repetition or imitation of the movements of another person). See Appendix C, Glossary of Technical Terms.

295.90 Schizophrenia, Undifferentiated Type

The person has symptoms that meet Criterion A of Schizophrenia but does not meet the criteria for the Paranoid, Disorganized, or Catatonic Type.

295.60 Schizophrenia, Residual Type

The person has had at least one episode of Schizophrenia but currently does not have prominent positive symptoms. However, negative symptoms or two or more limited positive symptoms are present.

Schizophreniform Disorder

Schizophreniform Disorder has the same positive and negative symptom requirements as Schizophrenia (Criterion A). The total duration of the disorder is at least one month, but less than six months, and the symptoms do not have to cause impaired social or occupational functioning, but impairment can be present. Schizophreniform Disorder is fully diagnosed if the person has already recovered completely from symptoms within a one- to six-month period. Schizophreniform Disorder is diagnosed as "Provisional" if the person has had the symptoms of Schizophrenia Criterion A for less than six months.

Schizoaffective Disorder

The main feature of Schizoaffective Disorder is an uninterrupted period of symptoms during which a Major Depressive, Manic, or Mixed Episode is concurrent with the Criterion A symptoms of Schizophrenia. This disorder has two subtypes:

Bipolar Type
Depressive Type

To make this diagnosis the reader should be familiar with the Mood Disorders section of the DSM-IV (pp. 317-391).

Delusional Disorder

Delusional Disorder involves the presence of one or more nonbizarre delusions that persist for at least one month in a person who has never had a set of symptoms that met Criterion A for Schizophrenia. Nonbizarre and bizarre delusions are difficult to distinguish and can be culture-bound. The primary criterion is that nonbizarre delusions are situations that can conceivably occur in real life, whereas bizarre delusions are implausible. For example, it is possible that a person could be slowly poisoned by a spouse who puts rat poison in the person's beverages, but implausible that the spouse is putting objects in the person's stomach with his/her hands without making an incision (see DSM-IV pp. 296-297 for more details of this differentiation).

Delusional Disorder has seven subtypes (see pp. 297-298 for explanations of these subtypes):

Erotomania Type
Grandiose Type
Jealous Type
Persecutory Type
Somatic Type
Mixed Type
Unspecified Type

Brief Psychotic Disorder

Brief Psychotic Disorder involves the sudden onset of positive psychotic symptoms that last at least one day but less than one month, and the person experiences full recovery to the level of functioning that existed prior to the onset of the symptoms.

Shared Psychotic Disorder (Folie à Deux)

Shared Psychotic Disorder is believed to be quite rare. In this disorder a person develops a delusion that he/she derives from being in a close relationship with a person who has psychotic delusions. The psychotic person is sometimes described as the "inducer" or "the primary case." The person comes to share, in whole or in part, the delusions of the "inducer."

Psychotic Disorder Due to . . . (Indicate GMC)

This disorder results when a person develops hallucinations or delusions that are clinically judged to be due to the direct physiological effects of a GMC. The history, physical examination, or laboratory findings must show evidence that the delusions or hallucinations are the direct consequence of the GMC. The two subtypes are coded on the basis of whether the person has predominantly delusions or hallucinations:

293.81 With Delusions
293.82 With Hallucinations

Substance-Induced Psychotic Disorder

Substance-Induced Psychotic Disorder results when a person develops hallucinations or delusions that are clinically judged to be due to the direct physiological effects of a substance. The two subtypes are based on whether the person has predominantly delusions or hallucinations (see pp. 175-272 for substance-specific codes):

With Delusions
With Hallucinations

Also, the diagnostician may further specify the context of the onset of the symptoms by using the following specifiers (see pp. 175-272 for coding):

With Onset During Intoxication
With Onset During Withdrawal

Tip: Appendix F, Numerical Listing of DSM-IV Diagnoses and Codes, can be helpful in coordinating the Substance-Related Disorders coding with Substance-Induced Psychotic Disorder.

Psychotic Disorder NOS

Psychotic Disorder NOS is used when the information is inadequate for diagnosis or is contradictory.

DIFFERENTIAL DIAGNOSIS

The primary differential diagnosis in this set of disorders involves the other disorders in this class. Other disorders that should be considered are PDDs, delirium, dementia, Substance-Related Disorders, Mood Episodes, Mood Disorders, Factitious Disorders, certain Personality Disorders, and Malingering.

RECOMMENDED STANDARDIZED MEASURES

- Minnesota Multiphasic Personality Inventory-2 (MMPI-2)
- Schizophrenia Index of the Rorschach Comprehensive System (SCZI)

RECOMMENDED READING

Andreasen, N. C. (1994). *Schizophrenia: From Mind to Molecule*. Washington, DC: American Psychiatric Press.

Keefe, R. S. E. and Harvey P. D. (1994). *Understanding Schizophrenia: A Guide to the New Research on Causes and Treatment*. New York: Free Press.

Mueser, K. T. (1994). *Coping with Schizophrenia: A Guide for Families*. Oakland, CA: New Harbinger.

Torrey, E. F. (1995). *Surviving Schizophrenia: A Manual for Families, Consumers, and Providers*. New York: HarperPerennial.

REFERENCE

American Psychiatric Association (1994). *Diagnostic and Statistical Manual of Mental Disorders,* Fourth Edition. Washington, DC: American Psychiatric Association.

Chapter 10

Mood Disorders

DISORDERS

Depressive Disorders

296.xx Major Depressive Disorder (see pp. 319-320 for recording procedures)
  .2x Single Episode
  .3x Recurrent
300.4 Dysthymic Disorder
311 Depressive Disorder NOS

Bipolar Disorders

296.xx Bipolar I Disorder (see pp. 319-320 for recording procedures)
  .0x Single Manic Episode
  .40 Most Recent Episode Hypomanic
  .4x Most Recent Episode Manic
  .6x Most Recent Episode Mixed
  .5x Most Recent Episode Depressed
  .7 Most Recent Episode Unspecified
296.89 Bipolar II Disorder (recurrent Major Depressive Episodes with Hypomanic Episodes)
301.13 Cyclothymic Disorder
296.80 Bipolar Disorder NOS

Other Mood Disorders

293.83 Mood Disorder Due to a GMC
___.__ Substance-Induced Mood Disorder (see p. 375 for Substance-Specific Codes)

Mood Disorders in Appendix B *

premenstrual dysphoric disorder
Alternative Criterion B for Dysthymic Disorder
minor depressive disorder
recurrent brief depressive disorder
mixed anxiety-depressive disorder

FUNDAMENTAL FEATURES

This class of disorders is one of the most researched sections in the DSM-IV.

The term mood, as defined in this section of the DSM-IV, means "a pervasive and sustained emotion that colors the person's perception of the world" (American Psychiatric Association, 1994, p. 768), and is limited to people with depressed, elevated, or irritable mood (Frances, First, and Pincus, 1995).

This class of disorders is divided into three sections and is structured somewhat differently from other classes of disorders (see Visual 10.1). The first section is a description of the mood episodes that make up the disorders in section two. People cannot be diagnosed with a mood episode, and mood episodes have no codes. The mood episodes serve as "building blocks" for the disorders in section two. It is important to read and understand the descriptions of the mood episodes before attempting to make a mood disorder diagnosis. Section three contains explanations of the specifiers that provide details of the most recent mood episode or the course of recurrent episodes. This section requires careful study to understand the multiple specifiers used to enhance the mood disorders.

The mood episodes are explained in Visual 10.2. The line in the visual referred to as "baseline stable mood" is the ideal state we would like to achieve on a daily basis, but rarely do, because of the vicissitudes of life. This represents the perfectly adjusted person in terms of unvarying mood. Below stable mood the criteria for Major Depressive Episodes are described. Most people have periodic depressive episodes based on life events, but the symptoms described in this section subside before the person meets the criteria to be diagnosed with depression. The Manic Episodes are described above the baseline. The distinction between Hypomanic Episodes

*Diagnosed under Mood Disorder NOS category

VISUAL 10.1. Mood Disorders Overview

Most thoroughly researched disorders in DSM

Mood disorders section is divided into three parts:

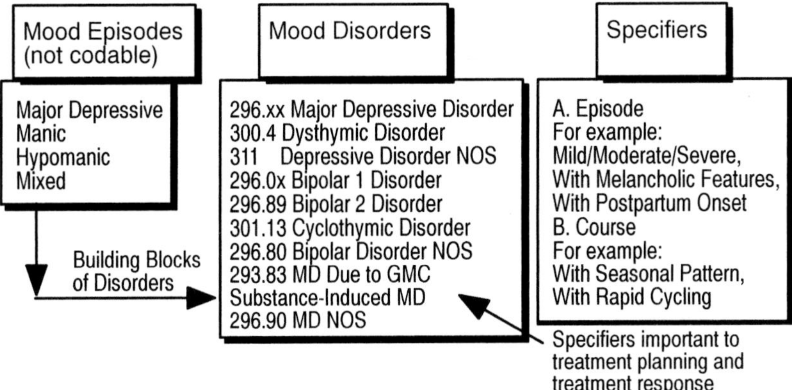

In Appendix B: . . . For Further Study Section

premenstrual dysphoric disorder
Depressed mood, anxiety, affect lability, and decreased activity interest during menstrual cycle

recurrent brief depressive disorder
Recurrence of brief episodes of depression identical to major depressive episodes that do not meet two-week duration criterion

Alternative Criterion B for Dysthymic Disorder

mixed anxiety-depressive disorder
Persistent or recurrent dysphoric mood for at least one month accompanied by anxiety symptoms

minor depressive disorder
Identical to Major Depressive Disorder, but involves fewer symptoms and less impairment

Source: American Psychiatric Association, 1994, pp. 317-391.

and Manic Episodes is minimal. Hypomanic Episodes were introduced in DSM-IV to offer an alternative to Manic Episodes and to provide a more precise diagnosis. Manic Episodes are manifested as unceasing energy, decreased need for sleep, and poor judgment that usually results in difficulty

VISUAL 10.2. Mood Episodes That Are the General Criteria for Mood Disorders

Manic Episode	*Criterion A and B* Distinct period of abnormal and persistent elevated, expansive, or irritable mood lasting at least 1 week and 3+: 1. inflated self-esteem, or grandiosity 2. decreased need for sleep 3. more talkative or pressured talking 4. flight of ideas or racing thoughts 5. distractibility 6. increased goal-directed activity or psychomotor agitation 7. excessive involvement in pleasurable activities with high potential for painful consequences *Criterion D* Causes impaired social or occupational functioning, or need for hospitalization to protect self and others, and psychotic features present	(Mixed Episode) Criteria met for Manic Episode and Major Depressive Episode nearly every day (for at least 1 week) Marked impairment in occupational or social functioning, need for hospitalization for safety of self or others, or psychotic features present
Hypomanic Episode	*Criterion A and B* Distinct period of persistent elevated, expansive, or irritable mood lasting at least 4 days and 3+: 1. inflated self-esteem or grandiosity 2. decreased need for sleep 3. more talkative or pressured talking 4. flight of ideas or racing thoughts 5. distractibility 6. increased goal-directed activity or psychomotor agitation 7. excessive involvement in pleasurable activities with high potential for painful consequences *Criterion C* Episode associated with uncharacteristic change not present before the person became symptomatic *Criterion D* Disturbance of mood and functioning change observable by others *Criterion E* Does not cause impaired social or occupational functioning, no need for hospitalization, and no psychotic features	
Baseline		
Stable Mood		
Depressive Episode	*Criterion A* At least 2 weeks when 5+ present: 1. depressed (in children mood can be irritable rather than sad) 2. loss of interest in nearly all activities 3. significant weight loss or gain 4. insomnia or hypersomnia 5. psychomotor agitation or retardation 6. fatigue or loss of energy 7. feelings of worthlessness or guilt 8. diminished ability to concentrate or make decisions 9. recurrent thoughts of death *Criterion C* Symptoms cause significant impairment in social, occupational, or other areas of functioning	(Mixed Episode) Criteria met for Manic Episode and Major Depressive Episode nearly every day (for at least 1 week) Marked impairment in occupational or social functioning, need for hospitalization for safety of self or others, or psychotic features present

Source: American Psychiatric Association, 1994, pp. 317-338. Reprinted with permission from the *Diagnostic and Statistical Manual of Mental Disorders,* Fourth Edition. Copyright 1994 American Psychiatric Association.

in interpersonal, social, and occupational relationships and can lead to legal problems if the symptoms are serious. You will notice that the set of seven symptoms for Manic and Hypomanic Episodes criteria are the same. Hypomanic and Manic Episodes are basically distinguished by Criterion D of Manic Episode, and Criteria C, D, and E for a Hypomanic Episode. In Criterion D of a Manic Episode, the person's symptoms cause severe impairment in relationships, the person may require hospitalization, and psychotic features are present. In Criteria C, D, and E of a Hypomanic Episode, the person's behavior change is noticeable to others but does not cause major disruption in relationships or require hospitalization, and no psychotic features are present. Mixed Episodes involve the person having the symptoms of mania and depression for at least one week so that the person meets the criteria for Manic and Major Depressive Episodes. The symptoms often include agitation, insomnia, eating dysfunction, psychotic features, and suicidal thinking. In Visual 10.2 the Hypomanic Episode is immediately above the baseline, and the Manic Episode is at the top. To the right of the visual, the criteria for a Mixed Episode are presented at the top and bottom.

Visual 10.3 presents the Mood Disorders, building on the episode criteria in Visual 10.2. One can develop a better understanding of the range of each disorder by following areas that are above and below the baseline. For example, Bipolar I Disorder ranges from the depressive low to the manic high areas of the visual, whereas Bipolar II Disorder ranges from the depressive area to the hypomanic, but not the manic, area, and, of course, depressive disorders never rise above the baseline in their range.

When you move from the building-block episodic features, the criteria for the individual mood disorders are fairly easy to comprehend. The key features are as follows.

Major Depressive Disorder

Major Depression Disorder is characterized by one or more depressive episodes without a history of manic, mixed, or hypomanic episodes. The specifiers for this disorder require special coding, which is illustrated in Visual 10.4.

Tip: A seventeen-page section beginning on page 375 contains a number of specifiers for the mood disorders. These specifiers allow more targeted diagnoses, create more homogeneous subgroupings, as well as aid in treatment planning and in estimating prognosis. A table on page 376 summarizes these specifiers and can aid the practitioner who is confused by the Mood Disorders specifiers.

VISUAL 10.3. Mood Disorders in Relation to Manic, Hypomanic, and Depressive Episodes

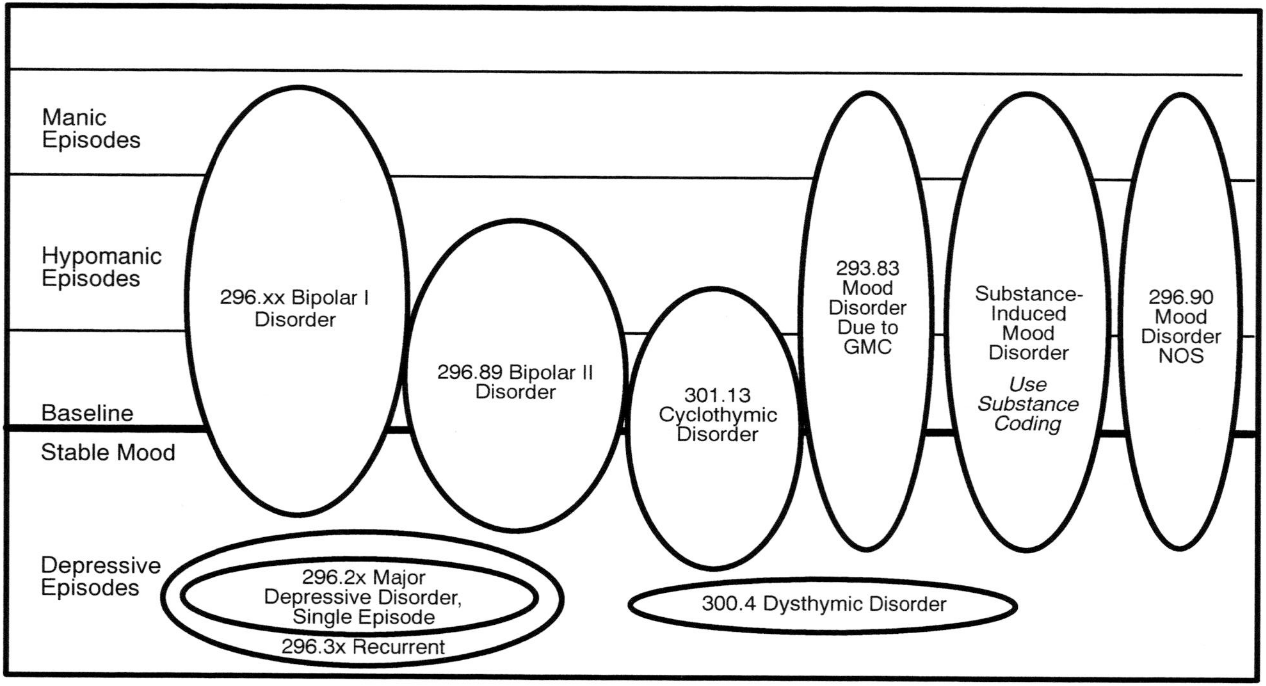

Manic Episodes

Hypomanic Episodes

Baseline

Stable Mood

Depressive Episodes

296.xx Bipolar I Disorder

296.89 Bipolar II Disorder

301.13 Cyclothymic Disorder

293.83 Mood Disorder Due to GMC

Substance-Induced Mood Disorder

Use Substance Coding

296.90 Mood Disorder NOS

296.2x Major Depressive Disorder, Single Episode

296.3x Recurrent

300.4 Dysthymic Disorder

Source: American Psychiatric Association, 1994, pp. 317-392.

VISUAL 10.4. Major Depressive Disorder Specifiers

4th Digit
2 = single depressive episode
3 = recurrent depressive episodes

5th Digit
1 = mild 2 = moderate
3 = severe w/o psychotic features
4 = severe with psychotic features
5 = partial remission 6 = in full remission
0 = unspecified

296.XX Major Depressive Disorder

Uncoded Specifiers
Chronic (p. 382)
With Catatonic Features (pp. 382-383)
With Melancholic Features (pp. 383-384)
With Atypical Features (pp. 384-385)
With Postpartum Onset (pp. 386-387)

Longitudinal Course Specifiers
With or Without Full Interepisode Recovery (pp. 387-388)
With Seasonal Pattern (pp. 389-390)
Used with Recurrent Major Depressive Disorder BPI and BPII

Source: American Psychiatric Association, 1994, pp. 339-340.

Dysthymic Disorder

Dysthymic Disorder has been referred to as a long-term, "low-grade depression" because the person must have "chronically depressed mood" (Criterion A) for most of the day, for most days, for at least two years. In children the mood may be irritable rather than depressed, and the duration of symptoms must be only one year. In Chapters 3 and 4, Dysthymic Disorder was used to illustrate diagnosis and treatment planning in Visuals 3.5, 4.4, and 4.5. The reader may want to refer back to these visuals to better comprehend Dysthymic Disorder.

Tip: People with Dysthymic Disorder can develop a Major Depressive Disorder and lapse back to the Dysthymic Disorder when the symptoms of Major Depressive Disorder have subsided.

Bipolar I Disorder

Bipolar I Disorder consists of a clinical course that is characterized by one or more Manic Episodes or Mixed Episodes. The same set of specifiers apply that are described in Visual 10.4, along with one additional specifier, **With Rapid Cycling** (p. 390). Rapid Cycling is defined as four episodes of a mood disturbance in the previous twelve months. The six separate criteria sets for this disorder are based on the episode type:

1. Single Manic Episode
2. Most Recent Episode Hypomanic
3. Most Recent Episode Manic
4. Most Recent Episode Mixed
5. Most Recent Episode Depressed
6. Most Recent Episode Unspecified

Visual 10.5 depicts the diagnosis of Bipolar I and Bipolar II Disorders based on the episodic features. In the visual, previous episodes are indicated by the symbol •, and the current/most recent episode is represented by the same symbol with a circle around it. Through studying this visual you can orient yourself to the complexities of Bipolar Disorder.

Bipolar II Disorder

Bipolar II Disorder is made up of the occurrence of one or more Major Depressive Episodes accompanied by at least one Hypomanic Episode. The specifiers in Visual 10.4 apply to Bipolar II Disorder, as do the specifiers **Hypomanic** or **Depressed** to indicate the nature of the current or most recent episode. The **Rapid Cycling** specifier also applies to this disorder. None of these specifiers is codable because the fifth digit is already taken for this disorder. The specifiers should be listed in the following order: specifiers indicating most recent episode, specifiers that apply to current or most recent depressive episode, and as many specifiers as apply to the course of the episodes.

Cyclothymic Disorder

Cyclothymic Disorder is composed of chronic, fluctuating mood disturbance with numerous periods of hypomanic symptoms and numerous

VISUAL 10.5. Bipolar I and II Disorders Overview

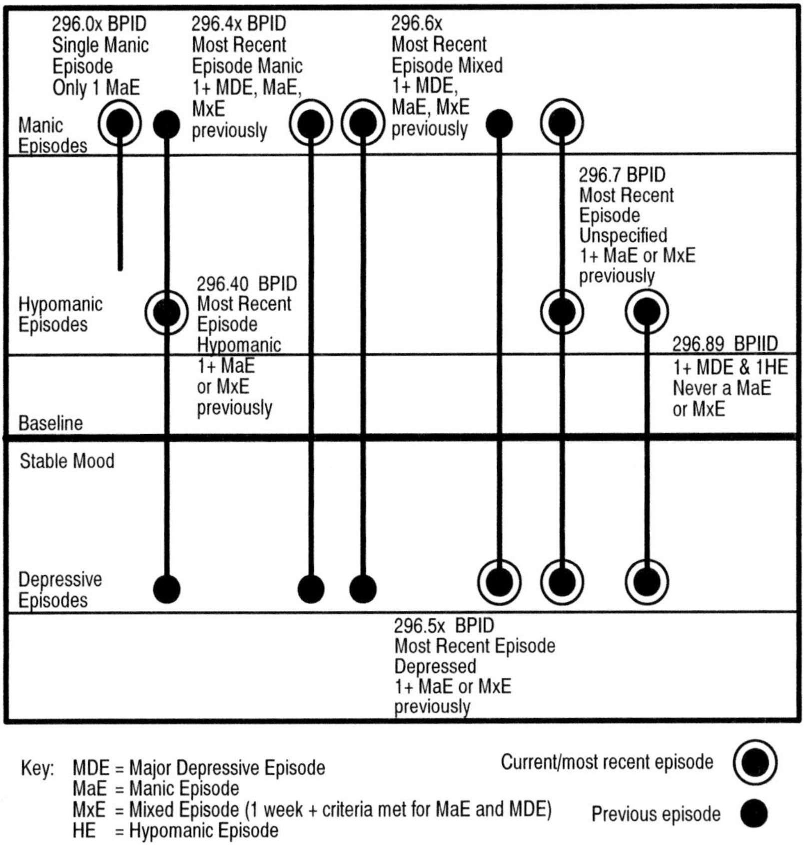

296.0x BPID
Single Manic
Episode
Only 1 MaE

296.4x BPID
Most Recent
Episode Manic
1+ MDE, MaE,
MxE
previously

296.6x
Most Recent
Episode Mixed
1+ MDE,
MaE, MxE
previously

Manic
Episodes

296.7 BPID
Most Recent
Episode
Unspecified
1+ MaE or MxE
previously

296.40 BPID
Most Recent
Episode
Hypomanic
1+ MaE
or MxE
previously

Hypomanic
Episodes

296.89 BPIID
1+ MDE & 1HE
Never a MaE
or MxE

Baseline

Stable Mood

Depressive
Episodes

296.5x BPID
Most Recent Episode
Depressed
1+ MaE or MxE
previously

Key: MDE = Major Depressive Episode
MaE = Manic Episode
MxE = Mixed Episode (1 week + criteria met for MaE and MDE)
HE = Hypomanic Episode

Current/most recent episode 

Previous episode

Source: American Psychiatric Association, 1994, pp. 350-363.

periods of depressive symptoms for at least two years (one year for children and adolescents). The symptoms do not meet the criteria for Hypomanic or Depressive Episodes.

Bipolar Disorder NOS

Bipolar Disorder NOS is reserved for disorders with bipolar features that do not meet the criteria for a specific Bipolar Disorder.

Mood Disorder Due to a General Medical Condition

This disorder is prominent and persistent disturbance in mood determined to be due to the direct physiological effects of a GMC. Subtypes include **With Depressed Features, With Major Depressive-Like Episode, With Manic Features,** and **With Mixed Features.** Visual 10.6 gives examples of the different ways to record diagnosis of depression as a direct physiological or psychological consequence of a GMC. The first diagnosis shown would be given when using Mood Disorder Due to a

VISUAL 10.6. Sample Diagnoses of Mood Disorder As Direct Physiological and Psychological Consequence of a GMC

DEPRESSION AS **DIRECT PHYSIOLOGICAL CONSEQUENCE** OF GMC

Axis I: 293.83 Mood Disorder Due to HIV Disease With Depressive Features

Axis II: V71.09 No Dx. on Axis II

Axis III: 042.2 AIDS, with specified malignant neoplasms as reported by Physician (Dr. R. U. Wright)

DEPRESSION AS **DIRECT PSYCHOLOGICAL CONSEQUENCE** OF GMC

Axis I: 296.23 Major Depressive Disorder, Single Episode, severe W/O Psychotic Features

Axis II: V71.09 No Dx. on Axis II

Axis III: 042.9 AIDS, unspecified as reported by IP and Physician (Dr. R. U. Wright)

DEPRESSION AS **DIRECT PSYCHOLOGICAL CONSEQUENCE** OF GMC

Axis I: 309.28 Adjustment Disorder with Anxiety and Depressed Mood, Acute

Axis II: V71.09 No Dx. on Axis II

Axis III: 042.9 AIDS, unspecified as reported by IP and Physician (Dr. R. U. Wright)

General Medical Condition. The second diagnosis would be given when the depression is a psychological consequence of the illness. The third is an example of a diagnosis when a person has depression and anxiety in the context of the early stage of the diagnosis of the GMC and the symptoms are deemed to be the result of an Adjustment Disorder.

Substance-Induced Mood Disorder

Substance-Induced Mood Disorder is characterized as prominent and persistent disturbance in mood determined to be due to the direct physiological effects of a substance. The subtypes include **With Depressive Features, With Manic Features, With Mixed Features,** and the context of the mood symptoms should be indicated by **With Onset During Intoxication** or **With Onset During Withdrawal.**

Mood Disorder NOS

Mood Disorder NOS covers disorders with mood symptoms that do not meet the criteria for a specific mood disorder.

Severity and Course Specifiers

The description of the Mood Disorders is followed by a third part that focuses on the range of specifiers associated with the Mood Disorders. This part has two sections titled Specifiers Describing Most Recent Episode and Specifiers Describing Course of Recurrent Episodes. These specifiers are illustrated in Visual 10.7.

Specifiers Describing Most Recent Episode

- Severity/Psychotic/Remission Specifiers for Major Depressive Episode
- Severity/Psychotic/Remission Specifiers for Manic Episode
- Severity/Psychotic/Remission Specifiers for Mixed Episode
- Catatonic Features Specifiers
- Melancholic Features Specifier
- Atypical Features Specifier
- Postpartum Onset Specifier

Specifiers Describing Course of Recurrent Episodes

- Longitudinal Course Specifiers (With and Without Full Interepisode Recovery)
- Seasonal Pattern Specifier
- Rapid-Cycling Specifier

VISUAL 10.7. Mood Disorders Specifiers

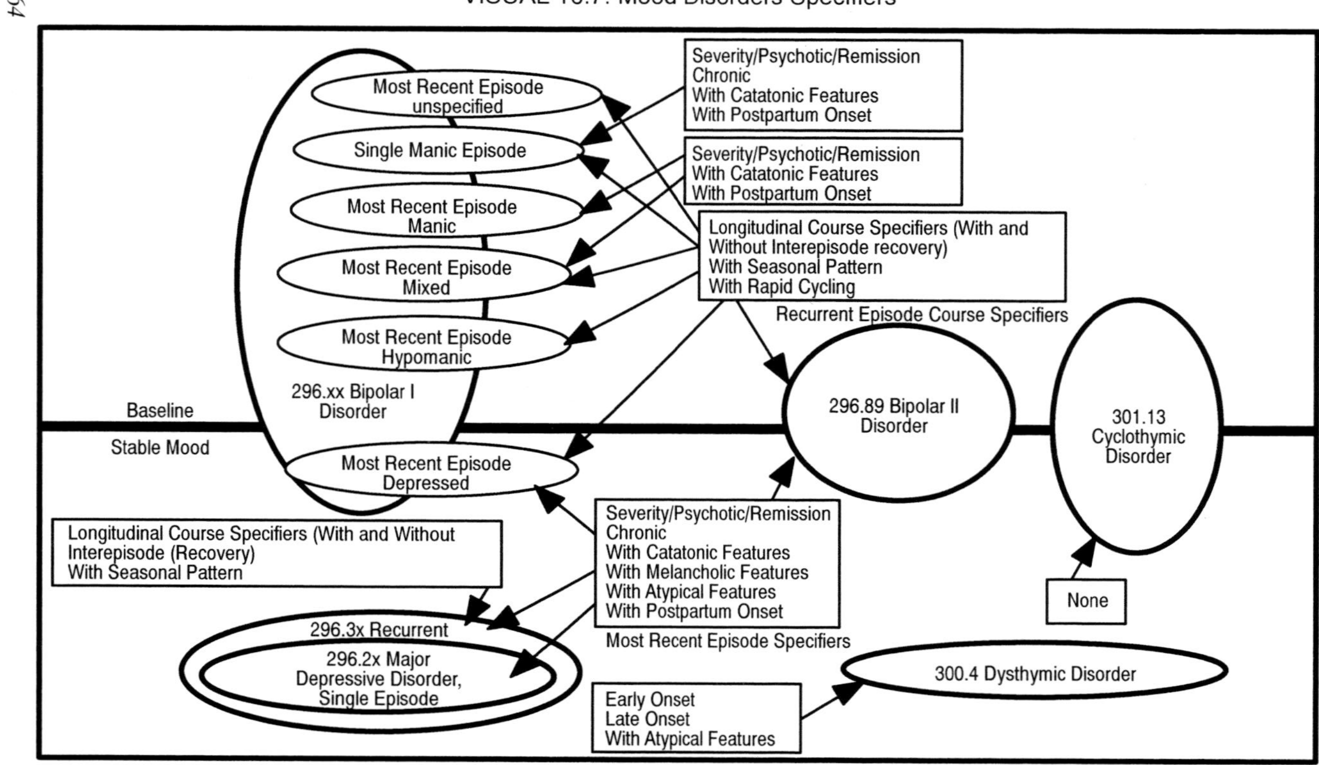

Source: American Psychiatric Association, 1994, pp. 375-392.

In Appendix B, several disorders are defined that can be diagnosed in the Mood Disorder NOS category. The first disorder is premenstrual dysphoric disorder. This disorder's essential features are depressed mood, anxiety, affect lability, and decreased interest in activities that have occurred during the last week of the luteal phase of most menstrual cycles. Minor depressive disorder involves one or more periods of depressive symptoms that are the same as Major Depressive Episodes in duration, but present with fewer symptoms and less impairment. Recurrent brief depressive disorder is characterized by recurring brief episodes of depressive symptoms that are the same as Major Depressive Disorder in number and severity, but do not meet the two-week duration criterion. The episodes last between two and fourteen days, but typically have a duration of two to four days. Mixed anxiety-depressive disorder has as its main feature persistent and recurrent dysphoric mood for one month that is accompanied by at least four of the following symptoms: difficulty concentrating or mind going blank, sleep disturbance, fatigue or low energy, irritability, worry, easily moved to tears, hypervigilance, anticipating the worst, hopelessness, or low self-esteem. For more details regarding these disorders, see Appendix B of the DSM-IV.

Visual 10.8 is an overview of the whole spectrum of Mood Disorders in the DSM-IV, including the disorders in Appendix B reserved for further study.

DIFFERENTIAL DIAGNOSIS

The individual disorders in this section have differential diagnosis requirements, and each section should be consulted when considering a particular diagnosis. In general, the disorders to be alert to when doing Mood Disorder differential diagnosis are primarily other disorders in this class (e.g., screening for Dysthymic Disorder when diagnosing Major Depressive Disorder, and vice versa). For all Mood Disorders, the diagnostician should screen for Mood Disorder Due to a GMC and Substance-Induced Mood Disorder. Other disorders that are common in differential diagnosis in this class are Dementia, ADHD, Adjustment Disorder with Depressed Mood, Bereavement, Schizoaffective Disorder, Schizophrenia, Psychotic Disorder NOS, and Personality Disturbance.

RECOMMENDED STANDARDIZED MEASURES

- Beck Depression Inventory II (BDI-II)
- Beck Scale of Suicidal Ideation (BSS)
- Hamilton Depression Inventory (HDI)

VISUAL 10.8. Spectrum of Mood Disorders

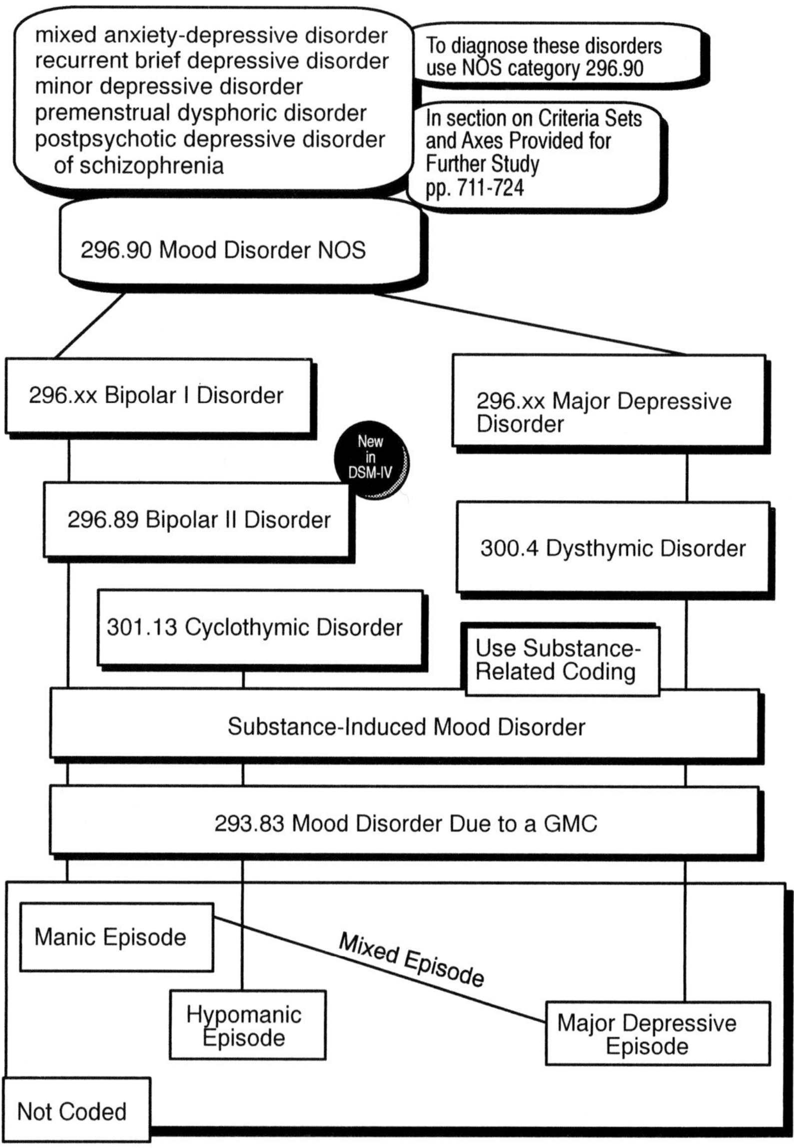

Source: American Psychiatric Association, 1994, pp. 317-391.

- Minnesota Multiphasic Personality Inventory-II (MMPI-II)
- Reynolds Adolescent Depression Scale (RADS)
- Reynolds Child Depression Scale (RCDS)
- Suicidal Behavior History Form (SBHF)

RECOMMENDED READING

Akiskal, H. S. and Cassano, G. B. (1997). *Dysthymia and the Spectrum of Chronic Depressions*. New York: Guilford.

Beck, A. T. (1967). *Depression: Causes and Treatment*. Philadelphia, PA: University of Pennsylvania Press.

Miklowitz, D. J. and Goldstein, M. J. (1997). *Bipolar Disorder: A Family-Focused Treatment Approach*. New York: Guilford.

REFERENCES

American Psychiatric Association (1994). *Diagnostic and Statistical Manual of Mental Disorders,* Fourth Edition. Washington, DC: American Psychiatric Association.

Frances, A., First, M. B., and Pincus, H. N. (1995). *DSM-IV Guidebook: The Essential Companion to the* Diagnostic and Statistical Manual of Mental Disorders. Washington, DC: American Psychiatric Association.

Chapter 11

Anxiety Disorders

DISORDERS

300.01 Panic Disorder Without Agoraphobia
300.21 Panic Disorder With Agoraphobia
300.22 Agoraphobia Without History of Panic Disorder
300.29 Specific Phobia (formerly Simple Phobia)
300.23 Social Phobia (Social Anxiety Disorder)
300.3 Obsessive-Compulsive Disorder
309.81 Posttraumatic Stress Disorder
308.3 Acute Stress Disorder
300.02 Generalized Anxiety Disorder
293.89 Anxiety Disorder Due to . . . (indicate GMC)
___.__ Substance-Induced Anxiety Disorder (see p. 443 for substance-specific codes)
300.00 Anxiety Disorder NOS

FUNDAMENTAL FEATURES

The Anxiety Disorders are, in part, based on the work of Sigmund Freud. Freud differentiated the disorders known during his era as neurasthenia. He described this syndrome as anxiety neurosis, and in his writings, he also described phobic neurosis, obsessive-compulsive neurosis, and posttraumatic stress (Frances, First, and Pincus, 1995). The conception of neurasthenia dates back to the 1700s when a Scottish neurologist, Robert Whytt, described the syndrome, and it was defined by a New York neurologist, George Beard, in the 1800s. Neurasthenia, referred to as "nervous exhaustion," involved studying the internal workings and subtle nature of "the nerves" (Stone, 1997). By the time the DSM-I was introduced, the term "neurosis" had become an organizing principle. The evolution of the DSM system has refined this class by dividing it into a number of discrete disorders.

The organization of this section is similar to the "Mood Disorders" section in that it begins by describing two categories of symptoms (Panic Attack and Agoraphobia), which can be a feature of some disorders in this section. Panic Attack (PA) and Agoraphobia are not codable or diagnosable disorders in the DSM-IV. The relationship between Panic Attack, Agoraphobia, and the disorders in this section is illustrated in Visual 11.1. The second part of this section describes the disorders (see Visual 11.2 for an overview of the disorders). There is no third section of specifiers as in the "Mood Disorders" section.

Panic Attacks (PAs)

Panic Attacks are characterized by a discrete period of intense fear or discomfort accompanied by at least four of the following thirteen somatic or cognitive symptoms:

- Palpitations, pounding heart, accelerated heart rate
- Sweating
- Trembling or shaking
- Sensations of shortness of breath or smothering
- Feeling of choking
- Chest pain
- Nausea or abdominal distress
- Feeling dizzy
- Derealization or depersonalization
- Fear of losing control or going crazy
- Fear of dying
- Numbness or tingling
- Chills or hot flushes

Agoraphobia

Agoraphobia consists of anxiety about being in places or situations in which escape may be difficult or embarrassing or in which help may not be available if a Panic Attack occurs. This anxiety leads to avoidance of perceived threatening situations, such as alone outside the home; home alone; in a crowd; in an automobile, a bus, a train, or an airplane; on a bridge; or in an elevator. Some people can tolerate being in these situations, but they feel extreme dread. Some people can tolerate these situations if they are accompanied by a companion.

VISUAL 11.1. Panic Attacks and Agoraphobia in Relation to Anxiety Disorders

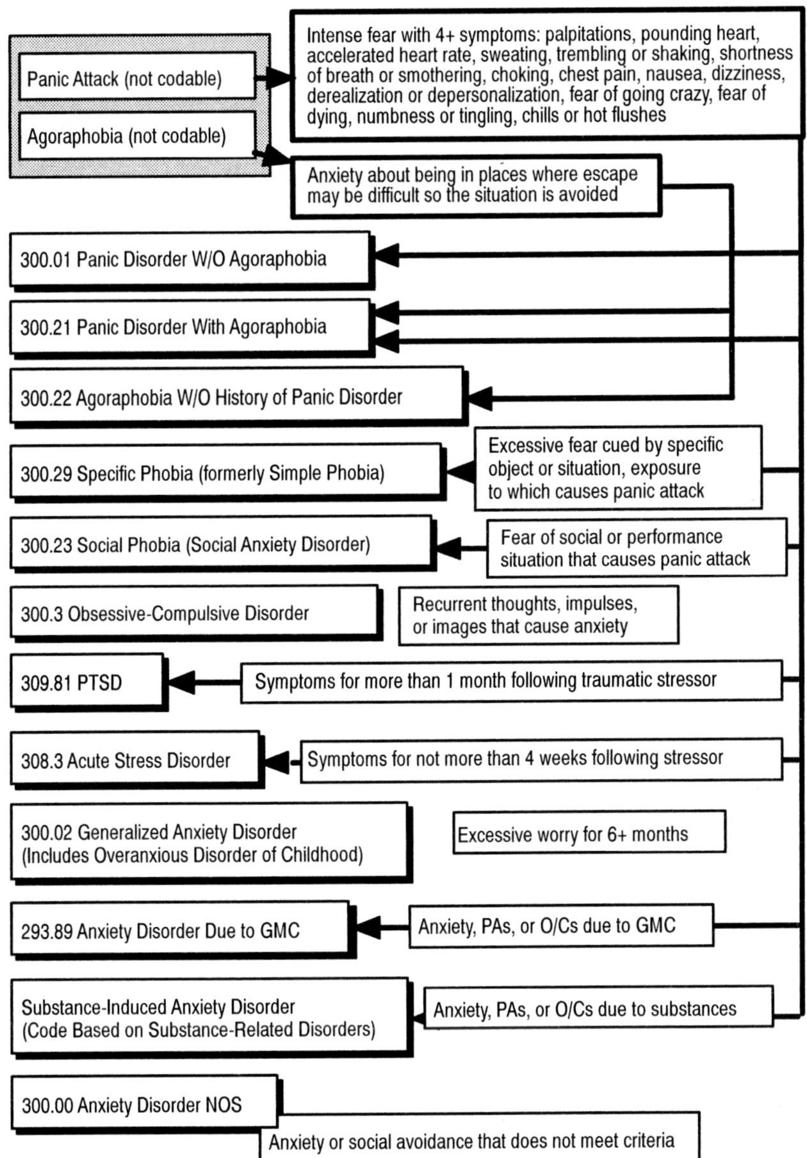

Source: American Psychiatric Association, 1994, pp. 393-444.

VISUAL 11.2. Anxiety Disorders Overview

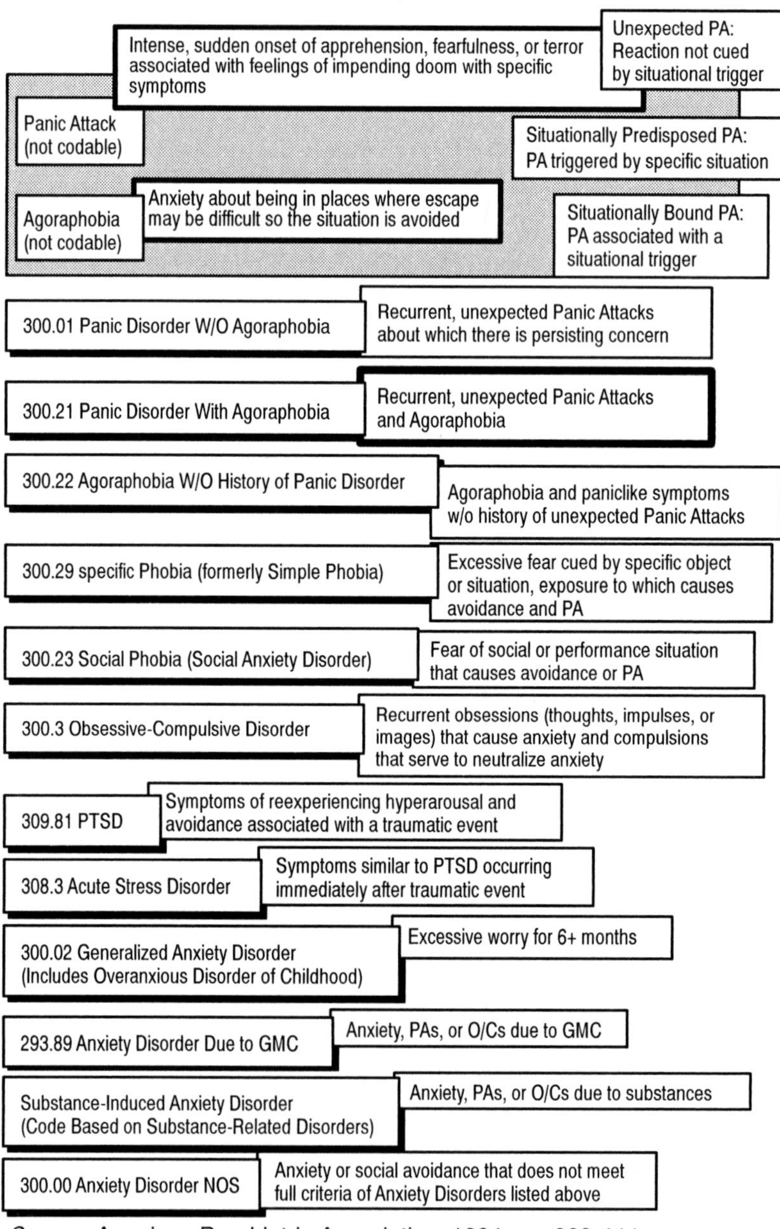

Source: American Psychiatric Association, 1994, pp. 393-444.

Panic Disorder

Panic Disorder's primary feature is recurrent, unexpected Panic Attacks, followed by at least one month of persistent concern about having another Panic Attack, worry about the possible implications of the Panic Attack, or a significant behavioral change related to the Panic Attacks. An unexpected Panic Attack is defined as a reaction that is not cued by a situational trigger event. A person must have at least two of these attacks to be diagnosed with Panic Disorder. People with this disorder also can have situationally predisposed Panic Attacks. These are Panic Attacks that are more likely triggered by a specific situation, but not necessarily so. Situationally bound Panic Attacks are usually associated with exposure to a situational trigger. The frequency and severity of Panic Attacks can vary significantly. People with Panic Disorder have concerns about the outcomes of the Panic Attacks and can be fearful the Panic Attacks are the result of an undiagnosed physical illness, and/or believe that they are going crazy. The two types of this disorder are Panic Disorder Without Agoraphobia and Panic Disorder With Agoraphobia. The separation of these disorders in the DSM-IV is related to the old "which came first" question. Some researchers believe that Panic Attacks lead to the avoidance of situations (Agoraphobia), and others believe that encountering the feared situations causes the Panic Attacks. Freud believed the Panic Attack took precedence, but the criteria in the ICD-10 give precedence to the feared situation (Agoraphobia). To circumvent this controversy, the DSM-IV lists the disorders separately.

Tip: Because of the lack of specificity about the etiological relationship between Panic Attacks and Agoraphobia, the clinician must carefully gather data regarding the onset of symptoms when both Panic Attacks and Agoraphobia are present so that treatment can be focused on the causative phenomena.

Agoraphobia Without a History of Panic Disorder

This form of Agoraphobia is similar to Panic Disorder With Agoraphobia except that the person focuses on fear of incapacitating or extremely embarrassing paniclike symptoms or limited symptom attacks rather than full Panic Attacks. The person must meet the criteria for symptoms of Agoraphobia (pp. 396-397).

Specific Phobia (Formerly Simple Phobia)

This disorder is the significant and persistent, excessive, unreasonable fear cued by the presence or anticipation of a specific object or situation. Exposure to the object or situation almost always provokes an immediate anxiety response. In children, the anxiety can be in the form of crying, tantrums, freezing, or clinging. The response may be situationally bound or situationally predisposed Panic Attack. Adults and adolescents recognize the fear as unreasonable, but children do not always have this understanding. The person avoids the phobic stimulus or endures it with significant dread. The response must be of a level that interferes with activities of daily living to diagnose the disorder. Five subtypes allow specification of the focus of fear or avoidance:

1. Animal Type
2. Natural Environment Type
3. Blood-Injection-Injury Type
4. Situational Type
5. Other Type

Social Phobia (Formerly Social Anxiety Disorder)

The distinctive feature of Social Phobia is significant and persistent fear of social or performance situations in which embarrassment may occur. Exposure to the feared situation usually produces an immediate anxiety response. The response can take the form of a situationally bound reaction or a situationally predisposed reaction. For children, there must be evidence of capacity for age-appropriate social relationships with familiar people, and anxiety must occur in peer settings, not just with adults. In children, the anxiety can be in the form of crying, tantrums, freezing, or clinging. Children may not recognize the fear as unreasonable, but adolescents and adults do. In some cases, the social performance situation is avoided or is endured, but significantly dreaded. The fear significantly impairs the person's functioning, and the person experiences marked distress about having the phobia. The only designated specifier for this disorder is Generalized, which is used if the person has this reaction in most social situations.

Obsessive-Compulsive Disorder

The distinguishing features of Obsessive-Compulsive Disorder are recurring obsessions or compulsions that are severe enough to be time-consuming (more than one hour a day) or cause significant distress or impairment. The person, at some time during the course of the disorder, has recognized that the obsessions or compulsions are excessive or unreasonable (this criterion does not apply to children). The only specifier for this disorder is With Poor Insight. This specifier is used when the person, during a current episode, does not recognize the excessiveness or unreasonableness of the obsessions and compulsions most of the time. For purposes of doing a DSM-IV diagnosis, obsessions and compulsions are defined as follows:

- *Obsessions* are persistent ideas, thoughts, impulses, or images which are experienced as intrusive and inappropriate and which cause marked anxiety or distress.
- *Compulsions* are repetitive behaviors or mental acts which are used to prevent or reduce anxiety or distress and which are not used for pleasure or gratification.

More detailed explanations and examples of obsessions and compulsions are provided on pages 418 and 419 in the DSM-IV.

Posttraumatic Stress Disorder (PTSD)

Posttraumatic Stress Disorder has its modern origins in combat reactions, and much research on this disorder was done with veterans of the Vietnam War. The stressors that form the basis of this disorder have expanded in the last twenty years. Much controversy surrounds the degree and intensity of symptoms that can be produced by traumatic stress. It is generally accepted that common symptoms of exposure to traumatic stressors include avoidance of the stimuli that remind the person of the trauma, reexperiencing the stressor directly and indirectly, and increased arousal when exposed to memories or triggers the person associates with the trauma. These common reactions form the basis of the criteria for PTSD. Much controversy exists regarding the effects of trauma because many people who suffer severe traumatic events show no long-term effects from the trauma, whereas others have significant, multiple, long-term symptoms.

The key components of PTSD are the definition of a traumatic event, the symptoms of the disorder, duration of symptoms, and degree of impairment. For a summary of the diagnostic criteria, see Visual 11.3.

In DSM-IV, the essential feature of PTSD is "development of characteristic symptoms following exposure to an extreme traumatic stressor involving direct personal experience of an event that involves actual or threatened death or serious injury, or other threat to one's physical integrity; or witnessing an event that involves death, injury, or a threat to the physical integrity

VISUAL 11.3. 309.81 Posttraumatic Stress Disorder Criteria Summary

REEXPERIENCING

A. Exposure to traumatic event in which:
   1. experienced, or witnessed an event(s) involving actual or threatened death, serious injury, or threat to physical integrity of self or others,
   2. response involved intense fear, helplessness, or horror (in children can be expressed as disorganized or agitated behavior).

B. Traumatic event persistently *reexperienced* in 1+ of:
   1. recurrent recollections of event
   2. recurrent dreams of event
   3. acting or feeling as if event were recurring
   4. psychological distress at exposure to internal/external cues symbolizing the trauma
   5. physiological distress at exposure to internal/external cues symbolizing the trauma

AVOIDANCE

C. *Avoidance* of stimuli associated with trauma and numbing with 3+ of:
   1. avoidance of thoughts, feelings, conversations associated with trauma
   2. avoidance of activities, places, people that cause recollection of trauma
   3. inability to recall parts of trauma
   4. diminished interest in activities
   5. detachment or estrangement from others
   6. restricted range of affect
   7. sense of limited future

AROUSAL

D. Symptoms of increased *arousal* with 2+ of:
   1. difficulty falling or staying asleep
   2. irritability or outbursts of anger
   3. difficulty concentrating
   4. hypervigilance
   5. exaggerated startle response

E. Duration of B, C, D criteria for more than one month

F. Disturbance causes clinically significant distress or impairment in social, occupational, or other areas of functioning.

Specify if:
Acute: duration of symptoms is less than 3 months
Chronic: duration of symptoms is more than 3 months

Specify if:
With Delayed Onset: onset of symptoms 6 months after stressor

Source: American Psychiatric Association, 1994, pp. 424-429. Reprinted with permission from the *Diagnostic and Statistical Manual of Mental Disorders,* Fourth Edition. Copyright 1994 American Psychiatric Association.

of another person; or learning about unexpected or violent death, serious harm, or threat of death or injury experienced by a family member or other close associate (Criterion A1)" (American Psychiatric Association, 1994, p. 424, reprinted with permission from the *Diagnostic and Statistical Manual of Mental Disorders,* Fourth Edition, copyright 1994 American Psychiatric Association). This is an expanded definition from the DSM-III definition of "development of characteristic symptoms following a psychologically traumatic event that is generally outside the range of usual human experience (DSM-III, 1980, p. 336, reprinted with permission from the *Diagnostic and Statistical Manual of Mental Disorders,* Third Edition, copyright 1980 American Psychiatric Association). Traumatic events have become so widespread and frequent that some forms of traumatic experience are not "outside the realm of usual human experience"; hence, the definition for DSM-IV needed to be more precise.

"The person's response to the traumatic event must involve intense fear, helplessness, or horror (in children, disorganized or agitated behavior) (Criterion A2)." Symptoms from exposure to trauma include "persistent reexperiencing of the traumatic event (Criterion B), persistent avoidance of stimuli associated with trauma and numbing of general responsiveness (Criterion C), and persistent symptoms of increased arousal (Criterion D)." The symptoms "must be present for more than one month (Criterion E), and the disturbance must cause clinically significant distress or impairment in social, occupational, or other . . . areas of functioning (Criterion F)" (American Psychiatric Association, 1994, p. 424, reprinted with permission from the *Diagnostic and Statistical Manual of Mental Disorders,* Fourth Edition, copyright 1994 American Psychiatric Association.).

The DSM-IV provides examples of traumatic events, such as military combat, violent personal assault (sexual assault, physical attack, robbery, mugging), being kidnapped or taken hostage, terrorist attack, torture, incarceration as a prisoner of war or in a concentration camp, natural or human disasters, severe automobile accidents, or being diagnosed with a life-threatening illness. For children, sexually traumatic events include developmentally inappropriate sexual experiences without threatened or actual violence or injury. Witnessed events are included in the definition and can include observing serious injury or unnatural death of another person due to violent assault, accident, war, or disaster, or unexpectedly witnessing a dead body or body parts. Events experienced by others of which a person learns are also part of the definition, including violent personal assault, serious accident, or serious injury experienced by family member or close friend; sudden, unexpected death of family member or close friend; or one's child having a life-threatening disease. The disorder may be severe or long-lasting when the stressor is of human design (e.g., torture, rape). Likelihood of developing PTSD may increase as intensity of and physical proximity to the stressor increase.

Tip: The DSM-IV definition of traumatic events was developed mainly with an adult population and does not take into account the effects of trauma on early childhood development. It is now known that trauma affects the child at the earliest stages of life and produces symptoms of sufficient duration and intensity to warrant a diagnosis of PTSD. I have devised a definition that can be added to the DSM-IV definition that will aid in treatment planning for children. When a small child is traumatized, the development processes are invariably involved and influenced. For these reasons, clinicians should consider this definition also when doing treatment planning for traumatized children: *Childhood trauma can result from any event or series of events that overwhelms, overstimulates, or creates extreme fear in the child, causing permanent or temporary interruption of normal developmental processes or tasks.*

In PTSD, the following associated features can be quite significant:

- Guilt feelings about surviving
- Phobic fears of events and relationships that resemble or symbolize the trauma
- Impaired affect modulation
- Self-destructive behavior
- Impulsive behavior
- Dissociative symptoms
- Somatic complaints
- Feelings of ineffectiveness, shame, despair, hopelessness
- Feelings of permanent damage
- Loss of previously sustained beliefs
- Hostility
- Withdrawal
- Feeling constantly threatened
- Impaired relationships
- Change of personality characteristics
- Increased risk of Panic Disorder, Agoraphobia, Obsessive-Compulsive Disorder, Social Phobia, Specific Phobia, Major Depressive Disorder, Somatization Disorder, and Substance-Related Disorders. Incidence of these disorders preceding or following the onset of PTSD is not known.

- Increased arousal, measured by autonomic functions (heart rate, electromyography, sweat gland activity)

Differential Diagnosis

Because of the extensive associated features of PTSD, the differential diagnosis can be complex. PTSD differential diagnosis should include the following:

- Adjustment Disorder: stressor must be extreme (life-threatening) for PTSD; in Adjustment Disorder it can be of any severity.
- Mood Disorder: avoidance, numbing, and hyperarousal preceding trauma.
- Anxiety Disorder: avoidance, numbing, and hyperarousal preceding trauma
- Brief Psychotic Disorder: consider Dual Diagnosis.
- Conversion Disorder: consider Dual Diagnosis.
- Major Depressive Disorder: consider Dual Diagnosis.
- Obsessive-Compulsive Disorder: inappropriate thoughts that are not associated with the traumatic event.
- Schizophrenia: differentiate flashbacks from illusions, hallucinations, and other perceptual disturbances.
- Malingering: should be ruled out where financial gain, benefits eligibility, or forensics are involved.

ACUTE STRESS DISORDER

Acute Stress Disorder is new to the DSM-IV. Frances, First, and Pincus (1995), in their excellent DSM study guide, point out that DSM-I had a similar category titled "Gross Stress Reaction" and that features of this disorder were covered in the DSM-III under PTSD. This disorder was included to cover people who have immediate and intense stress reactions to traumatic events and need immediate clinical attention rather than waiting more than a month to offer intervention based on the symptoms of PTSD. The criteria and symptom complex are similar to those for PTSD, but focus more on dissociative symptomology, and the duration criterion differs from PTSD in that the disturbance lasts at least two days, a maximum of four weeks, and occurs within four weeks of the traumatic event.

GENERALIZED ANXIETY DISORDER

Generalized Anxiety Disorder has been significantly revised for DSM-IV. Its basic feature is excessive anxiety and worry (apprehensive expectation) that occurs more days than not for a period of at least six months regarding a number of events or activities. The person has difficulty controlling the worry. The anxiety and worry produce at least three of six symptoms (in children, only one symptom is required):

1. Restlessness or feeling keyed up or on edge
2. Easily fatigued
3. Difficulty concentrating or mind going blank
4. Irritability
5. Muscle tension
6. Sleep disturbance

The focus of the anxiety and worry associated with this disorder is not limited to worry about fears experienced as part of a Panic Disorder, Social Phobia, Obsessive-Compulsive Disorder, Separation Anxiety Disorder, Anorexia Nervosa, Somatization Disorder, Hypochondriasis, or PTSD.

Anxiety Disorder Due to a GMC

This disorder is distinguished by clinically significant anxiety that is the direct physiological consequence of a GMC. The specifiers for this disorder are With Generalized Anxiety, With Panic Attacks, and With Obsessive-Compulsive Symptoms. The GMC is recorded on Axis I as part of the disorder diagnosis, and it is recorded on Axis III with the coding from Appendix G and the disclaimer if the person making the diagnosis is not a medical professional.

Substance-Induced Anxiety Disorder

Substance-Induced Anxiety Disorder has as its main feature significant anxiety symptoms that are the direct physiological consequence of a substance. The history, physical examination, or laboratory findings must show that the symptoms developed during or within one month of Substance Intoxication or Substance Withdrawal; otherwise, medication use is related to etiology. The full criteria for another Anxiety Disorder do not have to be met. The disturbance does not occur exclusively during the course of a delirium. The specifiers are With Generalized Anxiety, With Panic Attacks, With Obsessive-Compulsive Symptoms, With Phobic Symptoms, and the clinician should specify With Onset During Intoxication or With Onset During Withdrawal.

Anxiety Disorder NOS

Anxiety Disorder NOS covers disorders with prominent anxiety and phobic avoidance that do not meet the criteria of any of the Anxiety Disorders in this section or the Adjustment Disorders with anxiety features (Adjustment Disorder With Anxiety or Adjustment Disorder with Mixed Anxiety and Depressed Mood).

DIFFERENTIAL DIAGNOSIS

The differential diagnosis for most of the disorders in this class involves other disorders in the class. Other common differential diagnoses include Delusional Disorder, Major Depressive Disorder, Separation Anxiety Disorder, Hypochrondiasis, Anorexia Nervosa, Schizophrenia, Psychotic Disorder, PDD, Schizoid Personality Disorder, Avoidant Personality Disorder, Body Dysmorphic Disorder, Trichotillomania, Tic Disorders, Stereotypic Movement Disorder, Eating Disorders, Pathological Gambling, and Somatization Disorder.

RECOMMENDED STANDARDIZED MEASURES

- Davidson Trauma Scale (DTS)
- Hamilton Anxiety Rating Scale (HARS)
- Multidimensional Anxiety Questionnaire (MAQ)
- Social Phobia and Anxiety Inventory for Children (SPAI-C)
- Trauma Symptom Checklist for Children (TSCC)
- Trauma Symptom Inventory (TSI)
- Yale-Brown Obsessive-Compulsive Scale (YBOCS)

RECOMMENDED READING

Beck, A. T. and Emery, G. (1985). *Anxiety Disorders and Phobias: A Cognitive Perspective*. New York: Basic Books.

De Silva, P. and Rachman, S. (1998). *Obsessive-Compulsive Disorder: The Facts,* Second Edition. New York: Oxford University Press.

Swinson, R. P., Antony, M. M., Rachman, S., and Richter, M. A. (1998). *Obsessive-Compulsive Disorder: Theory Research and Treatment*. New York: Guilford.

Van der Kolk, B. A., McFarlane, A. C., and Weisbeth, L. (1996). *Traumatic Stress: The Effects of Overwhelming Experience on Mind, Body, and Society*. New York: Guilford.

REFERENCES

American Psychiatric Association (1980). *Diagnostic and Statistical Manual of Mental Disorders,* Third Edition. Washington, DC: American Psychiatric Association.

American Psychiatric Association (1994). *Diagnostic and Statistical Manual of Mental Disorders,* Fourth Edition. Washington, DC: American Psychiatric Association.

Frances, A., First, M. B., and Pincus, H. B. (1995). *DSM-IV Guidebook: The Essential Companion to the* Diagnostic and Statistical Manual of Mental Disorders. Washington, DC: American psychiatric Association.

Stone, M. H. (1997). *Healing the Mind: A History of Psychiatry from Antiquity to the Present.* New York: Norton.

Chapter 12

Somatoform Disorders

DISORDERS

300.81 Somatization Disorder
300.82 Undifferentiated Somatoform Disorder
300.11 Conversion Disorder
307.xx Pain Disorder
  307.80 Associated With Psychological Factors
  307.89 Associated With Both Psychological Factors and a GMC
300.7 Hypochondriasis
300.7 Body Dysmorphic Disorder
300.82 Somatoform Disorder NOS

FUNDAMENTAL FEATURES

The key feature of this class of disorders is the presence of physical complaints that suggest a General Medical Condition (GMC), but the physical complaints cannot be completely explained by a GMC, substances, or another mental disorder. The symptoms must be clinically significant and cause distress and functional impairment. With Somatoform Disorders, unlike Malingering and Factitious Disorders, the physical symptoms are not intentional. These disorders should be ruled out before diagnosing a Somatoform Disorder (see Visuals 13.1, 13.2, and 13.3). Somatoform Disorders differ from Psychological Factors Affecting Medical Condition (see "Other Conditions That May Be a Focus of Clinical Attention," in DSM-IV, pp. 675-676) in that they lack a GMC to account for the physical symptoms. The disorders in this section are commonly seen in medical settings.

People presenting with symptoms of this disorder should have a thorough medical screening before the diagnosis is made. In some cases, people receive extensive medical intervention before this diagnosis is made. Sometimes after the diagnosis is made, it is later discovered that the mental health professional and health care professionals misdiagnosed what was actually an existing General Medical Condition. The distinction of the disorders in this class is often difficult to make because of the mixture of imagined and intentional physical symptoms and psychological responses. Culture can play a role in the appearance of physical symptoms (Frances, First, and Pincus, 1995) making it a significant factor in this class of disorders. Diagnosis of this class of disorders requires close interdisciplinary cooperation between mental health and health care practitioners. (See Visual 12.1 for criteria summary.)

Somatization Disorder

Somatization Disorder was once referred to as "hysteria" or "Briquet's syndrome," which is named after Paul Briquet (1796-1881), who treated people suffering from illness for which no medical explanation could be found. He was methodical in his research to distinguish these disorders from medical conditions. He was also well known for his willingness to listen to his patients, and he saw the need for psychotherapy as a means to assist people with this disorder (Stone, 1997). The criteria used in the DSM-IV for this disorder are slightly more restrictive than the criteria used for Briquet's syndrome. The primary feature of this disorder is recurring, multiple, clinically significant somatic complaints. A somatic complaint is considered clinically significant if it results in medical treatment or causes significant impairment in functioning. The complaints must begin before thirty years of age and must endure for several years. A person must suffer from a particular number of physical complaints from four categories to be diagnosed with this disorder: four pain symptoms, two gastrointestinal symptoms, one sexual symptom, and one psuedoneurological symptom. (The number of symptoms may seem excessive, but in the DSM-III, women had to have at least fourteen symptoms and men twelve symptoms from a list of thirty-seven possible symptoms to qualify for this disorder. In DSM-III-R, the list was reduced to thirty-five symptoms, and the person had to have at least thirteen of the symptoms.) See the diagnostic dialogue box for a listing of the nature of these symptoms (pp. 449-450). These symptoms cannot be explained by a GMC, or if a GMC is present, the symptoms are in excess of what would be expected medically.

VISUAL 12.1. Somatoform Disorders Criteria Summary

Fundamental Features

Presence of physical symptoms suggesting GMC but not explained by a GMC. Symptoms must cause clinically significant impairment. Symptoms not due to Factitious Disorder or Malingering.

300.81 Somatization Disorder
A. History of many physical complaints before age 30, lasting several years, resulting in treatment or impaired functioning
B. Must have following pain symptoms: 4 pain, 2 gastrointestinal, 1 sexual, 1 pseudoneurological
C. Symptoms cannot be explained by GMC; if GMC present, complaints beyond expected for disorder
D. Symptoms not intentional or feigned

300.11 Conversion Disorder
A. 1+ symptoms/deficits of voluntary motor or sensory function suggesting neurological or other GMC
B. Psychological factors associated because of stressors
C. Not intentionally produced or feigned
D. Not fully explained by GMC, substances, or culture
E. Causes clinically significant impairment
F. Not better accounted for by other MD

300.81 Undifferentiated Somatoform Disorder
A. 1 or more physical complaints
B. Symptoms cannot be explained by GMC; if GMC present, complaints beyond expected for disorder
C. Causes clinically significant impairment
D. Longer than 6 months
E. Not better accounted for by other MD
F. Symptoms not intentional or feigned

Pain Disorder
A. Pain in 1+ anatomical sites
B. Clinically significant distress or impairment
C. Psychological factors important to onset
D. Not intentional or feigned
E. Not better accounted for by other MD

Coding:
307.80 Pain Disorder Associated With Psychological Factors (specify: acute/chronic)
307.89 Pain Disorder Associated With Both Psychological Factors and GMC (specify: acute/chronic)
(use GMC code) Pain Disorder Associated With GMC

300.7 Hypochondriasis
A. Preoccupation with fears of having serious disease based on misinterpretation of symptoms
B. Persists despite medical evaluation
C. Not delusional in intensity
D. Causes clinically significant distress or impairment
E. Duration 6+ months
F. Not better accounted for by other MD

300.7 Body Dysmorphic Disorder
A. Preoccupation with imagined defect in appearance
B. Causes clinically significant distress or impairment
C. Not better accounted for by other MD

300.81 Somatoform Disorder NOS
Symptoms that do not meet criteria for specific Somatoform Disorder

Source: American Psychiatric Association, 1994, pp. 445-469. Reprinted with permission from the *Diagnostic and Statistical Manual of Mental Disorders,* Fourth Edition.

Undifferentiated Somatoform Disorder

Undifferentiated Somatoform Disorder was introduced in the DSM-III-R because of the high level of symptoms and duration of symptoms required to meet the criteria for Somatoform Disorder. Though almost eliminated from the DSM-IV because of its lack of specificity, it was retained because of its relevance to primary health care settings (Frances, First, and Pincus, 1995). The main feature of this disorder is one or more physical complaints lasting for more than six months that cannot be explained by a GMC. The other criteria for this disorder are the same as those for Somatization Disorder.

Conversion Disorder

Conversion Disorder has as its essential feature the presence of symptoms or deficits affecting voluntary motor or sensory function that suggests a neurological or other GMC. Psychological factors are judged to be associated with the symptom or deficit because the onset of the symptoms or worsening of the symptoms is preceded by conflicts or other stressors. The symptoms are not intentional and cause clinically significant distress and dysfunction. The subtypes of this disorder are as follows:

With Motor Symptom or Deficit
With Sensory Symptom or Deficit
With Seizures or Convulsions
With Mixed Presentation

Pain Disorder

Pain Disorder is characterized by pain in one or more parts of the body that is of sufficient intensity to need intervention. The pain causes significant distress and dysfunction and is not intentional. Psychological factors are judged to have played a role in onset of the pain, and the pain is not better accounted for by another mental disorder. This disorder has two subtypes:

307.80 Pain Disorder Associated With Psychological Factors
307.89 Pain Disorder Associated With Both Psychological Factors and a GMC

Another designation, Pain Disorder Associated With a GMC, is not coded but is recorded on Axis III. This condition is pain due to a GMC and is included in the diagnostic dialogue box to aid in differential diagnosis of this disorder.

Hypochondriasis

Hypochondriasis involves fear of having a serious disease based on misinterpretation of bodily signs and symptoms. The person's concerns persist after medical evaluation and reassurance and are not of delusional intensity, and the person can acknowledge the lack of a medical cause of the concern. Clinically significant distress or dysfunction is present, and the duration of the disturbance is more than six months. The disorder is not better accounted for by another mental disorder. There is one specifier:

With Poor Insight

Body Dysmorphic Disorder

Body Dysmorphic Disorder (historically called "dysmorphophobia') is a preoccupation with an imagined defect in appearance. If a defect is present, the preoccupation must be markedly excessive. The preoccupation is clinically distressful and causes functional impairment.

Somatoform Disorder NOS

Somatoform Disorder NOS is reserved for disorders that do not meet the full criteria of other disorders in this section. Some conditions that can be included under this category are a false belief of being pregnant associated with objective signs of pregnancy, nonpsychotic hypochondriacal symptoms, and unexplained physical symptoms for less than six months.

DIFFERENTIAL DIAGNOSIS

Differential diagnosis includes other disorders within this class as well as GMCs, Schizophrenia and Other Psychotic Disorders, Anxiety Disorders, Mood Disorders, Factitious Disorders, Malingering, Adjustment Disorders, Dissociative Disorders, Dyspareunia (pain associated with sexual intercourse), and geriatric health concerns.

RECOMMENDED STANDARDIZED MEASURES

No specific psychological measures are recommended for this class of disorders. The key measures are standard medical evaluation and medical testing focused on the symptom presentation of the person.

RECOMMENDED READING

Morrison, J. (1997). *When Psychological Problems Mask Medical Disorders*. New York: Guilford.

REFERENCES

American Psychiatric Association (1994). *Diagnostic and Statistical Manual of Mental Disorders,* Fourth Edition. Washington, DC: American Psychiatric Association.

First, M. B., Frances, A., and Pincus, H. N. (995). *DSM-IV Guidebook: The Essential Companion to the* Diagnostic and Statistical Manual of Mental Disorders. Washington, DC: American Psychiatric Association.

Stone, M. H. (1997). *Healing the Mind: A History of Psychiatry from Antiquity to the Present.* New York: Norton.

Chapter 13

Factitious Disorders

DISORDERS

300.xx Factitious Disorder
- .16 With Predominantly Psychological Signs and Symptoms
- .19 With Predominantly Physical Signs and Symptoms
- .19 With Combined Psychological Signs and Physical Symptoms
- .19 Factitious Disorder NOS

FUNDAMENTAL FEATURES

Factitious Disorders are defined by physical and psychological symptoms that are intentionally produced or feigned to assume the sick role. The judgment that symptoms are intentionally produced is based on direct evidence and the exclusion of other causes. (See Visual 13.1 for the criteria summary.)

Factitious Disorder

Factitious Disorder is the key disorder in this section and has the following criteria:

- Intentional production/feigning of physical or psychological signs/symptoms.
- Motivation is to assume sick role.
- External incentives (e.g., economic gain) are absent.

The subtypes of this disorder are as follows:

With Predominantly Psychological Signs and Symptoms
With Predominantly Physical Signs and Symptoms
With Combined Psychological Signs and Physical Symptoms
(*Note:* See pages 472-473 for descriptions of these subtypes.)

VISUAL 13.1. Factitious Disorders Criteria Summary

Diagnostic Criteria for Factitious Disorder:

A. Intentional production/feigning of physical or psychological signs/symptoms.
B. Motivation is to assume sick role.
C. External incentives (e.g., economic gain) are absent.

Code based on type:

300.16 With Predominantly Psychological Signs/Symptoms

300.19 With Predominantly Physical Signs/Symptoms

Munchausen syndrome recorded here

300.19 With Combined Psychological and Physical Signs/Symptoms

300.19 Factitious Disorder NOS

e.g., A person applies the signs/symptoms to another person, usually a child (by proxy). See page 725 (Criteria Sets and Axes Provided for Further Study).

Differential Dx. of:

In section "Other Conditions That May Be a Focus of Clinical Attention," page 683

V65.2 Malingering

Intentional production of false and grossly exaggerated physical or psychological symptoms motivated by external incentives such as avoiding military, avoiding work, obtaining financial gain, evading criminal prosecution, or obtaining drugs.

Differentiated from Conversion Disorder and Somatoform Disorders by intentional production and external incentives

In Appendix B: . . . For Further Study

factitious disorder by proxy

Deliberate production or feigning of physical/psychological signs/symptoms in another person who is under the individual's care.

Source: American Psychiatric Association, 1994, pp. 471-475. Reprinted with permission from the *Diagnostic and Statistical Manual of Mental Disorders,* Fourth Edition.

Factitious Disorder NOS

Factitious Disorder NOS includes factitious symptoms that do not meet the threshold criteria for a Factitious Disorder. Factitious disorder by proxy is one disorder that can be diagnosed under the NOS category.

Factitious Disorder by Proxy

Factitious Disorder by Proxy is in Appendix B: Criteria Sets and Axes Provided for Further Study. The nature of this disorder is the deliberate production of physical or psychological symptoms in another person who is under an individual's care. The symptoms are usually produced in a child by the mother. The motivation for these acts is assumed to be for the perpetrator to assume the sick role by proxy. Motivation for the behavior is not based on incentives or economic gain. The behavior is not accounted for by another mental disorder. After inducing the symptoms, the perpetrator presents the victim for medical treatment and denies any knowledge of the origin of the symptoms. This disorder often coexists with Factitious Disorder and can be associated with life stress. The Factitious Disorder usually is not predominant as long as the perpetrator has access to a victim, and there is usually only one victim at a time. It is common for the perpetrator to have experience in health-related areas and to be stimulated by the medical environment. When confronted, the person may lie extensively, become angry with medical personnel, or become depressed and even suicidal. This disorder cannot be officially diagnosed in the DSM-IV system, but it can be listed under the Factitious Disorder NOS category (A. Frances, personal communication, August 13, 1997). The victim, if also seen by the mental health professional, would be diagnosed using the V code condition of **995.54 Physical Abuse of Child,** contained in the "Other Conditions That May Be a Focus of Clinical Attention" (p. 682).

DIFFERENTIAL DIAGNOSIS

Differential diagnosis includes review for GMCs, MD, Somatoform Disorders, and Malingering.

Malingering

Factitious Disorders are distinguished from Malingering (V65.2). Malingering involves feigning symptoms, but the motivation is in the form of incentives, including economic gain, avoiding military service, avoiding work, evading criminal prosecution, or obtaining drugs. The criteria for Malingering are contained in the section "Other Conditions That May Be a Focus of Clinical Attention" (p. 683). Visuals 13.2 and 13.3 document and illustrate the differences between Somatoform Disorders, Factitious Disorders, and Malingering.

RECOMMENDED STANDARDIZED MEASURES

- Structured Interview for Reported Symptoms (SIRS)
- Test of Memory Malingering (TMM)

RECOMMENDED READING

Hall, H. V. and Pritchard, D. A. (1996). *Detecting Malingering and Deception*. Boca Raton, FL: CRC Press.

Kaplan, H. I. and Sadock, B. J. (1998). *Synopsis of Psychiatry: Behavioral Sciences/Clinical Psychiatry,* Eighth Edition. Baltimore, MD: Williams and Wilkins.

REFERENCE

American Psychiatric Association (1994). *Diagnostic and Statistical Manual of Mental Disorders,* Fourth Edition. Washington, DC: American Psychiatric Association.

VISUAL 13.2. Somatoform Disorders, Factitious Disorders, and Malingering General Criteria Comparison

Somatoform Disorders (p. 445)
Presence of physical symptoms suggesting a GMC, but not explained by a GMC, a substance, or another mental disorder.
Unlike Factitious Disorder and Malingering, physical symptoms are not intentional (under patient's control).

Differs from Psychological Factors Affecting Medical Condition in that the disorder cannot be explained by a GMC.

Disorders:
300.81 Somatization Disorder
Polysymptoms before age 30 continuing for years with combination of pain, gastro-intestinal, sexual, and pseudoneurological symptoms.
300.81 Undifferentiated Somatoform Disorder
Unexplained symptoms for 6 months below threshold for Somatization Disorder.
300.11 Conversion Disorder
Unexplained symptoms/deficits affecting voluntary motor or sensory functions that suggest neurological or GMC with associated psychological factors.
Pain Disorder
307.80 Pain Disorder Associated With Psychological Factors
307.89 Pain Disorder Associated With Both Psychological Factors and GMC
Pain Disorder Associated with GMC (Not considered MD and coded on Axis III. Use coding of GMC.)
Pain is main focus of clinical attention, with psychological factors and GMC important in onset and continuation of pain.
300.7 Hypochondriasis
Preoccupation with fear of having a serious disease based on misinterpretation of bodily symptoms or functions.
300.7 Body Dysmorphic Disorder
Preoccupation with imagined defect in physical appearance.
300.81 Somatoform Disorder NOS
Symptoms that do not meet the criteria for a specific Somatoform Disorder.

Factitious Disorders (p. 471)
Physical/psychological symptoms intentionally produced/feigned to assume sick role. External incentives are absent (e.g., economic gain, avoiding legal responsibility, improving physical well-being).

Disorders:
Factitious Disorder:
300.16 With Predominantly Psychological Signs and Symptoms
300.19 With Predominantly Physical Signs and Symptoms
300.19 With Combined Psychological and Physical Signs and Symptoms
300.19 Factitious Disorder NOS

factitious disorder by proxy (p. 725)
Physical/psychological symptoms intentionally produced/feigned in another person who is under one's care so the perpetrator can assume the sick role by proxy.

Note: Refer to Appendix B: Criteria Sets and Axes Provided for Further Study. Use code 300.19 Factitious Disorder NOS to diagnose this disorder for the perpetrator. Victim is coded 995.54 Physical Abuse of Child.

V65.2 Malingering (p. 683)
Intentional production of false/grossly exaggerated physical/psychological symptoms motivated by external incentives.
In section "Other Conditions That May Be a Focus of Clinical Attention."

Not considered an MD

Source: American Psychiatric Association, 1994, pp. 471-475.

VISUAL 13.3. Somatoform Disorders, Factitious Disorders, and Malingering Fundamental Features Comparison

Somatoform Disorders (p. 445)

Presence of physical symptoms *suggesting a GMC, but not explained* by a GMC, a substance, or another mental disorder.
Unlike Factitious Disorder and Malingering, physical symptoms are not intentional (under patient's control).
Differs from Psychological Factors Affecting Medical Condition in that the disorder cannot be explained by a GMC.

Factitious Disorders (p. 471)

Physical/psychological symptoms *intentionally* produced/feigned *to assume sick role.* External incentives are absent (economic gain, avoiding legal responsibility, improving physical well-being).

factitious disorder by proxy (p. 725)

Physical/psychological symptoms intentionally produed/feigned in *another person* who is under one's care *to assume sick role by proxy for perpetrator.*

In Appendix B: Criteria Sets and Axes Provided for Further Study. Use 300.19 Factitious Disorder NOS to diagnose this disorder for perpetrator. Use 995.54 Physical Abuse of Child for victim.

V65.2 Malingering (p. 683)

Intentional production of false/grossly exaggerated physical/psychological symptoms *motivated by external incentives.*

In section "Other Conditions That May Be a Focus of Clinical Attention."

Not considered an MD

Chapter 14

Dissociative Disorders

DISORDERS

300.12 Dissociative Amnesia (formerly Psychogenic Amnesia)
300.13 Dissociative Fugue (formerly Psychogenic Fugue)
300.14 Dissociative Identity Disorder (formerly Multiple Personality Disorder)
300.6 Depersonalization Disorder
300.15 Dissociative Disorder NOS

FUNDAMENTAL FEATURES

The simplicity of this class of disorders is made up for by the controversy surrounding it. The DSM-IV Task Force Chairperson has questioned whether these disorders exist (Frances, 1995). The essential component of this class of disorders is disruption in the usually integrated functions of consciousness, memory, identity, or perception of the environment. The disturbance can be sudden, gradual, transient, or chronic. (See Visual 14.1 for an overview of this class.)

Dissociative Amnesia

Dissociative Amnesia (formerly Psychogenic Amnesia) is an inability to recall important personal information that is usually of a traumatic or stressful nature and is too extensive to be explained by normal forgetfulness. The memory loss is usually reversible. The criteria include ruling out a series of other possible disorders and assessment that the disturbance causes clinically significant distress or impairment. Five types of memory disturbance are associated with this disorder; these are summarized in Visual 14.2.

VISUAL 14.1. Dissociative Disorders Overview

Fundamental Feature

Disruption in normally integrated functions of consciousness, memory, identity, or perception of the environment

300.12 Dissociative Amnesia (formerly Psychogenic Amnesia)
Inability to recall personal information from trauma

300.13 Dissociative Fugue (formerly Psychogenic Fugue)
Sudden travel from home or work associated with inability to recall past, confusion about personal identity, or assumption of new identity

300.14 Dissociative Identity Disorder (formerly MPD)
Two or more identities that control behavior accompanied by inability to recall personal information

300.6 Depersonalization Disorder
Recurrent feeling of detachment from mental processes or body that is accompanied by intact reality testing

300.15 Dissociative Disorder NOS
Dissociative symptom that does not meet criteria for a Dissociative Disorder

In Appendix B: . . . For Further Study

dissociative trance disorder
Involuntary trance state that causes impairment

Source: American Psychiatric Association, 1994, pp. 477-491.

VISUAL 14.2. Memory Disturbance Associated with Dissociative Amnesia

Localized Amnesia
Failure to recall traumatic events within hours or days of the event

Selective Amnesia
Recall of *some* aspects of traumatic events within hours or days of the event

Generalized Amnesia
Failure to recall entire life/Report to police, ER, hospitals

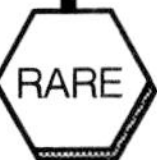

Continuous Amnesia
Inability to recall events from a specific time to the present

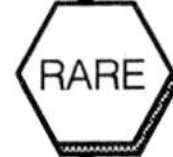

Systematized Amnesia
Memory loss for specific categories of information

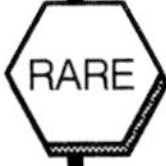

These amnesias are differentiated from amnesias in section 2, Delirium, Dementia, and Amnestic, and Other Cognitive Disorders. Section 2 amnesias are due to GMCs or substances and are related to the ability to remember new information and inability to recall previously learned information or past events.

If ability to repeat a sequence of information is present or aphasia, apraxia, agnosia, or disturbance of executive function is present, the diagnosis is more likely delirium.

Source: American Psychiatric Association, 1994, p. 478.

Dissociative Fugue

Dissociative Fugue (formerly Psychogenic Fugue) involves sudden, unexpected travel from home or place of work associated with the inability to recall one's past, confusion about personal identity, or assumption of new identity. The criteria include ruling out a series of other possible disorders and assessment that the disturbance causes clinically significant distress or impairment.

Dissociative Identity Disorder

Dissociative Identity Disorder (formerly Multiple Personality Disorder) is quite controversial and involves the presence of two or more distinct identities or personality states that frequently take control of behavior. Each personality state can be experienced as if it has a distinct history and identity and can have a separate name. The inability to recall personal information is beyond ordinary forgetfulness. In children, the symptoms cannot be attributed to imaginary playmates or other fantasy. This disorder represents the failure to integrate various aspects of identity, memory, and consciousness. People with this disorder suffer memory gaps for recent and past personal history.

Depersonalization Disorder

Depersonalization Disorder is distinguished by persistent episodes of depersonalization with a feeling of detachment or estrangement from one's self. The person can feel like an "automaton," as if living in a dream or in a film, or have the sense of being outside one's body. Realty testing remains intact. Depersonalization is a common experience and should be diagnosed when there is marked distress or impairment. Other mental disorders, substances, and GMCs should be ruled out.

Dissociative Disorder NOS

Dissociative Disorder NOS is reserved for dissociative symptoms that do not meet the full criteria for a Dissociative Disorder. Dissociative trance disorder can be diagnosed in this category; its criteria are contained in Appendix B.

Visual 14.3 is a summary of the symptoms that can be a part of this disorder and observed during the clinical interview. These symptoms can be applied in the context of the specific criteria for Dissociative Disorders.

VISUAL 14.3 Cues to Dissociation

Yawning
Appearing sleepy
Lengthy pauses in responding
Vagueness
Rolls head back
"I don't know" response to simple questions
Requests for breaks
Trancelike appearance
Hypnotic eye movements
Arm and leg gestures change
Facial expression changes
"We" statements (e.g., "We all live together." "We come as a package.")
Saying hello or good-bye in middle of session
Ambivalent or strong response regarding dissociative symptoms
Alteration in demeanor or identity
Spontaneous age regression
Inconsistencies/fluctuations in levels of functioning
Intra-interviewing depersonalization
Derealization or amnesia

Source: Steinberg, M. (1995). *Handbook for the Assessment of Dissociation: A Clinical Guide*. Washington, DC: American Psychiatric Press.

DIFFERENTIAL DIAGNOSIS

Differential diagnosis includes the disorders internal to the dissociative class. Other common differential diagnoses are Amnestic Disorder Due to a GMC, seizure disorders, delirium, dementia, Substance-Related Disorders, PTSD, Acute Stress Disorder, Somatization Disorder, Malingering, Age-Related Cognitive Decline, nonpathological forms of amnesia, and Schizophrenia.

RECOMMENDED STANDARDIZED MEASURES

- Structured Clinical Interview for DSM-IV Dissociative Disorders (SCID-D)
- Dissociative Experiences Scale (DES)

RECOMMENDED READING

Lynn, S. J. and Rhue, J. W. (1994). *Dissociation: Clinical and Theoretical Perspectives*. New York: Guilford.

Putnam, F. W. (1997). *Dissociation in Children and Adolescents: A Development Perspective*. New York: Guilford.

Shirar, L. (1996). *Dissociative Children: Bridging the Inner and Outer Worlds*. New York: Norton.

Steinberg, M. (1995). *Handbook for the Assessment of Dissociation: A Clinical Guide*. Washington, DC: American Psychiatric Press.

REFERENCES

American Psychiatric Association (1994). *Diagnostic and Statistical Manual of Mental Disorders,* Fourth Edition. Washington, DC: American Psychiatric Association.

Frances, A. (1995). *DSM-IV Audio Review.* Washington, DC: American Psychiatric Press.

Steinberg, M. (1995). *Handbook for the Assessment of Dissociation: A Clinical Guide*. Washington, DC: American Psychiatric Press.

Chapter 15

Sexual and Gender Identity Disorders

DISORDERS

Sexual Dysfunctions

Sexual Desire Disorders
- 302.71 Hypoactive Sexual Desire Disorder
- 302.79 Sexual Aversion Disorder

Sexual Arousal Disorders
- 302.72 Female Sexual Arousal Disorder
- 302.72 Male Erectile Disorder

Orgasmic Disorders
- 302.73 Female Orgasmic Disorder (formerly Inhibited Female Orgasm)
- 302.74 Male Orgasmic Disorder (formerly Inhibited Male Orgasm)
- 302.75 Premature Ejaculation

Sexual Pain Disorders
- 302.76 Dyspareunia (not due to a GMC)
- 306.51 Vaginismus (not due to a GMC)

Sexual Dysfunction Due to a GMC
- 625.8 Female Hypoactive Sexual Desire Disorder Due to . . . (indicate GMC)
- 608.89 Male Hypoactive Sexual Desire Disorder Due to . . . (indicate GMC)
- 607.84 Male Erectile Disorder Due to . . . (indicate GMC)
- 625.0 Female Dyspareunia Due to . . . (indicate GMC)
- 608.89 Male Dyspareunia Due to . . . (indicate GMC)
- 625.8 Other Female Sexual Dysfunction Due to . . . (indicate GMC)
- 608.89 Other Male Sexual Dysfunction Due to . . . (indicate GMC)
- ___.__ Substance-Induced Sexual Dysfunction (see p. 522 for substance-specific codes)
- 302.70 Sexual Dysfunction NOS

Paraphilias

302.4 Exhibitionism
302.81 Fetishism
302.89 Frotteurism
302.2 Pedophilia
302.83 Sexual Masochism
302.84 Sexual Sadism
302.3 Transvestic Fetishism
302.82 Voyeurism
302.9 Paraphilia NOS

Gender Identity Disorders

302.xx Gender Identity Disorder
.6 in Children
.85 in Adolescents or Adults
302.6 Gender Identity Disorder NOS
302.9 Sexual Disorder NOS

FUNDAMENTAL FEATURES

This class of disorders is divided into three sections: Sexual Dysfunctions, Paraphilias, and Gender Identity Disorders. Many disorders are included in this class, and the criteria for specific disorders are summarized in Visual 15.1. A brief description of each disorder is given in the following material.

Sexual Dysfunction Disorders

Sexual dysfunctions are related to disturbance in the sexual response cycle or pain associated with sexual intercourse. The sexual response cycle characteristics are divided into four areas in the DSM-IV:

1. *Desire:* Fantasies about sexual activity and the desire to have sexual activity.
2. *Excitement:* A subjective sense of sexual pleasure and accompanying physiological changes. During excitement or arousal, blood flow to the genital area increases, leading to erection in men and enlargement of the clitoris, engorgement of the vaginal walls, and increased vaginal

secretions in women. In the DSM-IV, this is explained as, in males, penile tumescence and erection and, in women, vasocongestion in the pelvis, vaginal lubrication, and expansion and swelling of the external genitalia.
3. *Orgasm:* The peaking of sexual pleasure, with release of semen from the penis and rhythmic contraction of the muscles around the vagina. At orgasm, men and women experience increased muscle tension throughout the body and contraction of the pelvic muscles.
4. *Resolution:* A sense of muscular relaxation and general well-being. During resolution men are unable to have another erection for a period of time. The time between erections (refractory period) usually increases with age. Many women can respond to additional stimulation almost immediately after orgasm.

Sexual response disorders can occur during one or more of these phases, and when more than one phase disorder are present, all are recorded.

Clinical judgment in these disorders is important, and the practitioner should consult the criteria closely when applying the words "persistent" and "recurrent."

Subtypes of this set of disorders include:

1. Nature of onset subtype:

   Lifelong Type: Present since the onset of sexual functioning.
   Acquired Type: Sexual dysfunction developed after a period of normal functioning.

2. Context subtype:

   Generalized Type: Sexual dysfunction not limited to certain types of stimulations, situations, or partners.
   Situational Type: Sexual dysfunction limited to certain types of stimulations, situations, or partners. Can be applied to masturbation.

3. Etiological Factors Subtype:

   Due to Psychological Factors: Condition judged to be due to psychological factors, and GMCs and substances have been ruled out.
   Due to Combined Factors: Condition judged to be due to a combination of psychological factors and GMCs and/or substances.

VISUAL 15.1. Sexual and Gender Identity Disorders Overview

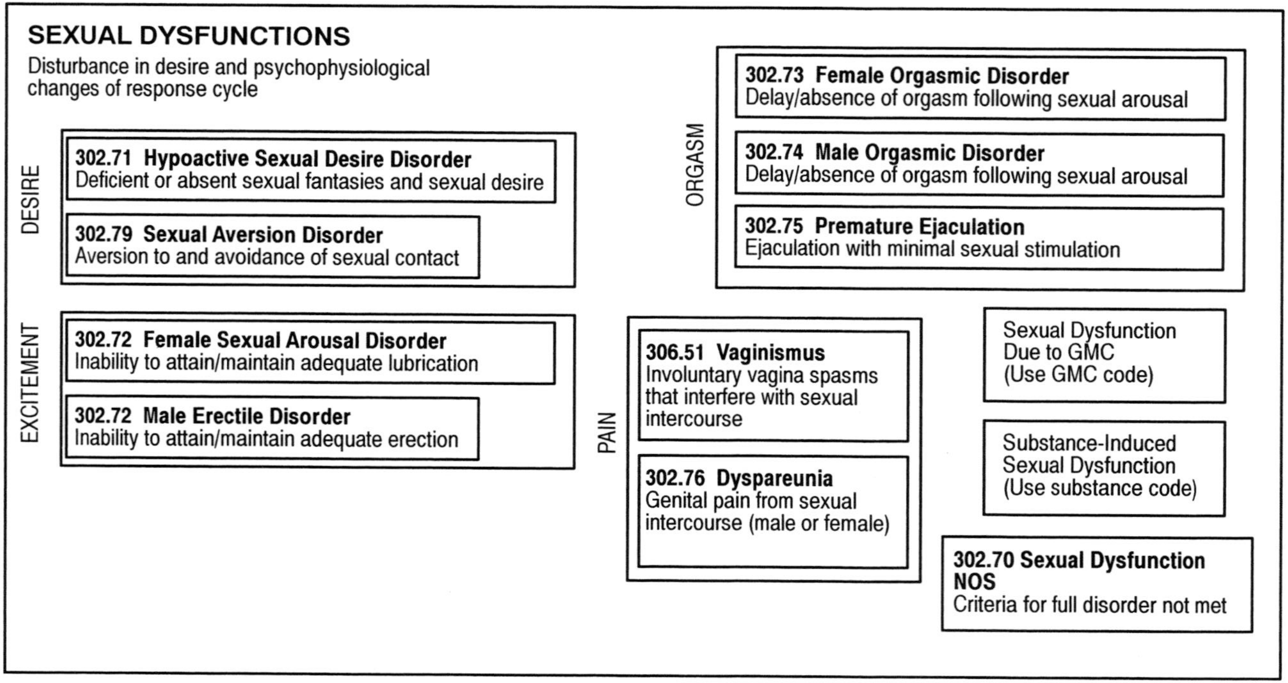

SEXUAL DYSFUNCTIONS

Disturbance in desire and psychophysiological changes of response cycle

DESIRE

302.71 Hypoactive Sexual Desire Disorder
Deficient or absent sexual fantasies and sexual desire

302.79 Sexual Aversion Disorder
Aversion to and avoidance of sexual contact

EXCITEMENT

302.72 Female Sexual Arousal Disorder
Inability to attain/maintain adequate lubrication

302.72 Male Erectile Disorder
Inability to attain/maintain adequate erection

ORGASM

302.73 Female Orgasmic Disorder
Delay/absence of orgasm following sexual arousal

302.74 Male Orgasmic Disorder
Delay/absence of orgasm following sexual arousal

302.75 Premature Ejaculation
Ejaculation with minimal sexual stimulation

PAIN

306.51 Vaginismus
Involuntary vagina spasms that interfere with sexual intercourse

302.76 Dyspareunia
Genital pain from sexual intercourse (male or female)

Sexual Dysfunction Due to GMC (Use GMC code)

Substance-Induced Sexual Dysfunction (Use substance code)

302.70 Sexual Dysfunction NOS
Criteria for full disorder not met

VISUAL 15.1 *(continued)*

PARAPHILIAS

Recurrent sexual urges, fantasies, behaviors involving the unusual

Duration criterion usually 6 months

302.4 Exhibitionism
Exposing genitals to strangers

302.81 Fetishism
Sex activity associated with nonliving objects

302.89 Frotteurism
Touching nonconsenting persons

302.2 Pedophilia
Sexual activity with children (under 13)

302.83 Sexual Masochism
Sexual activity with humiliation, beating, being bound, or made to suffer

302.84 Sexual Sadism
Sexual excitement from psychological or physical humiliation of others

302.3 Transvestic Fetishism
Heterosexual male cross-dressing

302.82 Voyeurism
Observing unsuspecting persons naked, disrobing, or in sexual activity

302.9 Paraphilia NOS
e.g., telephone scatologia, necrophilia, partialism, zoophilia

302.9 Sexual Disorder NOS
Criteria for specific disorder not met (e.g., inadequacy concerns, pattern of failed relationships, distress about sexual orientation)

GENDER IDENTITY DISORDERS

302.6 in Children
302.85 in Adolescents and Adults
Gender Identity Disorder
A. Cross-gender identification
B. Discomfort with sex and gender role

302.6 Gender Identity Disorder NOS
Gender identity not classifiable

Source: American Psychiatric Association, 1994, pp. 493-538.

Sexual Desire Disorders

Sexual Desire Disorders are of two types:

1. Hypoactive Sexual Desire Disorder involves a deficiency or absence of sexual fantasies and desire for sexual activity.
2. Sexual Aversion Disorder is characterized by aversion to and active avoidance of genital sexual contact with a sexual partner.

Sexual Arousal Disorders

Sexual Arousal Disorders have two types:

1. Female Sexual Arousal Disorder has as its main feature a persistent or recurrent inability to attain, or maintain until completion of sexual activity, an adequate lubrication-swelling response of sexual excitement.
2. Male Erectile Disorder is based on the criteria of a persistent or recurrent inability to attain, or maintain until completion of sexual activity, an adequate erection.

Orgasmic Disorders

Orgasmic Disorders are of three types:

1. Female Orgasmic Disorder (formerly Inhibited Female Orgasm) is conceptualized as a persistent or recurrent delay in, or absence of, orgasm following a normal sexual excitement phase.
2. Male Orgasmic Disorder (formerly Inhibited Male Orgasm) is presented as a persistent or recurrent delay in, or absence of, orgasm following a normal sexual excitement phase.
3. Premature Ejaculation consists of persistent or recurrent orgasm and ejaculation with minimal sexual stimulation before, on, or shortly after penetration, and before the person desires it.

Sexual Pain Disorders

Sexual Pain Disorders have two types:

1. Dyspareunia (Not Due to a GMC) is the experiencing of genital pain associated with intercourse.

2. Vaginismus (Not Due to a GMC) is the recurrent or persistent involuntary contraction of the perineal muscles surrounding the outer third of the vagina when vaginal penetration with penis, finger, tampon, or speculum (a medical instrument used to spread the walls of the vagina during a medical examination) is attempted.

Other Sexual Dysfunction Disorders

See pages 515-522 in the DSM-IV for details on coding, subtypes, and specifiers for the following categories of disorders:

1. Sexual Dysfunction Due to a GMC is diagnosed when the sexual dysfunction is judged to be due to the direct physiological effects of a GMC. The sexual dysfunction can be in one or more of the four types of this set of disorders: desire, arousal, orgasmic, and pain. The subtypes are based on the disorders listed previously (see p. 518 of the DSM-IV).
2. Substance-Induced Sexual Dysfunction is clinically significant sexual dysfunction with marked impairment based on evidence from the history, medical examination, or laboratory findings. The sexual dysfunction is explained by substance use, as shown by symptoms within a month of Substance Intoxication, or medication use on the basis of the disturbance. The specifiers for this disorder are With Impaired Desire; With Impaired Arousal; With Impaired Orgasm; and With Sexual Pain.
3. Sexual Dysfunction NOS is reserved for sexual dysfunctions that do not meet the criteria for a specific Sexual Dysfunction Disorder.

Paraphilias

Paraphilias are recurrent, intense, sexually arousing fantasies, sexual urges, or behaviors involving nonhuman subjects, suffering or humiliation of oneself or a partner, or children or nonconsenting adults, that occur over a period of at least six months. The following disorders in this section are based on the characteristics of the specific paraphilia:

1. Exhibitionism is the exposure of one's genitals to a stranger.
2. Fetishism is the use of nonliving objects. The more common fetish objects are underpants, bras, stockings, footwear, or other clothing.
3. Frotteurism is touching and rubbing against a nonconsenting person. This behavior usually occurs in crowded places where detection and apprehension are less likely to occur.

4. Pedophilia is involvement in sexual activity with a prepubescent child (usually age thirteen or younger). The person with pedophilia must be at least sixteen years of age and at least five years older than the child. For late adolescents with this disorder, no specific age criteria are applied, and the diagnostician's clinical judgment is used based on the sexual maturity of the child and the age difference between the perpetrator and the victim. Specifiers are Sexually Attracted to Males; Sexually Attracted to Females; Sexually Attracted to Both; Limited to Incest; Exclusive Type; and Nonexclusive Type.
5. Sexual Masochism involves the act, real or simulated, of being humiliated, beaten, bound, or otherwise made to suffer.
6. Sexual Sadism is the act, real or simulated, by which a person derives sexual excitement from psychological or physical suffering of a victim.
7. Transvestic Fetishism involves cross-dressing. Specify With Gender Dysphoria if the person has persistent discomfort with gender role or identity.
8. Voyeurism is observing unsuspecting individuals, usually strangers, while naked, disrobing, or engaging in sexual activity.
9. Paraphilia NOS is used to record disorders that do not meet the full criteria for the specific Paraphilia Disorders. Paraphilias that can be listed in the NOS category are telephone scatologia (obscene phone calls), necrophilia (corpses), partialism (exclusive focus on a body part), zoophobia (animals), coprophilia (feces), klismaphilia (enemas), and urophilia (urine).

Gender Identity Disorders

Gender Identity Disorders involve a strong and persistent cross-gender identification, which is the desire to be and/or insistence that a person is of the other sex. The cross-gender identification must not be a desire for a perceived cultural advantage of being the other sex:

1. Gender Identity Disorder in Children involves four or more of the following: repeated stated desire to be, or insists that he/she is another sex; males preferring cross-dressing or simulating female clothes; females insisting on wearing male-oriented clothing; strong, persistent preference for cross-sex roles in play or fantasies of being the other sex; intense desire to participate in the sex-typed games and pastimes; and strong preference for playmates of the other sex. The child also exhibits persistent discomfort with own sex or sense of inappropriateness in the gender role of that sex.

2. Gender Identity Disorder in Adolescents or Adults involves preoccupation with eliminating primary and secondary sex characteristics or the belief that he/she was born the wrong sex. Specifiers are Sexually Attracted to Males; Sexually Attracted to Females; Sexually Attracted to Both; and Sexually Attracted to Neither.
3. Gender Identity Disorder NOS is reserved for Gender Identity Disorders that are not classified as one of the two specific disorders. Examples of such disorders are intersex conditions; transient, stress-related cross-dressing; and persistent preoccupation with castration or penectomy without a desire to acquire the sex characteristics of the other sex.

Sexual Disorder NOS

Sexual Disorder NOS is used to code any Sexual and Gender Identity Disorder that does not meet the criteria of any disorder in this class of disorders including, but not limited to, feelings of inadequacy regarding sexual performance; traits related to self-imposed standards of masculine and feminine; distress about a pattern of successive unfeeling sexual relationships; or persistent and marked distress about sexual orientation.

DIFFERENTIAL DIAGNOSIS

Differential Diagnosis for each category is as follows:

1. Sexual Dysfunction: Other disorders within the Sexual and Gender Identity Disorders class, Personality Disorders, and Relational Problems (in "Other Conditions That May Be a Focus of Clinical Attention")
2. Paraphilias: Mental Retardation, Dementia, and Personality Change Due to a GMC
3. Gender Identity: Schizophrenia

RECOMMENDED STANDARDIZED MEASURES

- Hurlbert Index of Sexual Desire (HISD)
- Sexual Desire Interview Schedule (SDIS)
- Sexuality Interview Schedule (SIS)

- Sexual Orientation Scale (SOS)
- Golombok Rust Inventory of Sexual Satisfaction (male and female versions)
- Sexual Dysfunction Scale (SDS)
- Florida Sexual History Questionnaire (FSHQ)
- Sexual Self-Efficacy Scale (SSES)

RECOMMENDED READING

Seeman, M. V. (1995). *Gender and Psychopathology.* Washington, DC: American Psychiatric Press.

REFERENCE

American Psychiatric Association (1994). *Diagnostic and Statistical Manual of Mental Disorders,* Fourth Edition. Washington, DC: American Psychiatric Association.

Chapter 16

Eating Disorders

DISORDERS

307.1	Anorexia Nervosa
307.51	Bulimia Nervosa
307.50	Eating Disorder NOS

FUNDAMENTAL FEATURES

Two disorders are featured in this section of the DSM-IV, Anorexia Nervosa and Bulimia Nervosa, and both disorders are associated with a disturbance in perception of body shape and weight. (See Visual 16.1 for a criteria summary.)

Anorexia Nervosa

Anorexia Nervosa involves refusal to maintain a minimally normal body weight (measured by the person's weight being less than 85 percent of the body weight considered appropriate, based on age and height, as measured by standardized height and weight charts, body mass index calculations, or pediatric growth charts). This is accompanied by a significant fear of gaining weight. The person's fear of obesity does not decrease even following significant weight loss. In postmenarcheal females, amenorrhea (absence of menstrual periods) is present. The criterion for amenorrhea in eating disorder is the absence of at least three consecutive menstrual cycles (Criterion D). The specifiers for this disorder are *Restricting Type,* which indicates that regular binge-eating or purging behavior is not present, and *Binge-Eating/Purging Type,* indicating the person has regularly engaged in binge-eating or purging behavior, such as self-induced vomiting, misuse of laxatives, diuretics, or enemas.

VISUAL 16.1. Eating Disorders Criteria Summary

PRIMARY FEATURES

Severe disturbance in eating behavior with disturbed perception of body image and weight
Two disorders:
Anorexia Nervosa—refusal to maintain minimally normal body weight
Bulimia Nervosa—binge eating with inappropriate compensatory behaviors
Obesity in ICD as GMC not in DSM-IV

Two disorders distinguished primarily by failure to maintain normal body weight and presence of amenorrhea in Anorexia Nervosa

307.1 Anorexia Nervosa
A. Refusal to maintain minimally normal body weight or failure at normal growth weight gain (<85% of expected)
B. Fear of weight gain or obesity when underweight
C. Disturbance in way weight or shape experienced
D. In postmenarcheal, amenorrhea (absence of 3 cycles)

Specify Type:
Restricting
(no binges or purging)
Binge-Eating/Purging
(binge-eating/purging present)

307.51 Bulimia Nervosa
A. Recurrent binge-eating episodes
(Episode is eating unusual amounts of food in 2-hour period with no control of consumption)
B. Recurring compensatory behavior to prevent weight gain
C. Eating and compensation occurs twice a week for 3 months
D. Self-evaluation unduly influences body weight and shape
E. Does not occur exclusively during periods of Anorexia Nervosa

Purging behaviors:
self-induced vomiting, misuse of laxatives, diuretics, or enemas

Nonpurging behaviors:
fasting or excessive exercise

Specify Type:
Purging
Nonpurging

307.50 Eating Disorder NOS
Full criteria for eating disorder not met

Appendix B . . . For Further Study

Binge-eating disorder
A. Recurring binge-eating episodes
B. Eating large amounts rapidly with disgust and embarassment
C. Distress about eating is present
D. Occurs 2 days a week for 6 months
E. No regular use of compensatory behavior

pp. 729-731

Source: American Psychiatric Association, 1994, pp. 539-550. Reprinted with permission from the *Diagnostic and Statistical Manual of Mental Disorders,* Fourth Edition.

Tip: Severe physical problems can be associated with this disorder when significant weight loss occurs. Mental health professionals should seek medical intervention when the person is possibly at risk of serious physical disorders (see Associated Features and Disorders in the "Eating Disorders" section of the DSM-IV, pp. 541-542).

Bulimia Nervosa

Bulimia Nervosa involves repeated episodes of binge eating followed by compensatory behaviors to prevent weight gain. This disorder differs from Anorexia Nervosa in that the person is not grossly underweight; people with this disorder are usually of normal weight or are overweight. The eating occurs in a defined period of time, and the amount of food consumed is in excess of what would be considered normal for the time period. The person has no control over eating during the episode. The compensatory behavior to prevent weight gain can include self-induced vomiting, overuse of laxatives, misuse of diuretics or other medications, fasting, or excessive exercise. The binge-eating and compensatory behavior occur, on average, at least two times a week for three months. Self-evaluation is excessively influenced by body shape and weight. The disturbance does not occur exclusively during episodes of Anorexia Nervosa. The specifiers for this disorder are **Purging Type,** which is the regular engaging in purging behavior, such as self-induced vomiting and misuse of laxatives, diuretics, or enemas, and **Nonpurging Type,** indicating the person has regularly engaged in fasting and excessive exercise, but has not regularly engaged in self-induced vomiting and misuse of laxatives, diuretics, or enemas.

It is very difficult to distinguish these two disorders. People with Anorexia Nervosa and Bulimia Nervosa can engage in binge eating and purging, and the factors that distinguish the two disorders are the failure to maintain the boundary of normal body weight and the presence of amenorrhea.

Tip: Depressive features are common in Anorexia Nervosa and Bulimia Nervosa, and Personality Disorders are common in people with Bulimia Nervosa (DSM-IV, pp. 541-542 and 547-548). Eating Disorders have been found to be correlated with a history of childhood sexual abuse and dissociative symptoms (Steinberg, 1995). Clinicians should screen for these disorders and conditions that may coexist with an Eating Disorder.

Eating Disorder NOS

Eating Disorder NOS is used when a person does not meet the full criteria for an Eating Disorder. The following are some examples provided in the DSM-IV: females who meet all criteria for Anorexia Nervosa but have regular menses; criteria for Anorexia are met, but despite significant weight loss, the person's weight is in the normal range; criteria are met for Bulimia Nervosa, but binge-eating and compensatory behaviors do not meet the duration criterion of at least twice a week for three months; regular use of compensatory behavior by a normal body weight person after eating small amounts of food; repeated chewing and spitting out without swallowing of large amounts of food; and binge-eating disorder involving recurring episodes of binge eating without regular compensatory behaviors associated with Bulimia Nervosa (see p. 729).

DIFFERENTIAL DIAGNOSIS

Differential diagnosis for Anorexia Nervosa should include GMCs, Major Depressive Disorder, Social Phobia, OCD, and Body Dysmorphic Disorder. For Bulimia Nervosa, differential diagnosis involves screening for Kleine-Levin Syndrome, a rare form of periodic hypersomnia associated with bulimia, but without the concern with body shape and weight. Major Depressive Disorder and Borderline Personality Disorder should also be considered as part of the differential diagnosis.

Obesity is not included in the DSM-IV system because it has not been found to be associated with a psychological or behavioral syndrome. Obesity is included within the ICD as a GMC, defined as simple obesity. This disorder can be diagnosed on Axis III.

RECOMMENDED STANDARDIZED MEASURES

- Eating Inventory

RECOMMENDED READING

American Psychiatric Association (1993). *American Psychiatric Association Practice Guidelines for Eating Disorders*. Washington, DC: American Psychiatric Press.

Gordon, R. A. (1999). *Eating Disorders: Anatomy of a Social Epidemic.* Malden, MA: Blackwell.

REFERENCES

American Psychiatric Association (1994). *Diagnostic and Statistical Manual of Mental Disorders,* Fourth Edition. Washington, DC: American Psychiatric Association.

Steinberg, M. (1995). *Handbook for the Assessment of Dissociation: A Clinical Guide.* Washington, DC: American Psychiatric Press.

Chapter 17

Sleep Disorders

DISORDERS

Primary Sleep Disorders

Dyssomnias
- 307.42 Primary Insomnia
- 307.44 Primary Hypersomnia
- 347 Narcolepsy
- 780.59 Breathing-Related Sleep Disorder
- 307.45 Circadian Rhythm Sleep Disorder (formerly Sleep-Wake Schedule Disorder)
- 307.47 Dyssomnia NOS

Parasomnias
- 307.47 Nightmare Disorder (formerly Dream Anxiety Disorder)
- 307.46 Sleep Terror Disorder
- 307.46 Sleepwalking Disorder
- 307.47 Parasomnia NOS

Sleep Disorders Related to Another Mental Disorder

307.42 Insomnia Related to . . . (indicate Axis I or Axis II disorder)
307.44 Hypersomnia Related to . . . (indicate Axis I or Axis II disorder)

Other Sleep Disorders

780.xx Sleep Disorder Due to . . . (indicate GMC)
- 780.52 Insomnia Type
- 780.54 Hypersomnia Type
- 780.59 Parasomnia Type
- 780.59 Mixed Type

___.__ Substance-Induced Sleep Disorder (see p. 607 for substance-specific codes)

FUNDAMENTAL FEATURES

This section includes thirteen disorders divided into four categories based on suspected etiology of the disorder. The sleep disturbance must cause significant distress and involve clinical evaluation of the specific sleep complaints made by the client. The categories of the sleep class of disorders are as follows:

1. *Primary Sleep Disorders* are endogenous abnormalities in sleep-wake generating or timing of sleep. This category is divided into two types (see Visual 17.1 for their criteria summary):
   a. *Dyssomnias* involve abnormalities in amount, quality, or timing of sleep.
   b. *Parasomnias* are related to abnormal behavior or physiological events during sleep, specific sleep stages, or sleep-wake transitions (see Visual 17.2).
2. *Sleep Disorder Related to Another Mental Disorder* has as its main feature sleep disturbance that arises in the context of a diagnosable mental disorder. This form of sleep disturbance frequently occurs as part of a Mood or Anxiety Disorder, but is of sufficient magnitude to require independent clinical attention.
3. *Sleep Disorder Due to a GMC* is a sleep disturbance that occurs as a direct physiological consequence of a GMC.
4. *Substance-Induced Sleep Disorder* is a sleep disturbance caused by current use, or recent cessation of use, of a substance. (See Visual 17.3 for a criteria summary of categories 2, 3, and 4.)

This class of disorders is fairly complex and is the fourth longest section of the DSM-IV manual. The sleep disorders are viewed in the context of stages of sleep, and Visual 17.4 illustrates sleep stages that are related to sleep disturbances. Visual 17.5 shows the approximate hours of sleep, the stage-four sleep percentage, and the REM sleep percentage by age. This visual is included as a guide to judge age-appropriate variations in sleep patterns. Also, the sleep disorders are the only class of disorders that can be diagnosed through a standardized medical test. This test, called polysomnography, monitors multiple electrophysiological parameters during sleep, including measurement of the following:

- *Sleep latency:* the period of time from turning out lights until occurrence of stage-two sleep.
- *Early morning awakening:* the time of being continuously awake from the last stage of sleep until the end of the sleep record.

- *Sleep efficiency:* total sleep time/total time of the sleep record X 100.
- *Apnea index:* the total occurrences of apnea (cessation of airflow at the nose or mouth) longer than 10 seconds per hour of sleep.
- *Nocturnal myoclonus index:* a count of the number of periodic leg movements per hour during sleep.
- *REM latency:* the period of time from the onset of sleep until the first REM period of the night.
- *Sleep-onset REM period:* measurement of REM sleep during the first ten minutes of sleep. (Kaplan and Sadock, 1998)

Although polysomnography can serve as a measure of sleep disturbance, it was not included as a criterion for sleep disturbances in the DSM-IV because it is a lengthy, expensive procedure that requires the person be tested at a sleep center overnight. Despite the increase in sleep centers in the United States, it is difficult to get testing done in some parts of the country. The expense and variable accessibility of this testing ruled out its inclusion as a criterion in the DSM-IV. Possibly, polysomnography will be included in the next edition of the DSM manual, as research and technology advances reduce the costs associated with in-home sleep testing.

When evaluating sleep disturbance, the clinician must remember that what is considered "normal sleep" is highly variable in the population as a whole, and sleep patterns can vary significantly with age. Children are prone to certain sleep disturbances. Age-appropriate sleep disturbance should be ruled out in all sleep disturbances. Sleep disturbances can be a key factor in General Medical Conditions and substance use. For these reasons, sleep disorders can be quite serious and often require the intervention of primary health care systems in addition to mental health treatment.

Brief descriptions of the various sleep disorders are provided in the following material. For all disorders there must be clinically significant distress, impairment of functioning, ruling out of GMCs, and substances.

Primary Sleep Disorders: Dyssomnias

Primary Insomnia

Primary Insomnia involves complaints of difficulty initiating or maintaining sleep or nonrestorative sleep that lasts for a period of at least one month. The person usually has a history of easily disturbed sleep. Younger people are more likely to complain of difficulty falling asleep, whereas older individuals may have difficulty maintaining sleep and tend to awaken early. Most insomnias occur with a sudden onset associated with a

VISUAL 17.1. Dyssomnia and Parasomnia Sleep Disorders Criteria Summary

Fundamental Feature

Four categories based on etiology:
1. Primary Sleep Disorders are presented below

Visual 17.3 contains:

2. Sleep Disorder Related to Another Mental Disorder
3. Sleep Disorder Due to a General Medical Condition
4. Substance-Induced Sleep Disorder

DYSSOMNIAS Disturbance in amount, quality, or timing of sleep

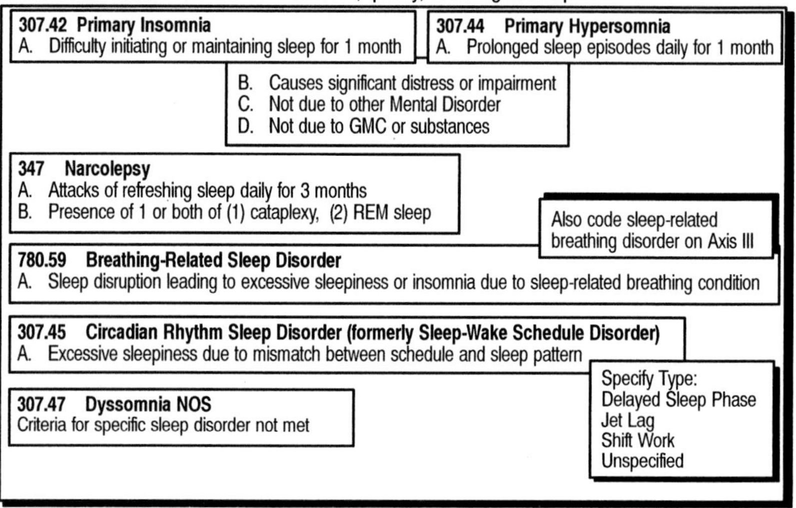

PARASOMNIAS Abnormal behavior or physiological events during sleep

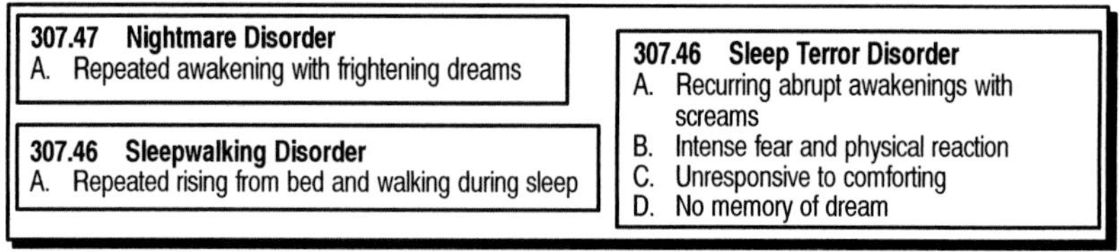

Source: American Psychiatric Association, 1994, pp. 551-607. Reprinted with permission from the *Diagnostic and Statistical Manual of Mental Disorders,* Fourth Edition.

VISUAL 17.2. Specific Aspects of Parasomnias

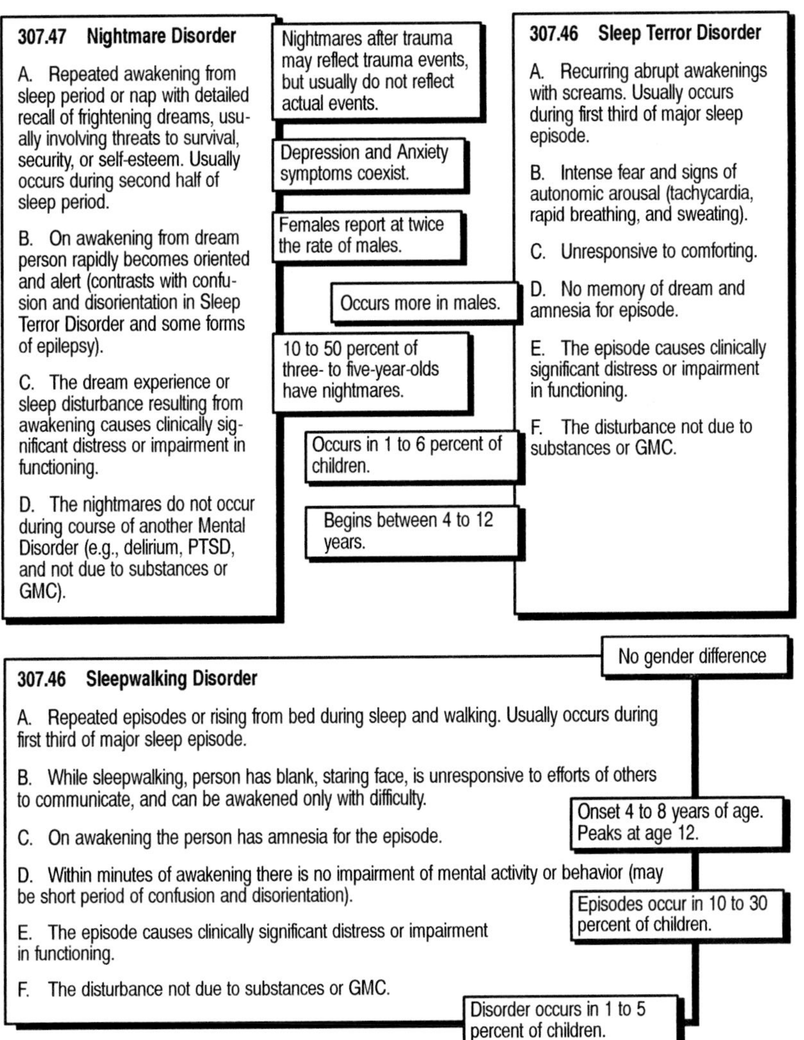

Source: American Psychiatric Association, 1994, pp. 579-592.

VISUAL 17.3. Sleep Disorders Due to Another Mental Disorder, GMC, or Substance-Induced Criteria Summary

Fundamental Feature

Four categories based on etiology:
1. Primary Sleep Disorders presented in Visual 17.1.

Presented below:

2. Sleep Disorders Related to Another Mental Disorder
3. Sleep Disorder Due to a General Medical Condition
4. Substance-Induced Sleep Disorder

Sleep Disorders Related to Another Mental Disorder

307.42 Insomnia Related to Another MD
A. Difficulty initiating or maintaining sleep for 1 month

307.44 Hypersomnia Related to Another MD
A. Prolonged sleep episodes daily for 1 month

B. Causes significant distress or impairment
C. Due to another Axis I or Axis II Mental Disorder
D. Disturbance not better accounted for by another sleep disorder
E. Not due to GMC or substances

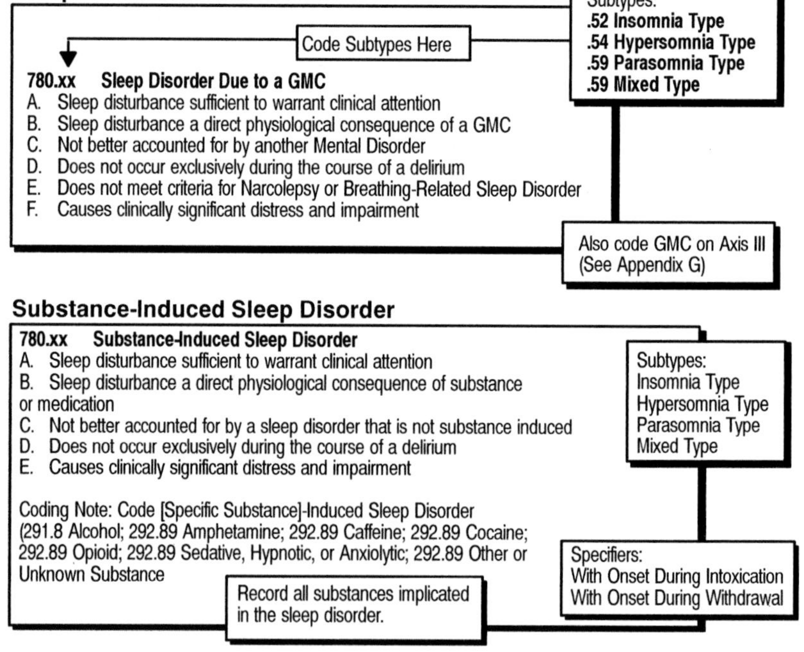

Sleep Disorder Due to a GMC

780.xx Sleep Disorder Due to a GMC
A. Sleep disturbance sufficient to warrant clinical attention
B. Sleep disturbance a direct physiological consequence of a GMC
C. Not better accounted for by another Mental Disorder
D. Does not occur exclusively during the course of a delirium
E. Does not meet criteria for Narcolepsy or Breathing-Related Sleep Disorder
F. Causes clinically significant distress and impairment

Substance-Induced Sleep Disorder

780.xx Substance-Induced Sleep Disorder
A. Sleep disturbance sufficient to warrant clinical attention
B. Sleep disturbance a direct physiological consequence of substance or medication
C. Not better accounted for by a sleep disorder that is not substance induced
D. Does not occur exclusively during the course of a delirium
E. Causes clinically significant distress and impairment

Coding Note: Code [Specific Substance]-Induced Sleep Disorder (291.8 Alcohol; 292.89 Amphetamine; 292.89 Caffeine; 292.89 Cocaine; 292.89 Opioid; 292.89 Sedative, Hypnotic, or Anxiolytic; 292.89 Other or Unknown Substance

Source: American Psychiatric Association, 1994, pp. 551-607.

VISUAL 17.4. Approximation of Stages of Sleep

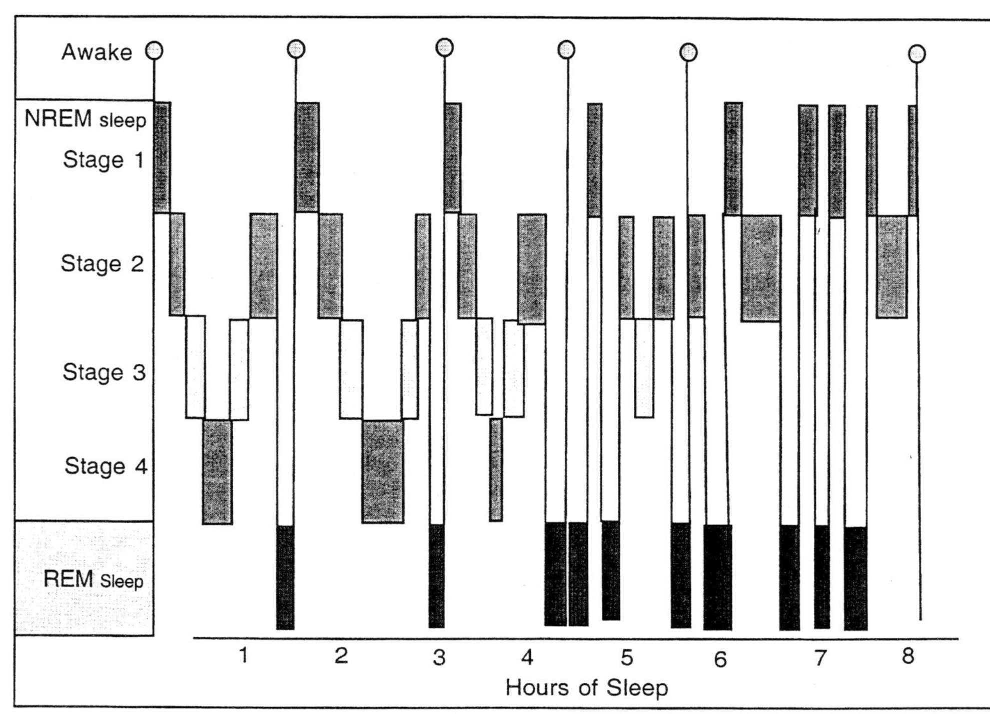

Source: American Psychiatric Association, 1994, pp. 551-552.

FIGURE 17.5. Average Daily Sleep Patterns by Age

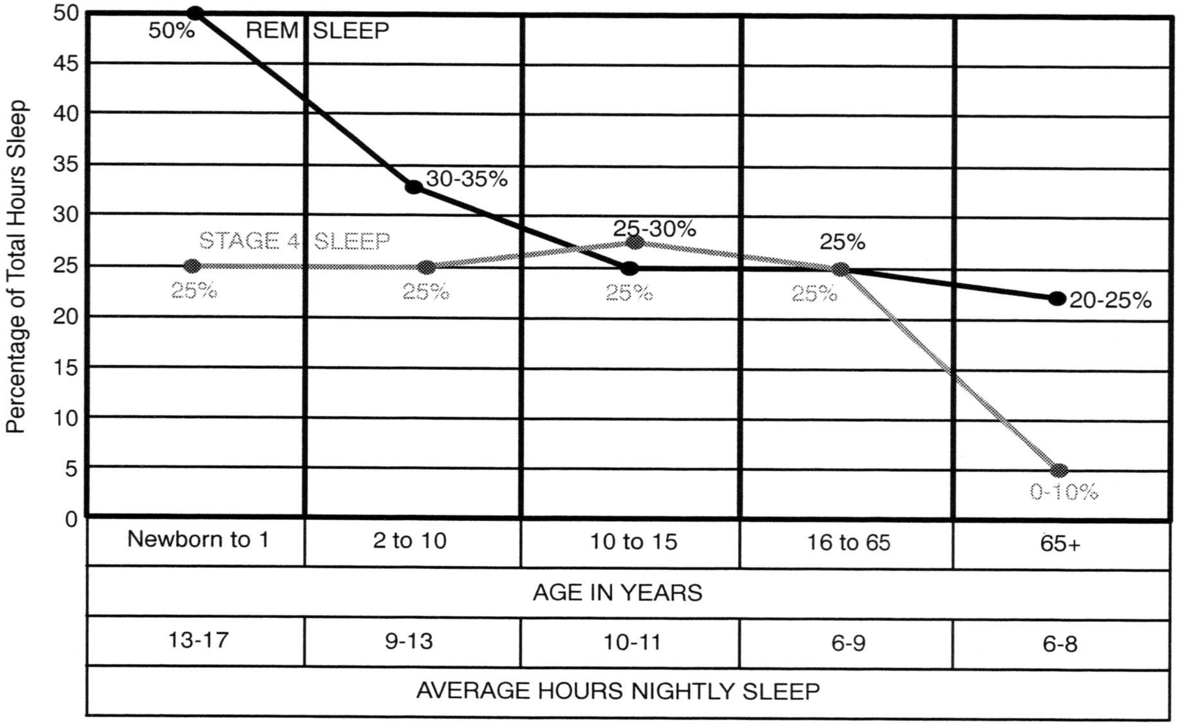

Percentage of Total Hours Sleep

50
45
40
35
30
25
20
15
10
5
0

50% REM SLEEP

30-35%

25-30%

25%

20-25%

STAGE 4 SLEEP

25%
25%
25%
25%
0-10%

Newborn to 1	2 to 10	10 to 15	16 to 65	65+
AGE IN YEARS				
13-17	9-13	10-11	6-9	6-8
AVERAGE HOURS NIGHTLY SLEEP				

stressor, and the sleep disturbance can endure long after the stress has subsided. For example, a person who is raped in a bed may have difficulty sleeping long after integration of the rape trauma. Prolonged sleep disturbance can lead to mood disturbance, decreased attention and concentration, and increased fatigue. The prevalence of this disorder is illustrated by the estimate that 30 to 40 percent of people suffered from Primary Insomnia during the past year.

Primary Hypersomnia

Primary Hypersomnia is excessive sleepiness for at least one month, with prolonged sleep episodes or with daytime sleep episodes occurring almost daily. For most people, these episodes can range from eight to twelve hours, followed by difficulty awakening. A rare form of this disorder, Kleine-Levin syndrome, results in recurrent, extended eighteen to twenty hours of sleep or staying in bed. Prevalence of Primary Hyperinsomnia in the general population is not known, but 5 to 10 percent of people who seek help for sleep disturbance are diagnosed with Primary Hypersomnia.

Narcolepsy

Narcolepsy is a rare disorder that involves repeated irresistible attacks of refreshing sleep, cataplexy (an immobile position that is constantly maintained), and recurrent intrusions of elements of rapid eye movement (REM) sleep during the transition time between sleep and wakefulness. The sleep episodes are not controlled by the individual and can occur in inappropriate situations that could result in danger, such as while driving a car or cooking. Usually two to six periods of intended and unintended sleep occur per day. Dreaming is frequently reported as part of the episodes. Dream imagery can be present before falling to sleep or after awakening. These pre- and poststates can take the form of mild hallucinations. A significant number of people report "sleep paralysis" before and after the episodes. People have described this state as being awake but unable to move or speak. The presence of cataplexy can be subtle, taking the form of sagging jaw or drooping eyelids, or more dramatic, resulting in the person dropping objects or falling to the ground. Acute psychosocial stressors or acute alterations in the sleep-wake schedule are associated with onset of this disorder in 50 percent of cases.

Breathing-Related Sleep Disorder

Breathing-Related Sleep Disorder has as its essential feature excessive sleepiness or insomnia that is considered to be due to abnormalities of ventilation during sleep. Three forms of Breathing-Related Sleep Disorder have been identified: obstructive sleep apnea syndrome, central sleep apnea syndrome, and central alveolar hypoventilation syndrome (see p. 568 of the DSM-IV for detailed descriptions of these syndromes). Excessive sleepiness is the most common presenting symptom of this disorder. In extreme forms of excessive sleepiness, the person complains of falling asleep during normal everyday activities. Naps usually are not refreshing, and the person complains of dull headache on awakening. The person often experiences nighttime chest discomfort, choking, suffocation, anxiety, and violent body movements and can suffer from memory disturbance, poor concentration, irritability, and personality change. The condition is more common in obese, aging males with mild hypertension. The onset is insidious, with gradual progression and chronicity. Note that for this disorder, also code the sleep-related breathing disorder on Axis III (p. 573).

Tip: Breathing-Related Sleep Disorder, although not considered a mental disorder, is included in the DSM-IV because of its importance to doing differential diagnosis of insomnia and hypersomnia and its clinical significance (Frances, First, and Pincus, 1995). This can be a medically significant disorder. When a person meets the criteria for this disorder in a mental health setting, the person should be referred for medical evaluation.

Circadian Rhythm Sleep Disorder

Circadian Rhythm Sleep Disorder (formerly Sleep-Wake Schedule Disorder) is a persistent or recurrent sleep disruption that occurs as a result of a conflict between the individual's internal circadian sleep-wake system and external demands regarding the timing and duration of sleep. The disorder does not arise essentially from the mechanisms that generate sleep or wakefulness. People with this disorder can have difficulty awakening, confusion and inappropriate behavior associated with the disorder, as well as excessive use of alcohol, substances, and medications to combat the problem. This disorder has the following four subtypes:

> **Delayed Sleep Phase Type.** This subtype results from an internal sleep-wake cycle delayed relative to the demands of society. People with this subtype sleep into daylight hours and cannot adjust to daytime schedules because of the delayed sleep cycle. This subtype has been found to be associated with schizoid, schizotypal, and avoidant personality features, especially in adolescents.

Jet Lag Type. This subtype relates to people with normal sleep-wake cycles, but disturbance arises when the person is required to adjust to a new time zone. Adjustment to time zones is more difficult when traveling eastward than when going westward.

Shift Work Type. This subtype is associated with sleep disturbance in normal sleep-wake cycles caused by the necessity to work evening, night, or rotating shifts. Rotating shift work produces the most disturbance in sleep.

Unspecified Type. This subtype is indicated if another circadian sleep disturbance is present, such as advanced sleep phase (the opposite of Delayed Sleep Phase Type), non-twenty-four-hour sleep-wake pattern (following a twenty-four- to twenty-five-hour circadian rhythm sleep pattern rather than a twenty-four-hour pattern with progressive delay of the sleep-wake pattern in relation to the twenty-four-hour clock), or an irregular sleep-wake pattern (absence of an identifiable sleep-wake pattern).

Dyssomnia NOS

Dyssomnia NOS is used for insomnias and hypersomnias or circadian rhythm disturbances that do not meet the criteria for a specific Dyssomnia. This can include disturbance related to environmental factors, such as noise, light, and frequent interruptions; excessive sleepiness due to sleep deprivation; unusual "restless leg syndrome"; unusual periodic limb movements ("nocturnal myoclonus"); and when a Dyssomnia is present but it cannot be determined if it is primary, due to a GMC, or substance induced.

Primary Sleep Disorders: Parasomnias

Nightmare Disorder

Nightmare Disorder (formerly Dream Anxiety Disorder) is the repeated experience of frightening dreams that lead to awakening from sleep. The nightmares usually occur in a lengthy, elaborate dream sequence that is anxiety producing and terrifying. Nightmares after traumatic events may reflect aspects of the original event, but the actual events of the trauma are not relived. The person becomes fully alert upon awakening and can remember the content of the nightmare. The nightmare usually ceases upon awakening, with a residual sense of anxiety. The significance attributed to nightmares can vary in different cultures. Nightmares in childhood can be common, and this diagnosis should not be used with children unless the occurrence is persistent and requires clinical intervention. Clinically significant nightmares in children are usually associated with psychosocial stressors.

Sleep Terror Disorder

Sleep Terror Disorder is characterized by the repeated occurrence of sleep terrors that are an abrupt awakening from sleep frequently preceded by a panicked scream or cry. Sleep terrors normally begin during the first third of the major sleep period and last one to ten minutes. The sleep terror is accompanied by autonomic arousal and signs of intense fear. During the episode, the person frequently sits up abruptly in bed and screams, yells, or cries. The person may experience racing heart, rapid breathing, flushing of the skin, sweating, pupil dilation, and increased muscle tone. The person is difficult to awaken or comfort. If the person awakens after the episode, he or she has no memory of the terror or the images involved and shows resistance to being touched or comforted. The individual usually returns to sleep after the episode. When the person awakens the following morning, he or she does not have any memory of the event. Usually, only one episode occurs per night. The episodes can be embarrassing, and people often avoid situations in which others may observe the episodes. Children with this disorder do not have a higher incidence of psychopathology than the general population, but in adults, an association between this disorder and psychopathology is more likely.

Sleepwalking Disorder

Sleepwalking Disorder involves repeated episodes of complex motor behavior during sleep that includes leaving bed and walking about. This disorder occurs most often during the first third of the sleep period. During an episode the person exhibits reduced alertness, a blank stare, and unresponsiveness. If awakened, the person has limited recall of the event, and this usually is true upon awakening the following morning. The person may experience a brief period of confusion and disorientation after awakening from the episode, but normal awareness returns rapidly. Some people wake the following morning in a different location or recognize the results of activity during the night but have no memory of the events. The person may talk or respond to others during the episode, but genuine dialogue is rare. Sleepwalking is common in children (10 to 20 percent have had at least one episode), but it usually does not reach the level of clinical significance.

Parasomnia NOS

Parasomnia NOS is reserved for disturbances that involve abnormal behavioral or physiological events during sleep or sleep-wake transitions, but do not meet the criteria for a specific Parasomnia. Some examples are REM sleep behavior disorder in the form of motor activity that arises during sleep and can be violent; sleep paralysis, which is an inability to perform voluntary movement during the period from sleep to wakefulness; and when a Parasomnia is present, but the clinician is unable to establish whether it is primary, due to a GMC, or substance induced.

Sleep Disorders Related to Another Mental Disorder

Insomnia Related to Another Mental Disorder

Insomnia Related to Another Mental Disorder is the presence of insomnia when another mental disorder is present and clinical judgment has been used to determine that the insomnia is temporally and causally related to that mental disorder. The diagnostic statement begins with the sleep disturbance type followed by the specific Axis I or Axis II mental disorder to which the insomnia is related, for example, *307.42 Insomnia Related to Dysthymic Disorder.*

Hypersomnia Related to Another Mental Disorder

Hypersomnia Related to another Mental Disorder is the coexistence of hypersomnia with another mental disorder that clinical judgment has determined to be temporally and causally related to the hypersomnia. The diagnostic statement begins with the sleep disturbance type, followed by the specific Axis I or Axis II mental disorder to which the hypersomnia is related, for example, *307.44 Hypersomnia Related to Major Depressive Disorder.*

Other Sleep Disorders

Sleep Disorder Due to a General Medical Condition

Sleep Disorder due to a GMC results when sleep disturbance is sufficient to require clinical attention and has been found to be the direct physiological consequence of a GMC. The symptoms can consist of insomnia, hypersomnia, a Parasomnia, or any combination of these. The GMC must be confirmed in making this diagnosis. This disorder has four subtypes with "subcodes" (entered as the fourth and fifth digits) that must be supplied by the clinician when making this diagnosis:

.52 Insomnia Type. This subtype is used when difficulty falling asleep, problems maintaining sleep, or a feeling of nonrestorative sleep are present.
.54 Hypersomnia Type. This subtype refers to complaints of excessive nocturnal sleep periods or excessive sleep periods during waking hours.
.59 Parasomnia Type. This subtype is used when abnormal behavioral events occur in relation to sleep or sleep transitions.
.59 Mixed Type. When the sleep problem is attributed to a GMC, and multiple sleep symptoms exist, this subtype is used.

This disorder is recorded by coding the sleep disorder on Axis I and then listing the GMC. The GMC is also recorded on Axis III. For example, on Axis I the clinician would record *780.52 Sleep Disorder Due to Arthritis, rheumatoid, Insomnia Type,* and on Axis III, *714.0 Arthritis, rheumatoid, as reported by Dr. R. U. Wright.*

Substance-Induced Sleep Disorder

Substance-Induced Sleep Disorder is diagnosed when a sleep disturbance is sufficient to require clinical attention and has been found to be the direct physiological consequence of a substance, alcohol, medication, or toxin. The symptoms can consist of insomnia, hypersomnia, a Parasomnia, or any combination of these. Insomnia and hypersomnia are common in this disorder, and Parasomnias are less common. Substance intoxication or withdrawal must be confirmed in making this diagnosis.

This disorder has the same four subtypes, with the same characteristics as Sleep Disorder Due to a GMC, although for Substance-Induced Sleep Disorder, these subtypes are not assigned numeric codes. The disorder is recorded using substance-specific codes (see diagnostic dialogue box on p. 607). This disorder also has the following two specifiers related to intoxication and withdrawal:

With Onset During Intoxication. Use this subtype when the onset of symptoms is during the intoxication phase.
With Onset During Withdrawal. Use this subtype when the criteria for withdrawal are met and the onset of symptoms is during or shortly after a withdrawal syndrome.

This disorder is recorded by entering the substance that is associated with the sleep disturbance, followed by the subtype, for example, *291.8 Alcohol-Induced Sleep Disorder, Insomnia Type, With Onset During Intoxication.* When more than one substance is judged to contribute to the sleep disturbance, each is listed as a separate diagnosis.

To better understand the complexity of sleep disturbance in relation to specific substances, see pages 603-605 of the DSM-IV for a summary of the types of sleep disturbance for each class of substances. Visual 17.6 provides a summary of sleep disturbances and the substance classes discussed in the DSM-IV.

VISUAL 17.6. Classes of Substances and Related Sleep Disturbances

Substance	Intoxication				Withdrawal			
	Insomnia	Hypersomnia	BRSD	Parasomnia	Insomnia	Hypersomnia	BRSD	Parasomnia
Alcohol	High	No Data	Moderate	No Data	High	No Data	No Data	No Data
Amphetamines	High	No Data	No Data	No Data	No Data	High	No Data	No Data
Caffeine	High	No Data	No Data	No Data	High	Moderate	No Data	No Data
Cocaine	High	No Data	No Data	No Data	No Data	High	No Data	No Data
Opioids	Moderate	High	No Data	No Data	No Data	High	No Data	No Data
Sedatives Hypnotics Anxiolytics	Moderate	High	Mild	No Data	High	Moderate	No Data	No Data

Symbols: High Occurrence; Moderate Occurrence; Mild Occurrence; No Data Reported ●

BRSD=Breathing-Related Sleep Disorder

Source: American Psychiatric Association, 1994, pp. 603-605.

DIFFERENTIAL DIAGNOSIS

Differential diagnosis is mostly within the sleep disorders' class, with much overlap among the different types of sleep disorders, and is particularly important in this class of disorders. Other disorders to be alert to are Mood Disorders, Anxiety Disorders, Malingering, and delirium.

RECOMMENDED STANDARDIZED MEASURES

- Sleep History Questionnaire

RECOMMENDED READING

Reite, M., Ruddy, J., and Nagel, K. (1997). *Concise Guide to Evaluation and Management of Sleep Disorders,* Second Edition. Washington, DC: American Psychiatric Press.

REFERENCES

American Psychiatric Association (1994). *Diagnostic and Statistical Manual of Mental Disorders,* Fourth Edition. Washington, DC: American Psychiatric Association.

Frances, A., First, M. B., and Pincus, H. N. (1995). *DSM-IV Guidebook: The Essential Companion to the* Diagnostic and Statistical Manual of Mental Disorders. Washington, DC: American Psychiatric Association.

Kaplan, H. I. and Sadock, B. J. (1998). *Synopsis of Psychiatry: Behavioral Sciences/Clinical Psychiatry,* Eighth Edition. Baltimore, MD: Williams and Wilkins.

Chapter 18

Impulse-Control Disorders Not Elsewhere Classified

DISORDERS

312.34	Intermittent Explosive Disorder
312.32	Kleptomania
312.33	Pyromania
312.31	Pathological Gambling
312.39	Trichotillomania
312.30	Impulse-Control Disorder NOS

FUNDAMENTAL FEATURES

This section covers impulse-control disorders that are not classified with other DSM-IV disorders that feature impulse control. Other sections of the DSM-IV that have disorders with impulse-control features are Substance-Related Disorders, Paraphilias, Antisocial Personality Disorder, Conduct Disorder, Schizophrenia, and Mood Disorders. (See Visual 18.1 for an overview of this class of disorders.)

The basic feature of Impulse-Control Disorders is failure to resist an impulse, drive, or temptation to perform an act that can be harmful to oneself or others.

The disorders in general involve an increased sense of tension or arousal before committing the act, and the person experiences pleasure, gratification, or relief at the time of committing the act. Following the act, the person may or may not experience regret or guilt.

The individual disorders in this class are covered in the following material.

VISUAL 18.1. Impulse-Control Disorders Overview

Fundamental Feature

Section of impulse-control disorders not in other DSM-IV sections. Fundamental feature is failure to resist an impulse, drive, or temptation to perform an act that is harmful to the person or others.

See: Antisocial Personality Disorder, Conduct Disorder, Schizophrenia, Substance-Related Disorders, Mood Disorders, and Paraphilias

312.43 Intermittent Explosive Disorder

Episodes of failure to resist aggressive impulses resulting in serious assault/destruction of property

312.32 Kleptomania

Recurring failure to resist impulses to steal objects not needed for personal use or for their monetary value

312.33 Pyromania

Deliberate, repeated fire setting; tension or affective arousal before the act; fascination, interest, curiosity, or attraction to fire; pleasure, gratification, or relief when setting fires or witnessing/participating in aftermath; fire setting not for economic gain, as part of socio-political ideology, to conceal criminal activity, to express anger or vengeance, to improve living circumstances, as part of delusion or hallucination, or result of impaired judgment (dementia, Mental Retardation, or Substance Intoxication)

312.31 Pathological Gambling

Recurrent maladaptive gambling behavior involving five or more of:

- Gambling preoccupation
- Need to increase gambling to achieve excitement
- Unsuccessful attempt to control gambling
- Restless/irritable when trying to decrease gambling
- Gambling a form of escape or relieving dysphoric mood
- "Chases losses" through increased gambling
- Lies to others about extent of gambling
- Has committed illegal acts to finance gambling
- Jeopardized/lost relationships/career/other opportunities because of gambling
- Relies on others for money to cover financial problems resulting from gambling

312.29 Trichotillomania

Recurrent hair pulling resulting in noticeable hair loss; increasing tension before pulling out hair; pleasure, gratification, or relief when pulling out hair

312.30 Impulse-Control Disorder NOS

Reserved for impulse control symptoms/behavior not meeting criteria for specific Impulse-Control Disorder

Source: American Psychiatric Association, 1994, pp. 609-621. Reprinted with permission from the *Diagnostic and Statistical Manual of Mental Disorders,* Fourth Edition. Copyright 1994 American Psychiatric Association.

Intermittent Explosive Disorder

Intermittent Explosive Disorder is the presence of discrete episodes of failure to resist aggressive impulses that result in serious assaults or destruction of property. A chief criterion based on clinical judgment is that the aggressive behavior is grossly out of proportion to any provocation or precipitating psychosocial stressor. Other DSM-IV disorders that may have precipitated the episode must be ruled out. Disorders that should be ruled out are Antisocial Personality Disorder, Borderline Personality Disorder, a Psychotic Disorder, a Manic Episode, Conduct Disorder, and ADHD. Substance use and GMCs should be ruled out as part of the diagnostic assessment. Cultural features can be present, such as the amok syndrome contained in the Glossary of Culture-Bound Syndromes (Appendix I), which involves episodes of unrestrained violent behavior about which the person claims amnesia after the episode.

Differential Diagnosis includes delirium; dementia; Personality Change Due to a GMC, Aggressive Type; Substance Intoxication; Substance Withdrawal; Oppositional Defiant Disorder; Conduct Disorder; Antisocial Personality Disorder; Borderline Personality Disorder; a Manic Episode; Schizophrenia; and Malingering.

Kleptomania

Kleptomania is the failure to resist recurring impulses to steal items even when the items are not needed for use or for monetary value. The person experiences a rising sense of tension before the theft and feels pleasure, gratification, or relief when committing the theft. The stealing is not done to express anger or vengeance and is not part of a delusion, hallucination, or another mental disorder.

Differential Diagnosis for Kleptomania consists of common shoplifting, Malingering, Antisocial Personality Disorder, Conduct Disorder, a Manic Episode, Schizophrenia, and dementia.

Pyromania

Pyromania involves multiple episodes of deliberate fire setting. The individual experiences tension or affective arousal before the fire setting and has a fascination, interest, curiosity, or attraction related to fire and its situational contexts. The individual frequently likes to watch fires and may set off false fire alarms and derive pleasure from association with fire-fighting personnel and working around fire apparatus. The individual receives pleasure, gratification, or tension release when setting fires, witnessing the effects of fire, or participating in the aftermath of the fire. The diagnosis is not made if the fire setting is done for monetary gain, as part of the activities of a sociopolitical ideology, to conceal criminal activity, to express anger or vengeance, to improve living circumstances, or as part of a delusion or hallucination. The diagnosis is not made if the fire setting is done as part of impaired judgment resulting from dementia, Mental Retardation, or Substance Intoxication. Individuals under the age of eighteen commit approximately 40 percent of fire-setting incidents in the United States. Childhood fire setting is rare and, in adolescence, is usually associated with Conduct Disorder, ADHD, or Adjustment Disorder.

Differential Diagnosis for Pyromania should take into account childhood developmental experimentation, Conduct Disorder, a Manic Episode, Antisocial Personality Disorder, Schizophrenia, dementia, Mental Retardation, or Substance Intoxication.

Pathological Gambling

Pathological Gambling is recurrent maladaptive gambling behavior that interferes with personal, family, or vocational activities. This diagnosis is not made if the gambling behavior occurs as part of a Manic Episode within a Mood Disorder. The person with this disorder is preoccupied with gambling through such activities as constantly thinking of past gambling acts, planning the next gambling activity, or plotting ways to get money to use for gambling. Most people with this disorder gamble more to reach a euphoric state than to get money. People develop a sort of tolerance and must increase the stakes of the gambling to achieve a "high." The gambling behavior cannot be stopped, despite efforts to do so, and efforts to stop produce anxiety. For some people, gambling becomes a way to escape other psychosocial stressors. Many people try to undo their losses by increasing gambling to win them back, and for people with this disorder, the "chase of losses" is a long-term strategy. The gambler often deceives family, friends, employers, and therapists about the extent of the gambling activity. The individual may resort to antisocial behavior to achieve funds to support gambling activity when traditional sources of funds are depleted. This can take the form of forgery, fraud, theft, or embezzlement. The person may have impaired family relationships or career opportunities because of gambling. This disorder can have devastating effects, such as loss of jobs, homes, and other possessions as a result of gambling. The person many cause significant disruption to personal relationships through borrowing money from others to support the gambling activity.

A number of traits and disorders can coexist with this disorder. These people often have distorted thinking, can be highly energetic, restless, easily bored, and competitive. They frequently are overachiever workaholics, with a strong desire for approval, and can be overgenerous. Common coexisting disorders are alcohol and substance disorders, Mood Disorders, ADHD, Narcissistic Personality Disorder, Antisocial Personality Disorder, Borderline Personality Disorder, and certain GMCs (hypertension, peptic ulcer disease, or migraine).

The actual number of people with this disorder is not known but has been estimated at 1 to 3 percent of the adult population. This disorder most likely will become more prevalent as U.S. society puts increasing emphasis on gambling to supplement government revenues, and clinicians should screen for gambling activity in clients.

Differential Diagnosis should include common social gambling, professional gambling, Manic Episode, and Antisocial Personality Disorder.

Trichotillomania

Trichotillomania is the recurrent pulling out of one's hair that produces noticeable hair loss. Body sites of hair pulling can be any part of the body that grows hair. The most common sites are the scalp, eyebrows, and eyelashes. Hair-pulling episodes can occur for brief periods throughout the day or in less frequent sustained periods. Hair pulling can increase during periods of stress, but also during times of relaxation. A sense of tension can precede hair pulling. In some cases, tension does not occur before the hair pulling but can be associated with attempts to resist the urge. This disorder is not diagnosed if the hair pulling is better accounted for by another mental disorder, such as during delusions or hallucinations, or as the result of a GMC. Hair pulling does not usually occur in the presence of others, except for family members, and the person, because of the disorder, may avoid social situations. The person may deny the hair pulling and attempt to conceal damaged body sites. Some people have urges to pull hair from other people. They may pull hair from pets, dolls, and other fibrous material. Nail biting, scratching, gnawing, and excoriation may be associated with this disorder. Coexisting disorders may be Mood Disorders, Anxiety Disorders, or Mental Retardation.

Differential Diagnosis includes other mental disorders that may include hair pulling: Obsessive-Compulsive Disorder, Stereotypic Movement Disorder, Factitious Disorder With Predominantly Physical Signs and Symptoms, and GMCs.

Impulse-Control Disorder NOS

Impulse-Control Disorder NOS is reserved for impulse-control behaviors that do not meet the criteria for a full-scale disorder in this category or for another mental disorder that has features involving impulse-control behaviors.

RECOMMENDED READING

Kaplan, H. I. and Sadock, B. J. (1998). *Synopsis of Psychiatry: Behavioral Sciences/Clinical Psychiatry,* Eighth Edition. Baltimore, MD: Williams and Wilkins.

REFERENCE

American Psychiatric Association (1994). *Diagnostic and Statistical Manual of Mental Disorders,* Fourth Edition. Washington, DC: American Psychiatric Association.

Chapter 19

Adjustment Disorders

DISORDERS

This class of disorders is coded based on six subtypes rather than discrete disorders.

309.xx Adjustment Disorder
- .0 With Depressed Mood
- .24 With Anxiety
- .28 With Mixed Anxiety and Depressed Mood
- .3 With Disturbance of Conduct
- .4 With Mixed Disturbance of Emotions and Conduct
- .9 Unspecified

FUNDAMENTAL FEATURES

The disorders in this section are defined by clinically significant emotional or behavioral symptoms in response to an identifiable psychosocial stressor or stressors. The symptoms in this class of disorders are designed to capture symptoms that are subthreshold for other DSM-IV disorders (mainly Mood and Anxiety Disorders), making this class of disorders a "residual category." This class is also unique in that it is one of the few classes of disorders in the DSM-IV that is diagnosed based on a presumed etiology of an identified stressor (Frances, First, and Pincus, 1995). Life is full of stresses, and the clinician must ensure that an adequate threshold of impairment and distress exists to assign an Adjustment Disorder diagnosis. Therefore, differential diagnosis is important whenever considering use of this class of disorders. The clinician should always review for the possibility that the person may meet the criteria for another DSM-IV disorder and consider whether the reaction to the stressor is out of proportion to the usual reaction to such a stressor. Also, the clinician should review for possible **Bereavement,** which is a reaction to the death of a loved one involving symptoms of a depressive disorder. This condition is in the section "Other Condition That May Be a Focus of Clinical Attention" (pp. 684-685) (for a criteria overview, see Visual 19.1). Symptoms must occur within three months after the onset of the stressor(s) and not persist more than six months after the stressor or its consequences have ended. Coding is based on subtypes selected according to predominant symptoms:

> **With Depressed Mood.** This subtype is used when the symptom presentation includes depressed mood, tearfulness, or feelings of hopelessness.
>
> **With Anxiety.** This subtype is used when the symptoms include nervousness, worry, or jitteriness. In children, fears of separation from attachment figures can be present.
>
> **With Mixed Anxiety and Depressed Mood.** This subtype is used when the presentation includes a combination of depression and anxiety.
>
> **With Disturbance of Conduct.** This subtype is used when the disturbance of conduct includes violation of others' rights or violation of age-appropriate societal norms and rules. Such violations can include truancy, vandalism, reckless driving, fighting, and default on legal responsibilities.
>
> **With Mixed Disturbance of Emotions and Conduct.** This subtype is diagnosed when the presentation includes emotional symptoms, such as anxiety and depression, and disturbance of conduct that meets the criteria for the subtype **With Disturbance of Conduct.**
>
> **Unspecified.** This subtype is used when maladaptive reactions, such as physical complaints, social withdrawal, work inhibition, or academic inhibition, are present in relation to psychosocial stressors that cannot be classified as one of the specific Adjustment Disorder subtypes.

The duration of Adjustment Disorder symptoms can be indicated by the following specifiers:

> **Acute.** This specifier is used if the symptoms persist for less than six months.

VISUAL 19.1. Adjustment Disorders Criteria Overview

Fundamental Feature

Clinically significant emotional or behavioral symptoms in response to an identifiable psychosocial stressor or stressors. Symptoms must occur within three months after the onset of the stressor(s).

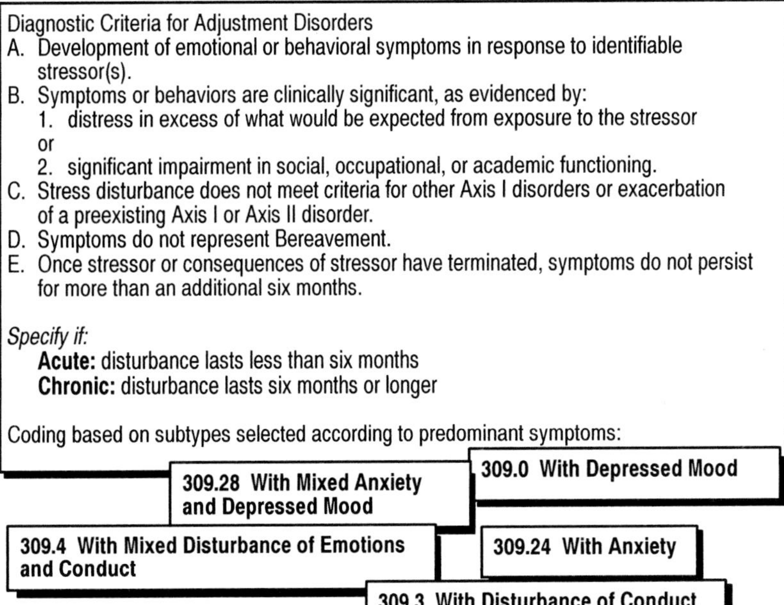

Diagnostic Criteria for Adjustment Disorders

A. Development of emotional or behavioral symptoms in response to identifiable stressor(s).
B. Symptoms or behaviors are clinically significant, as evidenced by:
   1. distress in excess of what would be expected from exposure to the stressor
   or
   2. significant impairment in social, occupational, or academic functioning.
C. Stress disturbance does not meet criteria for other Axis I disorders or exacerbation of a preexisting Axis I or Axis II disorder.
D. Symptoms do not represent Bereavement.
E. Once stressor or consequences of stressor have terminated, symptoms do not persist for more than an additional six months.

Specify if:
Acute: disturbance lasts less than six months
Chronic: disturbance lasts six months or longer

Coding based on subtypes selected according to predominant symptoms:

309.28 With Mixed Anxiety and Depressed Mood

309.0 With Depressed Mood

309.4 With Mixed Disturbance of Emotions and Conduct

309.24 With Anxiety

309.3 With Disturbance of Conduct

309.9 Unspecified

Differential Diagnosis:
Personality Disorders
PTSD and Acute Stress Disorder (require stressor)
Psychological Factors Affecting Medical Condition
Bereavement
Nonpathological reactions to stress

Source: American Psychiatric Association, 1994, pp. 623-627. Reprinted with permission from the *Diagnostic and Statistical Manual of Mental Disorders,* Fourth Edition. Copyright 1994 American Psychiatric Association.

Chronic. This specifier is used if the symptoms persist for more than six months. The symptoms for this disorder cannot persist for more than six months after the termination of the stressor or its consequences. The Chronic specifier is applied to the disorder when the duration of the disturbance is longer than six months in response to a chronic stressor or to a stressor that has enduring consequences.

DIFFERENTIAL DIAGNOSIS

As mentioned earlier, differential diagnosis is important in Adjustment Disorders. The key disorders to consider are Personality Disorders, PTSD and Acute Stress Disorder (require stressor), Psychological Factors Affecting Medical Condition, Bereavement, and nonpathological reactions to stress.

RECOMMENDED READING

Kaplan, H. I. and Sadock, B. J. (1998). *Synopsis of Psychiatry Behavioral Science/Clinical Psychiatry,* Eighth Edition. Baltimore, MD: Williams and Wilkins.

REFERENCES

American Psychiatric Association (1994). *Diagnostic and Statistical Manual of Mental Disorders,* Fourth Edition. Washington, DC: American Psychiatric Association.

Frances, A., First, M. B., and Pincus, H. N. (1995). *DSM-IV Guidebook: The Essential Companion to the* Diagnostic and Statistical Manual of Mental Disorders. Washington, DC: American Psychiatric Association.

Chapter 20

Personality Disorders

DISORDERS

Cluster A
- 301.0 Paranoid Personality Disorder
- 301.20 Schizoid Personality Disorder
- 301.22 Schizotypal Personality Disorder

Cluster B
- 301.7 Antisocial Personality Disorder
- 301.83 Borderline Personality Disorder
- 301.50 Histrionic Personality Disorder
- 301.81 Narcissistic Personality Disorder

Cluster C
- 301.82 Avoidant Personality Disorder
- 301.6 Dependent Personality Disorder
- 301.4 Obsessive-Compulsive Personality Disorder
- 301.9 Personality Disorder NOS

FUNDAMENTAL FEATURES

The Personality Disorders section includes ten dysfunctional personality types. The first portion of this section of the DSM-IV defines the general criteria for all Personality Disorders and then covers the specific criteria for each Personality Disorder. The disorders are clustered into three types, based on descriptive similarities (1) Cluster A: the odd and eccentric; (2) Cluster B: dramatic, emotional, and erratic behavior; and (3) Cluster C: the anxious and fearful (see Visual 20.1 for an overview of this class).

The most fundamental feature of the Personality Disorders is an enduring pattern of inner experience and behavior that deviates markedly from

VISUAL 20.1. Personality Disorders Overview

Fundamental Features and General Symptoms

A Personality Disorder is an enduring pattern of inner experience and behavior that deviates markedly from the expectations of the individual's culture, is pervasive and inflexible, has an onset in adolescence or early adulthood, is stable over time, and leads to distress or impairment.

The pattern of behavior is manifested in 2+ areas:

1. Cognition
2. Affectivity
3. Interpersonal functioning
4. Impulse control

Coded on Axis II

Controversial and Poorly Validated Clusters

Adolescent/Early Adult Onset
Diagnosed in Adults
Diagnosed in children/adolescents rarely and one year after symptom/behavior onset
Antisocial Personality Dx. only after 18.

Cluster A

Organized on the basis of odd and eccentric behavior

301.00 Paranoid
301.20 Schizoid
301.22 Schizotypal

Cluster B

Organized on the basis of dramatic, emotional, or erratic behavior

301.7 Antisocial
301.83 Borderline
301.50 Histrionic
301.81 Narcissistic

Cluster C

Organized on the basis of behaviors associated with fear and anxiety

301.82 Avoidant
301.60 Dependent
301.40 Obsessive-Compulsive
301.90 PD NOS

In Appendix B . . . For Further Study

depressive personality disorder
Pervasive pattern of depressive cognitions and behavior that begins by early adulthood and occurs in a variety of contexts.

passive-aggressive personality disorder
Pervasive pattern of negative attitudes and passive resistance to demands for adequate performance in social and occupational situations that begins by early adulthood.

R/O

Substances and GMCs. If symptoms existed prior to GMC/substance use, PD can be diagnosed.

Source: American Psychiatric Association, 1994, pp. 629-673.

the expectations of the person's culture. The person's personality dysfunction is pervasive and inflexible. Onset occurs in adolescence or young adulthood, and the disorder is stable over time, leading to distress and impairment. Because of the insidious and enduring nature of Personality Disorders, they are diagnosed on Axis II, and a person can receive more than one Personality Disorder diagnosis.

The Personality Disorders are one of the more controversial sections of the DSM-IV. Much research on Personality Disorders has been done recently, but it has produced no conclusive results about the clustering of Personality Disorders into three typologies, although some bizarre explanations of the historical basis of personality types have been offered (see Chapter 2). One topic of debate is whether personalities can be typed or should be measured through a dimensional approach. In the DSM-IV, the more common historical categorical approach has been continued. The Personality Disorders are also highly culture-bound, in that what is considered deviant in one culture can be expected behavior in another. Assessing personality is a complex task and requires a lengthy evaluation process. Diagnosis of a Personality Disorder can have serious lasting consequences for an individual. For these reasons, a Personality Disorder should only be diagnosed after a thorough evaluation, standardized testing, and a thorough differential diagnosis. In addition, a person must meet the general criteria of Personality Disorder before being diagnosed with a specific type.

Personality Disorders are rarely diagnosed in children because of the long-term enduring nature of the behaviors and symptoms required to diagnose these disorders. If a child is given a Personality Disorder diagnosis, the symptoms and behaviors must be present for at least one year. Antisocial Personality Disorder is never diagnosed in a person under eighteen years of age. A person under age eighteen with the symptoms of Antisocial Personality Disorder should be given a diagnosis of Conduct Disorder. Worthy of note here is that a person over eighteen years of age who is diagnosed with Antisocial Personality Disorder must have given evidence of Conduct Disorder behavior before age fifteen.

The general criteria for a Personality Disorder are listed in Visual 20.2. The specific criteria for each Personality Disorder in this class are discussed in the following material (see also Visuals 20.3, 20.4, and 20.5).

Cluster A Personality Disorders

Paranoid Personality Disorder

In this disorder, the person exhibits pervasive distrust and suspiciousness and four or more of the following characteristics: (1) feels exploited, harmed,

VISUAL 20.2. General Criteria for a Personality Disorder

A. An enduring pattern of inner experience and behavior that deviates markedly from the expectations of the person's culture. The person's personality dysfunction is pervasive and inflexible. The onset is in adolescence or young adulthood, and the disorder is stable over time, leading to distress and impairment. The pattern is evident in two or more of the following areas:

   1. Cognition is impaired, which can include distorted ways of perceiving self, others, and events.
   2. Affectivity can be dysfunctional, taking the form of abnormal range, intensity, lability, and appropriateness of emotional responses.
   3. Impaired and distressful interpersonal functioning.
   4. Poor impulse control.

B. The enduring pattern of dysfunction is inflexible and pervasive in a large number of personal and social situations.

C. The enduring pattern leads to clinically significant distress or impairment in social, occupational, or other areas of functioning.

D. The enduring pattern is stable over a long time period, and the onset can be established to have occurred in adolescence or early adulthood.

E. The enduring pattern of dysfunction is not better accounted for by another mental disorder.

F. The enduring dysfunctional pattern is not due to the direct physiological effects of a substance or a GMC.

Source: American Psychiatric Association, 1994, p. 633. Reprinted with permission from the *Diagnostic and Statistical Manual of Mental Disorders,* Fourth Edition. Copyright 1994 American Psychiatric Association.

or deceived by others without justification; (2) preoccupied with unjustified doubt about others' loyalty; (3) will not confide in others for fear information will be used to harm him or her; (4) reads hidden meaning into benign remarks; (5) persistently holds grudges; (6) perceives attacks on reputation or character that are not apparent to others; (7) has recurring doubts, without justification, about fidelity of spouse or others. The symptoms do not occur exclusively during the course of Schizophrenia, Mood Disorder With Psychotic Features, or a GMC.

Schizoid Personality Disorder

The person has detached social relationships and a restricted range of emotional expression with four or more of the following symptoms: (1) does

VISUAL 20.3. Cluster A Personality Disorders Criteria Summary

Cluster A: Odd or Eccentric Features

301.0 Paranoid PD

A. Pervasive distrust and suspiciousness, and 4+: (1) feels exploited, (2) doubts others' loyalty, (3) will not confide in others, (4) reads meaning into remarks, (5) holds grudges, (6) perceives attacks on reputation, (7) doubts fidelity of spouse/others

B. Not due to Schizophrenia, Mood Disorder, or a GMC

301.20 Schizoid PD

A. Detached social relations, restricted emotions, and 4+: (1) no desire for close relationships, (2) chooses solitary activities, (3) no sexual interests, (4) no pleasure from activities, (5) no close friends except relatives, (6) indifferent to praise and criticism, emotional coldness, detachment, flat affect

B. Not due to Schizophrenia, Mood Disorder, PDD, or a GMC

301.22 Schizotypal PD

A. Interpersonal deficits, no close relationships, cognitive/perceptual distortions, eccentric behavior, and 5+: (1) ideas of reference (excluding delusions), (2) odd beliefs/magical thinking, (3) unusual perceptions, (4) odd thinking and speech, (5) paranoid ideation, (6) inappropriate/constricted affect, (7) odd behavior/appearance, (8) no close friends, (9) excessive social anxiety

B. Not due to Schizophrenia, Mood Disorder, or PDD

Source: American Psychiatric Association, 1994, pp. 634-645. Reprinted with permission from the *Diagnostic and Statistical Manual of Mental Disorders,* Fourth Edition.

VISUAL 20.4. Cluster B Personality Disorders Criteria Summary

Fundamental Feature

Cluster B: Dramatic, Emotional, or Erratic Features

301.7 Antisocial PD

A. Violation of others' rights after age 15, and 3+: (1) nonconformity to norms and laws, (2) deceitfulness, (3) impulsivity, (4) irritability and aggressiveness, (5) disregard for safety of self and others, (6) irresponsibility in work and finances, (7) lack of remorse

B. Must be age 18

C. Conduct disorder before age 15

D. Not due to Schizophrenia or Manic Episode

301.83 Borderline PD

A. Unstable interpersonal relationships, self-image, and affects, and 5+: (1) frantic avoidance of abandonment (excluding suicidal or self-mutilating behavior), (2) unstable and intense relationships with extremes of idealization and devaluation, (3) unstable self-image or sense of self, (4) impulsivity (spending, sex, drugs, driving, eating) (exclude suicidal and self-mutilating behavior), (5) suicidal and self-mutilating behavior, (6) affective instability due to reactivity of mood, (7) chronic feelings of emptiness, (8) innappropriate anger, (9) paranoid/dissociative symptoms

301.50 Histrionic PD

A. Excessive emotionality and attention seeking, and 5+: (1) uncomfortable when not center of attention, (2) sexually seductive or provocative behavior, (3) shifting and shallow emotions, (4) uses physical appearance to draw attention, (5) impressionistic speaking style that lacks detail, (6) theatrical expression of emotion, (7) suggestible, (8) views relationships as more intimate than is realistic

301.81 Narcissistic PD

A. Pattern of grandiosity, need for admiration, and lack of empathy, and 5+: (1) grandiose sense of self-importance, expecting to be recognized as superior, (2) fantasies of unlimited success, power, brilliance, beauty, or ideal love, (3) believes he/she is "special" and should only associate with high-status people, (4) requires excessive admiration, (5) sense of entitlement, (6) interpersonally exploitive, (7) lacks empathy, (8) envious of others or believes others envious, (9) arrogant behaviors or attitudes

Source: American Psychiatric Association, 1994, pp. 645-661. Reprinted with permission from the *Diagnostic and Statistical Manual of Mental Disorders,* Fourth Edition.

VISUAL 20.5. Cluster C Personality Disorders Criteria Summary

Fundamental Feature

Cluster C: Anxious and Fearful Features

301.82 Avoidant PD

A. Social inhibition, inadequacy, hypersensitivity to negative evaluation, and 4+: (1) avoids occupational interpersonal activity, (2) gets involved with others only when certain of being liked, (3) restraint in intimate relationships, (4) preoccupied with possible criticism, (5) inhibited in new situations, (6) views self as socially inept, (7) reluctant to take personal risks

301.6 Dependent PD

A. Excessive need to be taken care of that leads to submissive and clinging behavior, and 5+: (1) difficulty making common decisions, (2) needs others to assume responsibility for major areas of life, (3) difficulty expressing disagreement with others, (4) difficulty initiating projects, (5) excessive efforts to get nurturance, (6) feels helpless when alone, (7) seeks constant relationships as source of care and support, (8) unrealistic fears of being left to care for self

301.4 Obsessive-Compulsive PD

A. Preoccupation with orderliness, perfectionism, and mental and interpersonal control at expense of flexibility, openness, and efficiency, and 4+: (1) irrational preoccupation with details, rules, lists, orders, organization, or schedules, (2) perfectionism that thwarts task completion, (3) excessively devoted to work, (4) overconscientious about morals and ethics, (5) cannot discard old and worthless objects, (6) reluctant to delegate tasks, (7) miserly spending style, (8) rigidity and stubbornness

301.9 Personality Disorder NOS

A. Does not meet criteria for specific PD or has a "Mixed" PD or has a PD provided for further study (e.g., depressive PD or passive-aggressive PD, pp. 732-733)

Source: American Psychiatric Association, 1994, pp. 662-673. Reprinted with permission from the *Diagnostic and Statistical Manual of Mental Disorders,* Fourth Edition. Copyright 1994 American Psychiatric Association.

not desire or enjoy close relationships, including family; (2) chooses solitary activities; (3) little or no sexual interest in others; (4) derives little pleasure from activities; (5) no close friends except close relatives; (6) appears indifferent to praise and criticism of others; and (7) shows emotional coldness, detachment, and flat affect. The symptoms are not due to Schizophrenia, Mood Disorder With Psychotic Features, PDD, or a GMC.

Schizotypal Personality Disorder

This type has social and interpersonal deficits, marked by acute discomfort, and diminished capacity for close relationships. Cognitive and perceptual distortions are common, as well as eccentric behavior and five or more of the following symptoms: (1) ideas of reference (excluding delusions); (2) odd beliefs or magical thinking that influences behavior; (3) unusual perceptual experiences; (4) odd thinking and speech; (5) suspiciousness or paranoid ideation; (6) inappropriate or constricted affect; (7) odd behavior or appearance that is considered eccentric or peculiar; (8) no close friends other than close relatives; and (9) excessive social anxiety that does not diminish with familiarity and tends to be associated with paranoid fears rather than negative self-judgment. The disorder is not due to Schizophrenia, Mood Disorder With Psychotic Features, another Psychotic Disorder, or PDD.

Cluster B Personality Disorders

Antisocial Personality Disorder

The person with this disorder has a pervasive pattern of disregard or violation of others' rights, occurring since age fifteen, and three or more of the following symptoms: (1) nonconformity to norms and laws by repeatedly committing acts that are grounds for arrest; (2) deceitfulness, as indicated by repeated lying, use of aliases, or conning others for profit or pleasure; (3) impulsivity or failure to plan ahead; (4) irritability and aggressiveness in the form of repeated fights or assaults; (5) reckless disregard for safety of self and others; (6) consistent irresponsibility in employment and finances; and (7) lack of remorse, as indicated by being indifferent to or rationalizing having hurt, mistreated, or stolen from another person. The person must be at least age eighteen and must have shown evidence of Conduct Disorder before age fifteen (see p. 90). The disorder is not due to Schizophrenia or a Manic Episode.

Borderline Personality Disorder

The person has a pattern of instability in interpersonal relationships, self-image, and affects, and marked impulsivity that begins by early adulthood and is present in a variety of contexts. The person has five or more of the following symptoms: (1) frantic efforts to avoid real or imagined abandonment (excluding suicidal or self-mutilating behavior); (2) a pattern of unstable and intense relationships with extremes of idealization and devaluation; (3) identity disturbance marked by unstable self-image or sense of self; (4) impulsivity in areas of functioning that can cause self-damage (e.g., spending, sex, drugs, driving, eating; suicidal and self-mutilating behavior are excluded from this symptom criterion); (5) recurrent suicidal and self-mutilating behavior; (6) affective instability due to marked reactivity of mood; (7) chronic feelings of emptiness; (8) inappropriate intense anger or difficulty controlling anger; and (9) transient, stress-related paranoid ideation or severe dissociative symptoms.

Histrionic Personality Disorder

This disorder is characterized by a pattern of excessive emotionality and attention seeking that is present in a variety of contexts, with an onset of early adulthood, and five or more of the following symptoms: (1) uncomfortable when not center of attention; (2) interaction with others involves sexually seductive or provocative behavior; (3) has shifting and shallow emotions; (4) consistently uses physical appearance to draw attention to self; (5) has an impressionistic speaking style that lacks detail; (6) prone to self-dramatization, theatrical, and exaggerated expression of emotion; (7) is suggestible and easily influenced by others and circumstances; and (8) views relationships as more intimate than is realistic.

Narcissistic Personality Disorder

This disorder involves a pervasive pattern of grandiosity (in fantasy or behavior), need for admiration, and lack of empathy, beginning in early adulthood, in a number of settings, and five or more of the following symptoms: (1) has grandiose sense of self-importance, expecting to be recognized as superior without appropriate achievement; (2) is preoccupied with fantasies of unlimited success, power, brilliance, beauty, or ideal love; (3) believes he or she is "special" or unique and should only associate with high-status people or institutions; (4) requires excessive admiration; (5) has a sense of entitlement, such as unreasonable expectation of favorable treatment or others' automatic compliance with his or her expectations; (6) is interpersonally exploitive, taking advantage of others to get needs met; (7) lacks empathy; (8) is often envious of others or believes others are envious of him or her; and (9) has arrogant, haughty behaviors or attitudes.

Cluster C Personality Disorders

Avoidant Personality Disorder

This disorder is a pervasive pattern of social inhibition, feelings of inadequacy, and hypersensitivity to negative evaluation, beginning in early adulthood and occurring in a number of contexts, plus four or more of the following symptoms: (1) avoids occupational activities that involve significant interpersonal activity because of fears of criticism, disapproval, or rejection; (2) is unwilling to get involved with others except when certain of being liked; (3) shows restraint in intimate relationships for fear of being shamed or ridiculed; (4) is preoccupied with possible criticism or rejection in social situations; (5) is inhibited in new interpersonal situations because of feelings of inadequacy; (6) views self as socially inept, personally unappealing, or inferior to others; and (7) is unusually reluctant to take personal risks or to engage in new activities because they may prove embarrassing.

Dependent Personality Disorder

People with this disorder have an excessive need to be taken care of that leads to submissive and clinging behavior and fear of separation, beginning in early adulthood and present in a variety of contexts, with five or more of the following symptoms: (1) has difficulty making common, everyday decisions without excessive advice and reassurance from others; (2) needs others to assume responsibility for most major areas of life; (3) has difficulty expressing disagreement with others because of fear of loss of support or approval (does not include realistic fears of retribution); (4) has difficulty initiating projects or doing things on own initiative because of lack of self-confidence; (5) makes excessive efforts to get nurturance and support from others to the point of volunteering for unpleasant tasks; (6) feels uncomfortable or helpless when alone out of fear the person will not be able to care for self; (7) urgently seeks another relationship as source of care and support when one relationship ends; and (8) has unrealistic fears of, and preoccupation with, being left to care for self.

Obsessive-Compulsive Personality Disorder

The main feature of this disorder is a pattern of preoccupation with orderliness, perfectionism, and mental and interpersonal control at the expense of flexibility, openness, and efficiency, with onset in early adulthood and occurring in a number of contexts, plus four or more of the following symptoms: (1) has an irrational preoccupation with details, rules, lists, orders, organization, or schedules to the extent that the major point of the activity is lost; (2) shows perfectionism that thwarts task completion; (3) is excessively devoted to work and productivity to the exclusion of leisure activity and friendships; (4) is overconscientious, scrupulous, and inflexible about morals, ethics, or values; (5) cannot discard old and worthless objects even when they have no sentimental value; (6) is reluctant to delegate tasks or to work with others unless they submit to exactly what he or she wants done; (7) adopts a miserly spending style toward self and others, with money being hoarded for future misfortune; and (8) shows rigidity and stubbornness.

Personality Disorder NOS

This diagnosis is used if the Personality Disorder symptoms do not meet criteria for a specific Personality Disorder, the person has a "Mixed" Personality Disorder, or the Personality Disorder is one designated for further study (e.g., depressive personality disorder or passive-aggressive personality disorder, pp. 732-733).

DIFFERENTIAL DIAGNOSIS

The differential diagnosis in this class primarily involves other disorders in this class, and some of the other diagnoses are specified in the criteria for individual Personality Disorders. Other common disorders to be aware of are Psychotic Disorders, Schizophrenia, Mood Disorders, Anxiety Disorders, Substance-Related Disorders, and Personality Change Due to a GMC.

RECOMMENDED STANDARDIZED MEASURES

- Adolescent Psychopathology Scale (APS)
- International Personality Disorder Examination (IPDE)

- Millon Index of Personality Styles (MIPS)
- Personality Assessment Inventory (PAI)
- Personality Assessment Screener (PAS)

RECOMMENDED READING

Brown, L. S. and Ballou, M. (1992). *Personality and Psychopathology.* New York: Guilford.

Denburg, E. V. and Choca, J. P. (1997). *Interpretive Guide to the Millon Clinical Multiaxial Inventory.* Washington, DC: American Psychological Association.

Ewen, R. B. (1998). *Personality: A Topical Approach.* Mahwah, NJ: Lawrence Erlbaum Associates.

Millon, T. (1997). *The Millon Inventories: Clinical and Personality Assessment.* New York: Guilford.

Millon, T. and Davis, R. (1995). *Disorders of Personality: DSM-IV and Beyond,* Second Edition. New York: Wiley.

Robinson, D. J. (1999). *Disordered Personalities,* Second Edition. Port Huron, MI: Rapid Psychler Press.

REFERENCE

American Psychiatric Association (1994). *Diagnostic and Statistical Manual of Mental Disorders,* Fourth Edition. Washington, DC: American Psychiatric Association.

Chapter 21

Other Conditions That May Be a Focus of Clinical Attention

CONDITIONS

Psychological Factors Affecting Medical Condition

316 Psychological Factor Affecting Medical Condition
Mental Disorder Affecting . . . (indicate GMC)
Psychological Symptoms Affecting . . . (indicate GMC)
Personality Traits or Coping Style Affecting . . . (indicate GMC)
Maladaptive Health Behaviors Affecting . . . (indicate GMC)
Stress-Related Physiological Response Affecting . . . (indicate GMC)
Other or Unspecified Factors Affecting . . . (indicate GMC)

Medication-Induced Movement Disorders

The criteria for these disorders are in Appendix B, and the research criteria for the disorders are on pages 735-751.

332.1 Neuroleptic-Induced Parkinsonism
333.92 Neuroleptic Malignant Syndrome
333.7 Neuroleptic-Induced Acute Dystonia
333.99 Neuroleptic-Induced Acute Akathisia
333.82 Neuroleptic-Induced Tardive Dyskinesia
333.1 Medication-Induced Postural Tremor
333.90 Medication-Induced Movement Disorder NOS

Other Medication-Induced Disorder

995.2 Adverse Effects of Medication NOS

Relational Problems

V61.9 Relational Problem Related to an MD or a GMC
V61.20 Parent-Child Relational Problem
V61.10 Partner Relational Problem
V61.8 Sibling Relational Problem
V62.81 Relational Problem NOS

Problems Related to Abuse or Neglect

V61.21 Physical Abuse of Child (use code 995.54 if focus is on the victim)
V61.21 Sexual Abuse of Child (use code 995.53 if focus is on the victim)
V61.21 Neglect of Child (use code 995.52 if focus is on victim)
___.__ Physical Abuse of Adult
V61.12 (if by partner)
V62.83 (if by person other than partner) (code 995.81 if focus is on victim)
___.__ Sexual Abuse of Adult
V61.12 (if by partner)
V62.83 (if by person other than partner) (code 995.83 if focus is on victim)

Additional Conditions That May Be a Focus of Clinical Attention

V15.81 Noncompliance With Treatment
V65.2 Malingering
V71.01 Adult Antisocial Behavior
V71.02 Child or Adolescent Antisocial Behavior
V62.89 Borderline Intellectual Functioning
780.9 Age-Related Cognitive Decline
V62.82 Bereavement
V62.3 Academic Problem
V62.2 Occupational Problem
313.82 Identity Problem
V62.89 Religious or Spiritual Problem
V62.4 Acculturation Problem
V62.89 Phase of Life Problem

FUNDAMENTAL FEATURES

In this section, conditions are identified that can be a focus of clinical attention in relation to the major mental disorders in the DSM-IV (see pp. 675-686). The problem can be related to a mental disorder in the following ways:

1. The problem is a focus of treatment, but the person has no mental disorder.
2. The individual has a mental disorder, but it is unrelated to the problem.
3. The individual has a mental disorder related to the problem, but the problem warrants independent clinical attention.

The conditions and problems covered in this section are placed on Axis I, except Borderline Intellectual Functioning, which is recorded on Axis II because of its relationship to Mental Retardation.

There is a tendency to overlook many of these conditions when doing a diagnosis, but these conditions should be considered when conducting evaluations. The conditions described in the following material should be noted as part of the evaluation and entered in the multiaxial diagnosis if they become a focus of clinical attention. These conditions can play a significant role in the course and treatment of a mental disorder. Left undiagnosed and untreated, they can result in failure to relieve the symptoms of many mental disorders. (See Visual 21.1 for an overview of these conditions.)

Psychological Factors Affecting Medical Condition

Psychological Factors Affecting Medical Condition involves the presence of one or more specific psychological or behavioral symptoms that adversely affect a GMC. Psychological factors are present in most GMCs, but to assign this condition on Axis I, the psychological factor must have a significant impact on the GMC or affect the outcome of the GMC. The psychological factors that can influence a GMC are as follows:

- Axis I disorders
- Axis II disorders
- Psychological symptoms
- Personality traits that do not meet the full criteria for a specific mental disorder
- Maladaptive health behaviors
- Physiological responses to environmental or social stressors

VISUAL 21.1. Other Conditions That May Be a Focus of Clinical Attention Overview

PSYCHOLOGICAL FACTORS AFFECTING MEDICAL CONDITION

316 Psychological Factor Affecting Medical Condition

MEDICATION-INDUCED MOVEMENT DISORDERS

332.1 Neuroleptic-Induced Parkinsonism
333.92 Neuroleptic Malignant Syndrome
333.7 Neuroleptic-Induced Acute Dystonia
333.99 Neuroleptic-Induced Acute Akathisia
333.82 Neuroleptic-Induced Tardive Dyskinesia
333.1 Medication-Induced Postural Tremor
333.90 Medication-Induced Movement Disorder NOS

OTHER MEDICATION-INDUCED DISORDER

995.2 Adverse Effects of Medication NOS

The condition is entered on Axis I (Borderline Intellectual Functioning is entered on Axis II) if it is principal focus of clinical attention for person who may or may not have coexisting mental disorder. If the condition is not principal focus of clinical attention, it is listed on Axis IV.

RELATIONAL PROBLEMS

V61.9 Relational Problem Related to an MD or a GMC
V61.20 Parent-Child Relational Problem
V61.10 Partner Relational Problem
V61.8 Sibling Relational Problem
V62.81 Relational Problem NOS

If condition coexists with mental disorder, it is listed on Axis I when severity level warrants independent clinical attention.

PROBLEMS RELATED TO ABUSE OR NEGLECT

V61.21 Physical Abuse of Child (*Note:* Coded as 995.54 if victim is clinical focus)
V61.21 Sexual Abuse of Child (*Note:* Coded as 995.53 if victim is clinical focus)
V61.21 Neglect of Child (*Note:* Coded as 995.52 if victim is clinical focus)
V61.1 Physical Abuse of Adult (*Note:* Coded as V61.12 if focus of clinical attention is perpetrator and abuse is by partner, V62.83 if focus of clinical attention is perpetrator and abuse is by person other than partner, 995.81 if victim is clinical focus)

ADDITIONAL CONDITIONS THAT MAY BE A FOCUS OF CLINICAL ATTENTION

V15.81 Noncompliance with Treatment (e.g., discomfort, medication side effects, cost, religion, culture, personality traits, PDs)
V65.2 Malingering (e.g., intentional production of symptoms motivated by external inducements, e.g., avoidance of military, work, or to gain financial compensation)
V71.01 Adult Antisocial Behavior (antisocial behavior not due to an MD)
V71.02 Child or Adolescent Antisocial Behavior (antisocial behavior not due to an MD)
V62.89 Borderline Intellectual Functioning (IQ range 71-84) (*Note*: Coded on Axis II)
780.9 Age-Related Cognitive Decline
V62.82 Bereavement
V62.3 Academic Problem
V62.2 Occupational Problem
313.82 Identity Problem
V62.89 Religious or Spiritual Problem
V62.4 Acculturation Problem
V62.89 Phase of Life Problem

Source: American Psychiatric Association, 1994, pp. 675-686.

These factors are recorded by placing the psychological factor on Axis I, followed by the GMC, and the GMC is also listed on Axis III. The following are the categories for listing psychological factors.

Mental Disorder Affecting . . . (Indicate the GMC)

This is an Axis I or Axis II disorder that significantly affects the course or treatment of a GMC. The medical condition is listed on Axis I and on Axis III. Morrison (1995, p. 534) gives a nice example of how to record this condition:

> . . . A man with schizophrenia hears voices that tell him to refuse dialysis for his kidney disease. This would be coded as follows:
>
> | | | |
> |---|---|---|
> | Axis I: | 295.30 | Schizophrenia, Paranoid Type, Continuous |
> | Axis II: | 316 | Mental Disorder Affecting Renal Disease |
> | Axis III: | 585 | Chronic Renal Failure |

Psychological Symptom Affecting . . . (Indicate the GMC)

This involves symptoms that do not meet the full criteria for an Axis I mental disorder but significantly affect the course or treatment of a GMC.

Personality Traits or Coping Style Affecting . . . (Indicate the GMC)

This relates to a personality trait or maladaptive coping style that significantly affects course or treatment of a GMC. Personality traits can be subthreshold for an Axis II diagnosis or represent another pattern of behavior or symptoms that places the person at risk for certain illnesses. An example of this would be the person who is considered "type A" personality.

Maladaptive Health Behaviors Affecting . . . (Indicate the GMC)

This focuses on health behaviors that are maladaptive and significantly affect the course and treatment of a GMC. Some examples of these types of behaviors provided in the DSM-IV are sedentary lifestyle, unusual sex practices, overeating, excessive alcohol use, and substance use. It is important to keep in mind that you must rule out in this situation that the behavior may be better accounted for as the result of an Axis I mental disorder.

Stress-Related Physiological Response Affecting . . . (Indicate the GMC)

This is associated with a physiological response that is stress-related and significantly influences the course and treatment of a GMC.

Other or Unspecified Factors Affecting . . . (Indicate the GMC)

This is a category for factors not included in the previous subtypes listed above that influence the course or treatment of a GMC.

Tip: The nonmedical mental health professional working with the Psychological Factors Affecting Medical Condition should always do so with the cooperation of a physician. The subtle nature of these psychological factors often requires team effort to establish accurate diagnosis of GMCs, mental disorders, and conditions that may be contributing to the person's difficulties. The psychological factors must always be viewed in the light of a possible Axis I or Axis II Mental Disorder that may account for the psychological factor. It is important to rule out Mental Disorder Due to a GMC and Somatoform Disorders. Mental Disorder Due to a GMC is the opposite of Psychological Factors Affecting Medical Condition and Somatoform Disorders that involve both psychological and physiological symptoms.

Medication-Induced Movement Disorders

Medication-Induced Movement Disorders are included in the DSM-IV because of their importance in managing medications for mental disorders or GMCs, and their role in differential diagnosis of mental disorders. These diagnoses should be made by a physician. See pages 679-680 in the DSM-IV for brief descriptions of these disorders. The research criteria for these disorders are included in Appendix B, pages 735-751. These disorders are diagnosed on Axis I. The disorders included in this set are as follows:

1. Medication-Induced Movement Disorders
   - Neuroleptic-Induced Parkinsonism
   - Neuroleptic Malignant Syndrome
   - Neuroleptic-Induced Acute Dystonia
   - Neuroleptic-Induced Acute Akathisia
   - Neuroleptic-Induced Tardive Dyskinesia
   - Medication-Induced Postural Tremor
   - Medication-Induced Movement Disorder NOS
2. Other Medication-Induced Disorder
   - Adverse Effects of Medication NOS

Relational Problems

Relational Problems are defined as patterns of interaction involving members of a relational unit that are associated with clinically significant impairment in functioning, symptoms in one or more members of the relational unit, or impairment of the relational unit itself. Relational problems are often a factor in the presentation and treatment of a mental disorder, and the relational problems can be a significant focus of clinical attention in mental disorder treatment. If relational problems are the principal focus of clinical attention, they are listed on Axis I. If relational problems are identified but are not a principal focus of clinical attention, they are listed on Axis IV. The following Relational Problems are included in the DSM-IV.

Relational Problem Related to an MD or GMC

This category deals with clinical attention focused on impaired interaction that results from a mental disorder or a GMC in a family member.

Parent-Child Relational Problem

Parent-Child Relational Problem refers to a pattern of interaction between a parent and child that is associated with clinically significant impairment or development of clinically significant symptoms in the child or parent that become the focus of clinical attention. Examples of this type of interaction given in the DSM-IV are impaired communication, overprotection, and inadequate discipline.

Partner Relational Problem

Partner Relational Problem is indicated when clinical attention is focused on a pattern of negative communication between spouses or partners that is associated with clinically significant impairment in functioning of one or both partners or development of clinically significant symptoms in one or both partners. Examples of this type of interaction given in the DSM-IV are criticisms, distorted communication, unrealistic expectations, and withdrawal.

Sibling Relational Problem

Sibling Relational Problem is listed when the focus of clinical attention is a pattern of interaction involving siblings that is associated with clinically significant impairment in family functioning or development of symptoms in one or more siblings.

Relational Problem NOS

Relational Problem NOS is used when clinical attention is focused on problems in areas that are not included in the previous categories.

Problems Related to Abuse or Neglect

Problems Related to Abuse or Neglect include situations in which the focus of clinical attention is severe mistreatment of one individual by another. This mistreatment can take the form of neglect, sexual abuse, or physical abuse. Note that the coding is based on whether the victim or the perpetrator or the relational unit is the focus of clinical attention.

Tip: The abuse and neglect codes changed with the code revisions issued after the release of the DSM-IV. The 995 codes added a fifth digit, and V61.1 Sexual Abuse of Adult was deleted.

Physical Abuse of Child

Physical Abuse of Child is used when the focus of clinical attention is physical abuse of a child. This is coded as **V61.21** if the focus of clinical attention is on the perpetrator or family, and **995.54** if clinical focus is on the victim.

Sexual Abuse of Child

Sexual Abuse of Child is indicated when the focus of clinical attention is sexual abuse of a child. This is coded as **V61.21** if the focus of clinical attention is on the perpetrator or family, and **995.53** if clinical focus is on the victim.

Neglect of Child

Neglect of Child is used when the focus of clinical attention is child neglect. This is coded as **V61.21** if the focus of clinical attention is on the perpetrator or family, and **995.52** if clinical focus is on the victim.

Physical Abuse of Adult

Physical Abuse of Adult is recorded when the focus of clinical attention is physical abuse of an adult. This is coded as **V61.12** if focus of clinical attention is the perpetrator and abuse is by partner, **V62.83** if focus of clinical attention is the perpetrator and abuse is by person other than partner, and **995.81** if victim is the clinical focus.

Tip: It is recommended that the abuse or neglect conditions be entered as part of a diagnosis only after a designated social service agency finds that neglect or abuse has occurred or the perpetrator has acknowledged committing the abuse or neglect. A neglect or abuse condition should not be entered as part of a diagnosis based on the statements of third parties (a spouse, sibling, relatives) or the victim unless the abuse has been independently verified or substantiated.

Additional Conditions That May Be a Focus of Clinical Attention

Noncompliance With Treatment

Noncompliance With Treatment is used when the focus of clinical attention is on noncompliance with treatment for a mental disorder or a GMC. Discomfort with treatment, medication side effects, cost, religion, culture, personality traits, or a mental disorder itself can lead to resistance, and are examples of factors associated with this condition.

Malingering

Malingering is the intentional production of false or exaggerated symptoms motivated by external inducements (e.g., avoidance of military service, avoidance of work, or to gain financial compensation). This condition should be considered in the presence of medical or legal implications for the person, a marked discrepancy between objective findings and the person's manifest stress or disability, a lack of cooperation with evaluation and noncompliance with treatment, or an existing diagnosis of Antisocial Personality Disorder. See Chapter 13, "Factitious Disorders," for more details of Malingering and its relationship to other disorders.

Adult Antisocial Behavior

Adult Antisocial Behavior is listed when the focus of clinical attention is adult antisocial behavior that is not due to a mental disorder, such as

Conduct Disorder, Antisocial Personality Disorder, or Impulse-Control Disorder.

Child or Adolescent Antisocial Behavior

Child or Adolescent Antisocial Behavior is used when the focus of clinical attention is antisocial behavior by a child or adolescent that is not due to a mental disorder, such as Conduct Disorder, Antisocial Personality Disorder, or Impulse-Control Disorder.

Borderline Intellectual Functioning

This diagnosis is indicated when the focus of clinical attention is Borderline Intellectual Functioning, defined as an IQ score range between 71 and 84, as measured by standardized instruments. This condition is coded on Axis II.

Age-Related Cognitive Decline

Age-Related Cognitive Decline is noted on a diagnosis when the focus of clinical attention is an objectively identified decline in cognitive functioning related to the aging process that is within normal limits given the person's age. People with this condition will frequently report difficulty remembering names, addresses, numbers, and appointments, and may have difficulty performing complex mental tasks. Mental disorders and GMCs should be ruled out before assigning this condition.

Bereavement

Bereavement is recorded when the focus of clinical attention is reaction to the death of a loved one. Persons with this condition may have the symptoms of Major Depressive Episode and appear for treatment even though the person considers the reaction "normal." The diagnosis of Major Depressive Disorder is not given unless the bereavement symptoms endure longer than two months and meet the criteria for a depressive disorder. In some situations, bereavement can be differentiated from a depressive disorder based on the survivor's symptoms, such as guilt about things other than the acts by the survivor at the time of the death; thoughts of death other than wanting to be with the dead person, or feelings of being better off dead; morbid preoccupation with worthlessness; significant psychomotor retardation; significant functional impairments; and hallucinations other than thinking he or she has seen or heard the dead person.

Academic Problem

Academic Problem is used when clinical attention is focused on an academic problem that is not due to a mental disorder or, if due to a mental disorder, requires independent clinical attention.

Occupational Problem

Occupational Problem is noted when an occupational problem not due to a mental disorder is a focus of clinical attention and warrants independent clinical attention.

Identity Problem

Identity Problem is made part of the diagnosis when the focus of clinical attention is uncertainty about multiple concerns related to identity. The DSM-IV lists as examples such factors as long-term goals, career choice, friendship patterns, sexual orientation, moral values, and group loyalties.

Religious or Spiritual Problem

Religious or Spiritual Problem is used when the focus of clinical attention is a religious or spiritual problem. This can take the form of loss of faith, questioning faith, problems with conversion to a new faith, or questioning values or beliefs that are not part of an established religion.

Acculturational Problem

Acculturation Problem is listed when a problem adjusting to a different culture is a focus of clinical attention.

Phase of Life Problem

Phase of Life Problem is made part of the multiaxial diagnosis when the focus of clinical attention is a problem related to a particular developmental phase or another life circumstance that is not due to a mental disorder. If the Phase of Life Problem is due to a mental disorder, it is severe enough to require independent clinical attention.

REFERENCES

American Psychiatric Association (1994). *Diagnostic and Statistical Manual of Mental Disorders,* Fourth Edition. Washington, DC: American Psychiatric Association.

Morrison, J. (1995). *DSM-IV Made Easy: The Clinician's Guide to Diagnosis.* New York: Guilford.

Chapter 22

Appendix B of the DSM-IV: Criteria Sets and Axes Provided for Further Study

PROPOSALS

Postconcussional disorder
Mild neurocognitive disorder
Caffeine withdrawal
Alternative dimensional descriptors for Schizophrenia
Postpsychotic depressive disorder of Schizophrenia
Simple deteriorative disorder (simple Schizophrenia)
Premenstrual dysphoric disorder
Alternative Criterion B for Dysthymic Disorder
Minor depressive disorder
Recurrent brief depressive disorder
Mixed anxiety-depressive disorder
Factitious disorder by proxy
Dissociative trance disorder
Binge-eating disorder
Depressive personality disorder
Passive-aggressive personality disorder (negativistic personality disorder)
Medication-Induced Movement Disorders (included in the section "Other Conditions That May Be a Focus of Clinical Attention"; text and research criteria included in Appendix B)

- 332.1 Neuroleptic-Induced Parkinsonism
- 333.92 Neuroleptic Malignant Syndrome
- 333.7 Neuroleptic-Induced Acute Dystonia
- 333.99 Neuroleptic-Induced Acute Akathisia
- 333.82 Neuroleptic-Induced Tardive Dyskinesia
- 333.1 Medication-Induced Postural Tremor
- 333.90 Medication-Induced Movement Disorder NOS

Defensive Functioning Scale
Global Assessment of Relational Functioning (GARF) Scale
Social and Occupational Functioning Assessment Scale (SOFAS)

FUNDAMENTAL FEATURES

Over 100 new disorders were reviewed for inclusion in the DSM-IV. Twenty-six disorders and items were approved for appearance in Appendix B to allow further research on these "promising" disorders. The disorders are organized in the same fashion as the major disorders in the DSM-IV manual, with some minor variations. The titles of the disorders are not capitalized because they are not full-fledged disorders. Instead of having Diagnostic Features, they have Features, and the criteria are referred to as "research criteria." The sections Associated Features and Differential Diagnosis are also included for these disorders. New disorders were accepted in the DSM-IV based on an assessment of the amount of research available to support inclusion of the disorders. The disorders in Appendix B are considered impressive, but in need of more research validation before they can be considered full-scale mental disorders. These disorders are diagnosed in the NOS category for the class of disorders to which they apply. For example, people who meet the criteria for recurrent brief depressive disorder would be given the diagnosis Depressive Disorder NOS (this would be recorded as Depressive Disorder NOS, recurrent brief depressive disorder). The Medication-Induced Movement Disorders are diagnosed on Axis I. Visual 22.1 gives a summary of where each of these disorders would be diagnosed.

Brief descriptions of the research disorders are provided in the following material.

Postconcussional Disorder

Postconcussional disorder has as its main feature an acquired impairment in cognitive functioning, with specific neurobehavioral symptoms that occur as a consequence of a closed head injury, with severity sufficient to produce a significant cerebral concussion. The person must have three or more of the following symptoms occurring shortly after the trauma and lasting at least three months: easily fatigued, disturbed sleep, headache, vertigo, dizziness, irritability, aggression without provocation, anxiety, depression, affective lability, change in personality, apathy, or lack of spontaneity.

VISUAL 22.1. Coding and Recording of Disorders Provided for Further Study

Research Disorder	Code #	Diagnostic Class	Where Recorded
Postconcussional disorder	294.9	Cognitive Disorder NOS	Axis I
Mild neurocognitive disorder	294.9	Cognitive Disorder NOS	Axis I
Caffeine withdrawal	292.9	Caffeine-Related Disorder NOS	Axis I
Postpsychotic depressive disorder of Schizophrenia	311	Depressive Disorder NOS	Axis I
Simple deteriorative disorder (simple Schizophrenia)	300.9	Unspecified Mental Disorder (nonpsychotic)	Axis I
Premenstrual dysphoric disorder	311	Depressive Disorder NOS	Axis I
Minor depressive disorder	311 309.0	Depressive Disorder NOS Adjustment Disorder With Depressed Mood (if symptoms in response to psychosocial stressor)	Axis I Axis I
Recurrent brief depressive disorder	311	Depressive Disorder NOS	Axis I
Mixed anxiety-depressive disorder	300.00	Anxiety Disorder NOS	Axis I
Factitious disorder by proxy	300.19	Factitious Disorder NOS	Axis I
Dissociative trance disorder	300.15	Dissociative Disorder NOS	Axis I
Binge-eating disorder	307.50	Eating Disorder NOS	Axis I
Depressive personality disorder	301.9	Personality Disorder NOS	Axis II
Passive-aggressive personality disorder (negativistic personality disorder)	301.9	Personality Disorder NOS	Axis II
Neuroleptic-Induced Parkinsonism	332.1	—	Axis I
Neuroleptic Malignant Syndrome	333.92	—	Axis I
Neuroleptic-Induced Acute Dystonia	333.7	—	Axis I
Neuroleptic-Induced Acute Akathisia	333.99	—	Axis I
Neuroleptic-Induced Tardive Dyskinesia	333.82	—	Axis I
Medication-Induced Postural Tremor	333.1	—	Axis I
Medication-Induced Movement Disorder NOS	333.90	—	Axis I
Defensive Functioning Scale	None	—	Separate Form
Global Assessment of Relational Functioning (GARF) Scale	None	—	Axis IV
Social and Occupational Functioning Assessment Scale (SOFAS)	None	—	Axis I

Mild Neurocognitive Disorder

Mild neurocognitive disorder results from mild neurocognitive impairment due to a GMC, with at least two of the following symptoms most of the time for at least two weeks: memory impairment, disturbance in executive functioning, disturbance in attention, disturbance in speed of information processing, impaired perceptual-motor abilities, or impaired language. Objective evidence of the GMC or neurocognitive impairment and neuropsychological testing is necessary to establish the existence of these symptoms.

Caffeine Withdrawal

Caffeine withdrawal is a withdrawal syndrome due to the abrupt stopping or reduction of the use of products containing caffeine after a long period of significant daily use of these products. The symptoms of withdrawal are present, including one or more of the following: headache, fatigue, drowsiness, anxiety, depression, nausea, or vomiting.

Alternative Dimensional Descriptors for Schizophrenia

Alternative dimensional descriptors for Schizophrenia are a proposed alternative to the existing Schizophrenia subtypes. These alternative descriptors are proposed because of perceived limitations of the current subtyping of Schizophrenia (see pp. 286-290). The alternative descriptor model has three dimensions: (1) psychotic (hallucinations/delusions) dimension, (2) disorganized dimension, and (3) negative (deficit) dimension. Each dimension is given a rating based on a general severity specifier: *absent, mild, moderate, or severe*. The psychotic dimension refers to the degree to which hallucinations or delusions are present. The disorganized dimension covers the degree to which disorganized speech, disorganized behavior, or inappropriate affect are present. The negative dimension is the reporting of the degree to which negative symptoms such as affective flattening, alogia, or avolition have been present.

Postpsychotic Depressive Disorder of Schizophrenia

Postpsychotic depressive disorder of Schizophrenia is the diagnosis of a Major Depressive Episode, as defined in the "Mood Disorders" section of the DSM-IV, superimposed on, and occurring only during, the residual phase of Schizophrenia, which follows the active phase.

Simple Deteriorative Disorder (Simple Schizophrenia)

Simple deteriorative disorder (simple Schizophrenia) is characterized by the occurrence of prominent negative symptoms that clearly are a change from a preestablished baseline, and the symptoms are severe enough to cause marked impairment. Gradual, progressive onset of negative symptoms, such as affective flattening, alogia, or avolition, occurs over a one-year period in work or educational settings, and Criterion A for Schizophrenia has never been met (p. 285).

Premenstrual Dysphoric Disorder

Premenstrual dysphoric disorder is the regular occurrence during the last week of the luteal phase in most menstrual cycles of at least five or more symptoms, such as depressed mood, self-deprecating thoughts, hopelessness, anxiety, tension, feeling "on edge," affective lability, sudden feelings of tearfulness, increased sensitivity to rejection, irritability, anger, increased interpersonal conflicts, decreased interest in activities, difficulty concentrating, lethargy, fatigue, lack of energy, sleep disturbance, sense of being overwhelmed, or physical symptoms.

Alternative Criterion B for Dysthymic Disorder

Alternative Criterion B for Dysthymic Disorder is being considered because of controversy surrounding its current Criterion B. DSM-IV field trials suggest that the following is a more accurate criterion:

B. Presence, while depressed, of three (or more) of the following:

- low self-esteem or self-confidence, or feelings of inadequacy
- feelings of pessimism, despair or hopelessness
- generalized loss of interest or pleasure
- social withdrawal
- chronic fatigue or tiredness
- feelings of guilt, brooding about the past
- subjective feelings of irritability or excessive anger
- decreased activity, effectiveness, or productivity
- difficulty in thinking, as reflected by poor concentration, poor memory, or indecisiveness (p. 718) (Reprinted with permission from the *Diagnostic and Statistical Manual of Mental Disorders,* Fourth Edition. Copyright 1994 American Psychiatric Association.)

Minor Depressive Disorder

Minor depressive disorder is one or more periods of depressive symptoms that are identical to Major Depressive Disorder in duration but involve fewer symptoms and less degree of impairment. An episode includes sad or depressed mood or loss of interest in almost all activities. In total, at least two, but less than five, additional symptoms must be present. In other words, in this disorder, there is no alteration in the number of criteria for depression, but there is a lessening of the extent of the symptom complex to qualify for this form of depressive disorder. See the "Mood Disorders" section, pages 320-327, for the Major Depressive Episode criteria.

Recurrent Brief Depressive Disorder

Recurrent brief depressive disorder is used when the person meets the criteria for Major Depressive Episode in number and severity of symptoms but does not meet the two-week duration criterion (see pp. 320-327). Episodes last at least two days but less than two weeks. Episodes must recur at least once a month for at least twelve consecutive months and must not be associated exclusively with the menstrual cycle. The symptoms must cause impaired functioning in important areas of daily activity.

Mixed Anxiety-Depressive Disorder

Mixed anxiety-depressive disorder has as its main feature persistent or recurrent dysphoric mood, lasting at least one month, and the dysphoric mood is accompanied by at least four or more of the following symptoms: difficulty concentrating, mind going blank, sleep disturbance, fatigue, low energy, irritability, worry, being easily moved to tears, hypervigilance, anticipating the worst about situations, hopelessness, low self-esteem, or feelings of worthlessness. The symptoms cause distress or impairment in several important areas of functioning.

Factitious Disorder by Proxy

Factitious disorder by proxy is deliberately causing or feigning physical or psychological signs or symptoms in another person who is under an individual's care. Usually, the victim is a child and the perpetrator is the child's mother. The presumed motivation for the behavior is the need for the perpetrator to assume the sick role by proxy. External incentives, such as economic gain, are absent. This disorder can be triggered by life stresses. The perpetrator frequently has experience related to medical environments.

Dissociative Trance Disorder

Dissociative trance disorder is the occurrence of involuntary trance states that are not a part of one's cultural or religious belief system and cause clinically significant distress or impairment in functioning. Trance is the temporary marked alteration in state of consciousness or loss of sense of personal identity, without replacement by an alternative identity, associated with at least one of the following: narrowing of awareness of surroundings, unusually narrow and selective focus on environmental stimuli, or stereotyped behaviors or movements considered beyond one's control. In this disorder, the person can also experience possession trance, which is a single or episodic alteration of the state of consciousness with the replacement of the personal sense of identity by a new identity. This experience is attributed to the influence of a spirit, power, deity, or other person and is associated with at least one of the following: stereotyped and culturally determined behaviors or movements controlled by the possessing agent or full or partial amnesia for the event.

Binge-Eating Disorder

Binge-eating disorder is recurrent episodes of binge eating associated with subjective behavioral indicators of impaired control over, and distress about, the binge eating. Regular compensatory behaviors, such as self-induced vomiting, use of laxatives or other medications, fasting, and excessive exercise, are absent. The nature of the binge-eating episodes is the same as for Bulimia Nervosa (see p. 550). The criteria include eating large amounts of food in discrete time periods, lack of control over eating, eating more rapidly than usual, eating until uncomfortably full, eating large amounts of food when not hungry, eating alone because of embarrassment about the amount eaten, and disgust with self about eating problems. The binges occur, on average, at least two days a week for at least six months.

Depressive Personality Disorder

Depressive personality disorder is an extensive pattern of depressive cognitions and behaviors that begin by early adulthood and occur in a variety of contexts. The pattern does not occur exclusively during a Major Depressive Episode and cannot be accounted for by Dysthymic Disorder. Five or more of the following symptoms are present: usual mood is dominated by dejection, gloominess, cheerlessness, joylessness, or unhappiness; self-concept focuses on beliefs of inadequacy, worthlessness, and low self-esteem; critical, blaming, and derogatory toward self; brooding and prone to worry; negativistic, critical, and judgmental toward others; pessimistic; or prone to feeling guilty or remorseful.

Passive-Aggressive Personality Disorder

Passive-aggressive personality disorder (negativistic personality disorder) is a pattern of negative attitudes and passive resistance to demands for adequate performance, beginning by early adulthood and present in a variety of contexts. The person has four or more of the following characteristics: passively resists routine tasks in social and occupational situations; complains of being misunderstood and unappreciated by others; sullen or argumentative; unreasonably criticizes or scorns authority; expresses envy and resentment toward more fortunate people; heightened complaints of personal misfortune; or alternation between hostile defiance and contrition.

Medication-Induced Movement Disorders

Medication-Induced Movement Disorders are included in the section "Other Conditions That May Be a Focus of Clinical Attention," but the text and research criteria are in Appendix B. Only brief summaries of these disorders are given here. The reader should refer to pages 735-751 for the full criteria for these disorders.

Neuroleptic-Induced Parkinsonism is the presence of Parkinsonian signs or symptoms that are associated with the use of neuroleptic medication. The signs and symptoms are Parkinsonian tremor, Parkinsonian muscular rigidity, and akinesia (decreased spontaneous facial expressions, gestures, speech, or body movements).

Neuroleptic Malignant Syndrome involves severe muscle rigidity, elevated temperature, and a series of possible physical and psychological symptoms in a person using neuroleptic medication.

Neuroleptic-Induced Acute Dystonia is the development of sustained abnormal posture or muscle spasms associated with the use of neuroleptic medication.

Neuroleptic-Induced Acute Akathisia involves subjective complaints of restlessness and symptoms of unusual movements and agitation associated with the use of neuroleptic medication.

Neuroleptic-Induced Tardive Dyskinesia is associated with the abnormal, involuntary movements of the tongue, jaw, trunk, or extremities that develop in connection with the use of neuroleptic medications.

Medication-Induced Postural Tremor is a fine postural tremor that develops in association with the use of medication. This condition can develop with the use of a number of medications (see pp. 749-751).

Medication-Induced Movement Disorder NOS is reserved for medication-induced disorders that do not fit any of the previous disorders.

Defensive Functioning Scale

The Defensive Functioning Scale (DFS) is designed to measure defense mechanisms or coping styles that are automatic psychological processes protecting the person against anxiety and blocking the awareness of external dangers or stressors. The individual defense mechanisms are grouped according to defensive levels. In using the DFS, the clinician should list up to seven specific defenses or coping styles, starting with the most prominent defense and then indicating the most predominant level attained by the person. Specific defense mechanisms listed can be drawn from different Defense Levels. The defensive functioning is recorded on a form provided on page 754 of the DSM-IV. The form has an axis for recording the seven defense mechanisms and the predominant defensive level. A glossary of the specific defense mechanisms and coping styles is provided on pages 755-757 of the DSM-IV manual. The rating should reflect the person's level of functioning at the time of the evaluation. Visual 22.2 summarizes the DFS.

Global Assessment of Relational Functioning (GARF) Scale

The Global Assessment of Relational Functioning (GARF) Scale is used to do an overall assessment of the level of functioning of a family or other sustained relationship. Ratings are on a continuum ranging from competent, optimal relational functioning to disrupted, dysfunctional relationships. The scale and scoring are analogous to the Axis V Global Assessment of Functioning (GAF) Scale. The relational unit is assessed in the areas of problem solving, organization, and emotional climate. The scale is designed to rate functioning at the time of evaluation but can be used to rate periods in the past, such as the highest functioning level in the past three months or past year. The time period should be indicated after the GARF score is entered. Visual 22.3 summarizes the GARF Scale.

Tip: The GARF is the only measurement tool of its kind and can be useful in settings where DSM-IV diagnosis is not commonly used. It also can be used in conjunction with family therapy and couples therapy as an assessment and outcome measurement tool.

VISUAL 22.2. Defensive Functioning Scale Summary

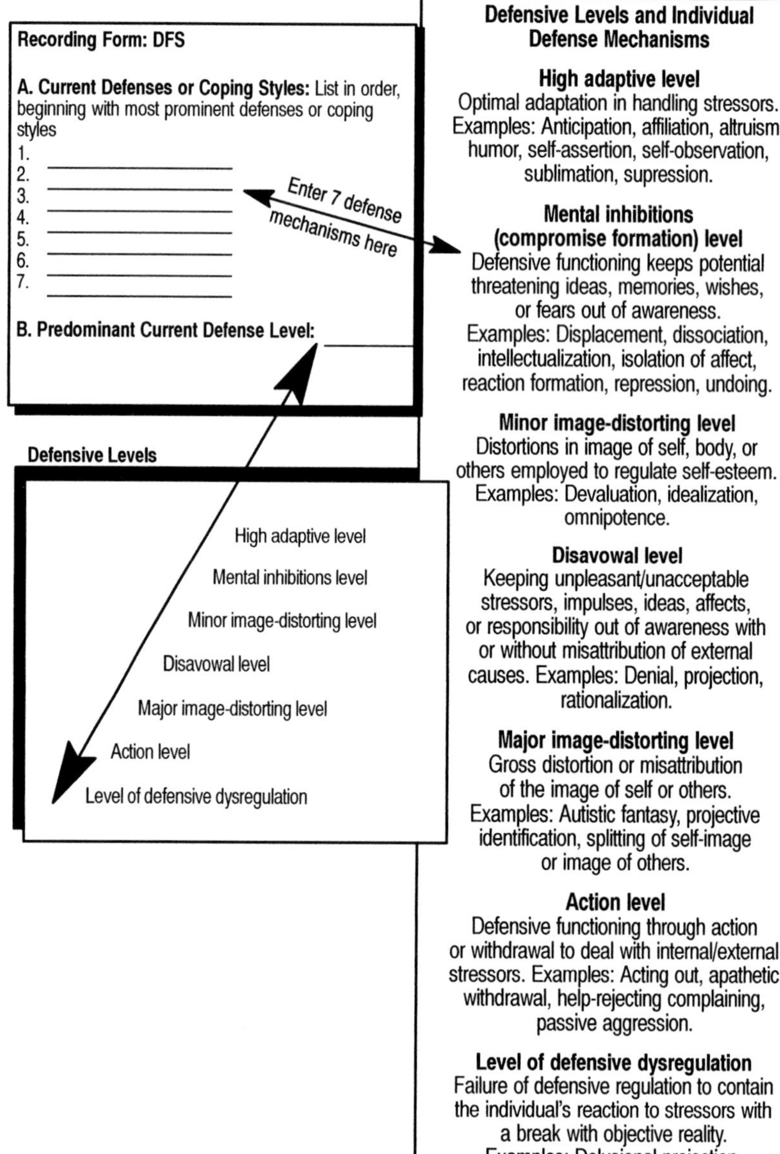

Source: American Psychiatric Association, 1994, pp. 751-753.

VISUAL 22.3. Global Assessment of Relational Functioning (GARF) Scale Summary

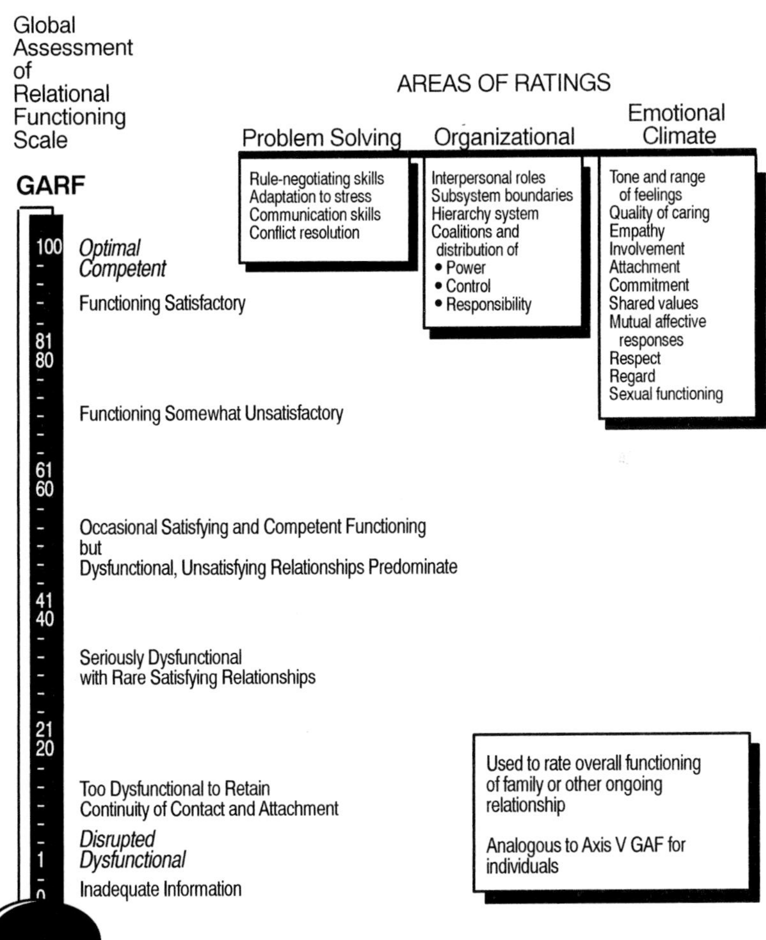

Source: American Psychiatric Association, 1994, pp. 758-759.

Social and Occupational Functioning Assessment Scale (SOFAS)

The Social and Occupational Functioning Assessment Scale (SOFAS) differs from the GAF scale in that it focuses exclusively on the person's level of social and occupational functioning and is not directly influenced by the person's overall severity of psychological problems. Unlike the GAF, any impairment in social and occupational functioning that is due to a GMC is taken into account when making the rating. The SOFAS is generally used to rate functioning at the time of evaluation but can be used to evaluate previous time periods. After assigning the SOFAS score, the time period should be entered. The SOFAS uses the same numeric scale as the GAF. This scale's criteria are on page 761 of the DSM-IV. Visual 22.4 summarizes the SOFAS Scale.

RECOMMENDED READING

American Psychiatric Association (1992). *DSM-IV Options Book.* Washington, DC: American Psychiatric Association.

REFERENCE

American Psychiatric Association (1994). *Diagnostic and Statistical Manual of Mental Disorders,* Fourth Edition. Washington, DC: American Psychiatric Association.

VISUAL 22.4. DSM-IV Social and Occupational Functioning Scale (SOFAS)

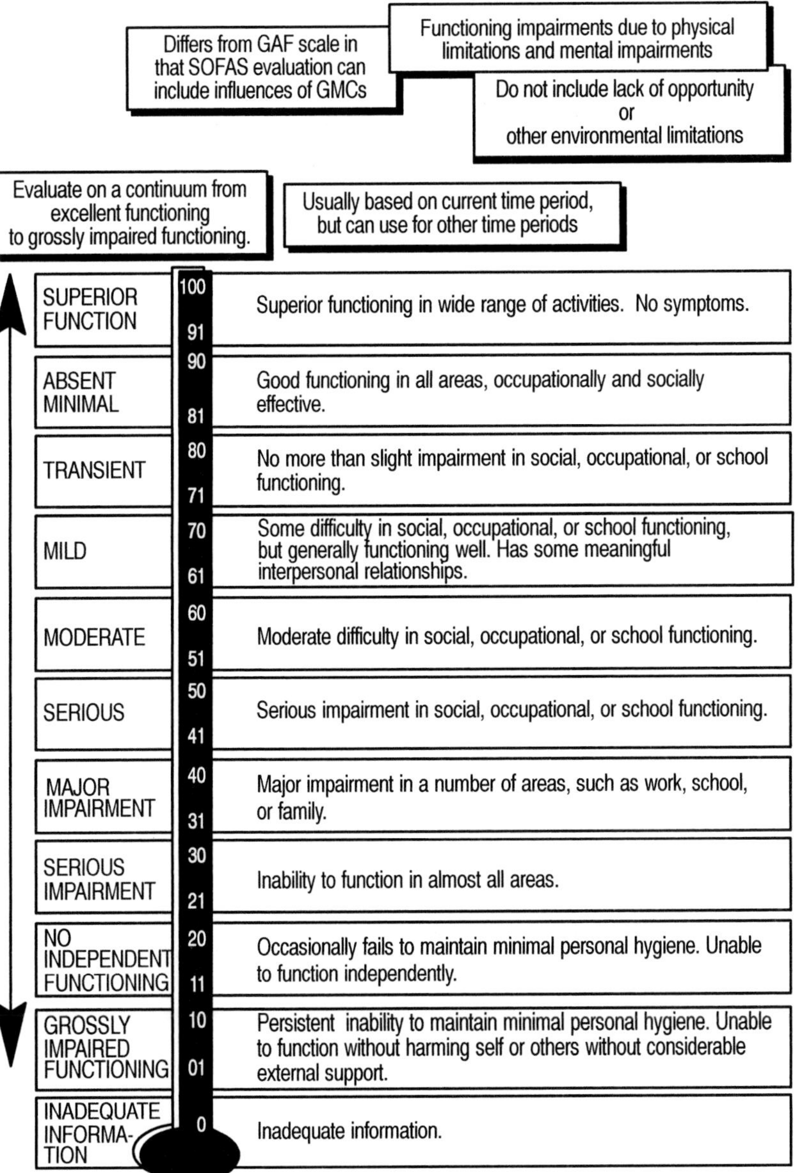

Source: American Psychiatric Association, 1994, pp. 760-761.

Chapter 23

Appendix I of the DSM-IV: Outline for Cultural Formulation and Glossary of Culture-Bound Syndromes

CULTURE-BOUND SYNDROMES

amok
ataque de nervios
bilis and colera (also referred to as muina)
boufée delirante
brain fag
dhat
falling-out or blacking out
ghost sickness
hwa-byung (also known as wool-hwa-byung)
koro
latah
locura
mal de ojo
nervios
pibloktoq
qi-gong psychotic reaction
rootwork
sangue dormido ("sleeping blood")
shenjing shuairuo ("neurasthenia")
shen-k'uei (Taiwan); shenkui (China)
shin-byung
spell
susto ("fright," or "soul loss")
taijin kyofusho
zar

FUNDAMENTAL FEATURES

The term "culture-bound syndrome" was coined in 1969 by a Western-trained Chinese psychiatrist named Pow Meng Yap (Mezzich et al., 1996). Some have argued that use of this term in the DSM-IV has limitations (Frances, First, and Pincus, 1995). However, inclusion of this section in the DSM-IV is an attempt to highlight the role of culture in functioning and make clinicians more aware of cultural factors in behavior. The inclusion of this appendix will hopefully lead to refinement of the culturally sensitive application of mental disorders to persons with different cultural backgrounds.

This Appendix is new to the DSM-IV and is the result of work done by a DSM-IV Task Force Work Group that met at the National Institutes of Health. Cultural influences on mental health diagnosis are included in the DSM-IV because the manual is used in many countries, the increasing cultural diversity of the United States requires consideration of the role of culture in production of symptoms, and the need exists for differentiation of cultural behaviors and mental disorders.

This appendix has two sections. The first section is an outline that is intended to supplement the multiaxial diagnosis through guidelines for evaluating and recording an individual's cultural context. The second section is a glossary of culture-bound syndromes. (See Visual 23.1 for the appendix summary.)

OUTLINE FOR CULTURAL FORMULATION

The following outline for cultural formulation supplements the multiaxial diagnostic assessment and addresses difficulties encountered in applying DSM-IV criteria in multicultural environments. This section provides an outline for systematic evaluation of cultural factors that may be influencing the person's functioning and may impact the relationship between the person and the mental health professional. Clinicians should take into account individual ethnic and cultural contexts in DSM-IV diagnosis.

Tip: This section can be especially helpful when the person being evaluated and the mental health professional are from different cultures and should be used whenever the practitioner is encountering difficulty understanding a person's cultural context.

VISUAL 23.1. Appendix I: Outline for Cultural Formulation and Glossary of Culture-Bound Syndromes Summary

Outline of Cultural Formulation

- Record data about person's culture through narrative summary in the following categories:

1. **Cultural Identity of Individual**
   - Ethnic/cultural reference groups (immigrants/ethnic minorities, note degree of involvement with culture of origin and host culture).
   - Language abilities, use, and preference (including multilingualism).
2. **Cultural Explanations of Illness**
   - Predominant distress idioms through which symptoms or need for social support are communicated.
   - Meaning and perceived severity of symptoms in relation to norms of cultural reference group.
   - Local illness category used by the individual's family and community to identify the condition (derived from section two, which contains the Culture-Bound Syndromes).
   - Perceived causes/explanations individual and reference group provide for illness.
   - Current preferences and past experiences with professional and popular sources of care.
3. **Cultural Factors in Psychosocial Environment and Levels of Functioning**
   - Interpretations of social stressors, social supports, and levels of functioning and disability.
   - Stresses in local social environment and role of religion and kin networks in providing support.
4. **Cultural Elements of Relationship Between Individual and Clinician**
   - Differences in culture and social status of client and clinician.
   - Problems differences may cause in diagnosis and treatment.
5. **Overall Cultural Assessment for Diagnosis and Care**
   - Explain how cultural considerations specifically influence comprehensive diagnosis and care.

Glossary of Culture-Bound Syndromes

Culture-bound syndrome means recurrent, locality-specific patterns of aberrant behavior and troubling experience that may or may not be linked to a particular DSM-IV diagnostic category.

Culture-Bound Syndromes

- amok
- ataque de nervios
- bilis and colera (also called muina)
- boufée delirante
- brain fag
- dhat
- falling-out or blacking out
- ghost sickness
- hwa-byung (also called wool-hwa-byung)
- koro
- latah
- locura
- mal de ojo
- nervios
- pibloktoq
- qi-gong psychotic reaction
- rootwork
- sangue dormido ("sleeping blood")
- shenjing shuairuo ("neurasthenia")
- shen-k'uei (Taiwan); shenkui (China)
- shin-byung
- spell
- susto ("fright," or "soul loss")
- taijin kyofusho
- zar

Tip: This section is helpful when person evaluated and mental health professional are from different cultures and should be used whenever practitioner encounters difficulty understanding person's cultural context.

Source: American Psychiatric Association, 1994, pp. 843-849.

The clinician can record the data gathered about a person's culture by writing a narrative summary for each of the following categories (see Visual 23.2 for an illustration of this outline).

Cultural Identity of Individual

The clinician should note the individual's ethnic or cultural reference groups. For immigrants and ethnic minorities, note the degree of involvement with culture of origin and host culture. Note language abilities, use, and preference (including multilingualism).

Cultural Explanations of Illness

The predominant idioms of distress (e.g., "nerves," possessing spirits, somatic complaints, inexplicable misfortune) through which symptoms or the need for social support are communicated by the individual should be noted. The meaning and perceived severity of symptoms in relation to cultural reference group norms and any local illness category used by the individual's family and community to identify the condition should be recorded. These are derived from section two, which contains the culture-bound syndromes. The perceived causes or explanations the individual and the reference group provide to explain the illness should also be described. Note also current preferences and past experiences with professional and popular sources of care.

Cultural Factors Related to Psychosocial Environment and Levels of Functioning

The practitioner should note interpretations of social stressors, social supports, and levels of functioning and disability. Include stresses in the local social environment and the role of religion and kin networks in providing support.

Cultural Elements of the Relationship Between Individual and Clinician

Describe differences in culture and social status of client and clinician and problems differences may cause in diagnosis and treatment (e.g., difficulty in communicating in first language, in eliciting symptoms or understanding their cultural significance, in negotiating an appropriate relationship or level of intimacy, in determining whether a behavior is normative or pathological).

VISUAL 23.2. Outline for Cultural Formulation Case Illustration

1. Cultural identity of individual

An evaluation was done today of Mary Sanchez in our mental health center. Mary is 34 years old. She immigrated to Houston five years ago from her home in Reynosa, Mexico. Mary came to the United States with her husband and three children. Mary's husband has not permitted Mary to leave the home for any extended period of time alone since living in Houston. Mary has learned very little English, most likely due to her forced isolation by the husband. Mary's children have not been isolated, and they attend public school. Mary was accompanied to the evaluation by her oldest son, who is age sixteen. Her son Carlos speaks good English and was able to describe most of Mary's symptoms to me.

2. Cultural explanations of illness

Mary's primary reference group remains her family in Mexico. She has been back to visit them several times since moving to the United States. Mary recently returned from a visit to Mexico. While in Mexico she had sudden onset of symptoms. She complains of stomachaches, headaches, sleep difficulty, and inexplicable crying spells. She has experienced a significant appetite loss and is unable to concentrate on her household chores. Mary says she has a bad case of "nerves" (nervios). Mary believes her "case of the nerves" is inherited and "runs in my family." She believes her symptoms are getting worse, and she does "not know what to do." She is fearful her husband will find out she came to the Center.

Mary will be further assessed for differential diagnosis of possible Adjustment Disorder, Anxiety Disorder, Mood Disorder, Somatoform Disorder, and Acculturation Problem. There is no evidence of Dissociative Disorder or Psychotic Disorder, but these disorders will continue to be reviewed as part of the rule-out process. The consideration of the Culture-Bound Syndromes of nervios and locura will be a key part of the comprehensive assessment.

3. Cultural factors in psychosocial environment and levels of functioning

Mary reported that she has become more active in the church in the last year, and when her husband found this out, he became very angry with her and ordered her to stay away from the church. Mary was planning to enroll in English classes that the church was sponsoring. Mary has no social supports or social contacts outside her family. During her return trip to Mexico, her family "pressured" her to do something about her situation with her husband. While in Mexico Mary visited a curandero and received some herbal treatments.

4. Cultural elements of the relationship between individual and clinician

I was able to communicate with Mary minimally, and my Spanish is not good enough to do ongoing intervention with Mary. If her son had not been present today, it would have been difficult for me to do the evaluation.

VISUAL 23.2 *(continued)*

5. Overall cultural assessment for diagnosis and care

It is difficult to give Mary a DSM-IV diagnosis at the present time. Stress-related factors in her life have been present for some time and could be indicative of a stress-related disorder. She denies her symptoms are due to the stresses produced by the relationship with her husband, or the pressure she is feeling from her family. I am concerned about the possibility of an eating disorder. I am reluctant to involve Mary in further appointments because of her fear of Mr. Sanchez finding out about her evaluation visit to the Center. I do not know to what degree Mary's situation may be made worse by acculturation issues. The role of religion needs to be considered in assisting Mary to get help, as well as the potential for religion to cause more difficulties if her husband objects to her involvement in religion and treatment. I am reluctant to encourage Mary to involve Mr. Sanchez in the treatment. I will contact Mary's priest about the religious issues, and I will familiarize myself with the Catholic religion in order to better understand Mary in relation to her religious beliefs and the supports provided by the church. I will contact a Spanish-speaking MSW therapist who works in an outreach facility that is part of our Center and is located in Mary's neighborhood. I will have the therapist arrange further appointments for Mary. I will refer Mary to a primary care physician in her neighborhood to follow up on the physical symptoms and to evaluate the herbal treatments that were provided by the curandero. I believe more assessment of Mary's family situation and relationships needs to be done before family intervention is implemented. Diagnosis will be deferred until the precipitating factors are clarified. The differential diagnosis process described in item 2 above will be completed as part of the ongoing evaluation. I will consult with the Spanish-speaking MSW social worker who will be doing the intervention. Mary was provided a consent-for-treatment form, and she signed release-of-information forms. These forms were given to Mary in Spanish and were read to her by her son in my presence. Mary understands the treatment and evaluation plans described in this formulation and did agree to them.

Overall Cultural Assessment for Diagnosis and Care

The clinician should conclude with a discussion of how cultural considerations specifically influence comprehensive diagnosis and care.

GLOSSARY OF CULTURE-BOUND SYNDROMES

Culture-bound syndrome (CBS) means recurrent, locality-specific patterns of aberrant behavior and troubling experience that may or may not be linked to a particular DSM-IV diagnostic category. These patterns can be considered indigenously to be "illnesses," or at least afflictions, and most have local names (p. 844). Presentations conforming to the major DSM-IV categories can be found throughout the world, but it must be recognized that the particular symptoms, course, and social response are very often influenced by local culture. Culture-bound syndromes are usually limited to specific societies or cultures and are localized, folk, diagnostic groupings that contain meanings for troubling symptoms and behaviors.

Rarely are culture-bound syndromes equivalent to a DSM-IV diagnostic entity. Strange behavior that might be observed by a clinician using DSM-IV and sorted into several categories may be included in a single folk category, and presentations that might be considered by a diagnostician using DSM-IV as belonging to a single category may be sorted into several categories by a clinician from the particular culture. Some conditions and disorders are culture-bound syndromes specific to industrialized societies (e.g., Anorexia Nervosa, Dissociative Identity Disorder), given their rarity or absence in other cultures. Industrialized societies include distinctive and varied subcultures, including diverse immigrant groups that may have culture-bound syndromes.

The following is a list and summary of the twenty-five culture-bound syndromes included in the DSM-IV. Where information is provided in the DSM-IV, the CBS has been described according to the categories of fundamental feature, CBS symptoms, relevant cultures, and the DSM-related disorder(s) having the most relevance for the CBS.

amok

Fundamental Feature: Dissociative episode with brooding and outburst of violent or homicidal behavior directed at people and objects. Precipitated by insult. Found mostly among males.

Cultures: Malaysia, Laos, Philippines, Polynesia *(cafard or cathard)*, Papua New Guinea, and Puerto Rico *(mal de pelea)*, and among the Navajo *(iich'aa)*.

DSM-Related Disorders: Brief psychotic episode or a chronic psychotic process.

ataque de nervios

Fundamental Feature: Sense of being out of control. Result of stressful event relating to family (e.g., news of the death of a close relative, a separation or divorce from a spouse, conflicts with a spouse or children, or witnessing an accident involving a family member).

Symptoms: Uncontrollable shouting, attacks of crying, trembling, heat in the chest rising into the head, and verbal or physical aggression. Dissociative experiences, seizurelike or fainting episodes, and suicidal gestures. People may experience amnesia for what happened during ataque de nervios, but they quickly return to their usual level of functioning.

Cultures: Latinos from the Caribbean, Latin American and Latin Mediterranean groups.

DSM-Related Disorders: Panic Attacks, Anxiety, Mood, Dissociative, or Somatoform Disorders.

bilis and colera (also referred to as muina)

Fundamental Feature: Strongly experienced anger or rage. Anger is powerful emotion that has direct effects on the body and can exacerbate existing symptoms. Anger disturbs the core body balances (balance between hot and cold valences in the body and between material and spiritual aspects of the body).

Symptoms: Acute nervous tension, headache, trembling, screaming, stomach disturbances, loss of consciousness, and chronic fatigue from the acute episode.

Cultures: Latin cultures.

boufée delirante

Fundamental Feature: French term refers to sudden outburst of agitated and aggressive behavior, marked confusion, and psychomotor excitement. May be accompanied by visual and auditory hallucinations or paranoid ideation.

Cultures: West Africa and Haiti.

DSM-Related Disorders: Can resemble Brief Psychotic Disorder.

brain fag

Fundamental Feature: Condition experienced by high school or university students in response to challenges of schooling.

Symptoms: Difficulties in concentrating, remembering, and thinking. Complaints that brains are "fatigued." Somatic complaints centered around head and neck that include pain, pressure or tightness, blurring of vision, heat, or burning.

Cultures: West Africa. "Brain tiredness" or fatigue from "too much thinking" in many cultures.

DSM-Related Disorders: Anxiety, Depressive, and Somatoform Disorders.

dhat

Fundamental Feature: Diagnostic term referring to severe anxiety and hypochondriacal concerns associated with discharge of semen, whitish discoloration of the urine, and feelings of weakness and exhaustion.

Cultures: India. Similar to *jiryan* (India), *sukra prameha* (Sri Lanka), and *shen-k'uei* (China).

falling-out or blacking out

Fundamental Feature: Sudden collapse that can occur without warning but sometimes is preceded by feelings of dizziness or "swimming" in the head.

Symptoms: Eyes are open, but person claims inability to see. The person hears and understands what is occurring but feels powerless to move.

Cultures: Southern United States and Caribbean groups.

DSM-Related Disorders: Conversion Disorder or Dissociative Disorder.

ghost sickness

Fundamental Feature: Preoccupation with death and the deceased (sometimes associated with witchcraft).

Symptoms: Bad dreams, weakness, feelings of danger, loss of appetite, fainting, dizziness, fear, anxiety, hallucinations, loss of consciousness, confusion, feelings of futility, and a sense of suffocation.

Cultures: Many American Indian tribes.

hwa-byung (also known as wool-hwa-byung)

Fundamental Feature: English translation is "anger syndrome" and attributed to suppression of anger.

Symptoms: Insomnia, fatigue, panic, fear of impending death, dysphoric affect, indigestion, anorexia, dyspnea, palpitations, generalized aches and pains, and a feeling of a mass in the epigastrium.

Cultures: Korean folk syndrome.

koro

Fundamental Feature: Sudden and intense anxiety that the penis or the vulva and nipples will recede into the body and possibly cause death.

Cultures: Malaysian origin, south and east Asia, where known by local terms, such as *shuk yang, shook yong,* and *suo yang* (Chinese); *jinjinia bemar* (Assam); or *rok-joo* (Thailand). Occasionally found in the West.

DSM-Related Disorders: In the *Chinese Classification of Mental Disorders,* Second Edition (CCMD-2).

latah

Fundamental Feature: Hypersensitivity to sudden fright, often with echopraxia, echolalia, command obedience, and dissociative or trancelike behavior.

Cultures: Malaysian or Indonesian origin, although found in many parts of the world. Other terms for this condition are *amurakh, irkunii, ikota, olan, myriachit,* and *menkeiti* (Siberian groups); *bah tschi, bah-tsi, baah-ji* (Thailand); *imu* (Ainu, Sakhalin, Japan); and *mali-mali* and *silok* (Philippines).

locura

Fundamental Feature: Severe form of chronic psychosis attributed to inherited vulnerability, to the effect of multiple life difficulties, or to a combination of both factors.

Symptoms: Incoherence, agitation, auditory and visual hallucinations, inability to follow rules of social interaction, unpredictability, and possible violence.

Cultures: Latinos in the United States and Latin America.

mal de ojo

Fundamental Feature: Spanish phrase translated into English as "evil eye." Children are especially at risk. Sometimes adults (especially females) have the condition.

Symptoms: Fitful sleep, crying without apparent cause, diarrhea, vomiting, and fever in a child or infant.

Cultures: Mediterranean cultures and elsewhere in the world.

nervios

Fundamental Feature: General state of vulnerability to stressful life experiences and to a syndrome brought on by difficult life circumstances.

Symptoms: Various symptoms of emotional distress, somatic disturbance, and inability to function. Headaches, "brain aches," irritability, stomach disturbances, sleep difficulties, nervousness, easy tearfulness, inability to concentrate, trembling, tingling sensations, and *mareos* (dizziness with occasional vertigo-like exacerbations). Nervios tends to be an ongoing problem.

Cultures: Latinos in the United States and Latin America. Other ethnic groups have related ideas of "nerves" (such as *nevra* among Greeks in North America).

DSM-Related Disorders: Adjustment, Anxiety, Depressive, Dissociative, Somatoform, or Psychotic Disorders.

pibloktoq

Fundamental Feature: Abrupt dissociative episode accompanied by extreme excitement of up to thirty minutes' duration and frequently followed by convulsive seizures and coma lasting up to twelve hours.

Symptoms: Withdrawn or mildly irritable for hours or days before the attack and typically complete amnesia for the attack. During attack, the person may tear off clothing, break furniture, shout obscenities, eat feces, flee from protective shelters, or perform other irrational or dangerous acts.

Cultures: Arctic and subarctic Eskimo communities, although regional variations in name exist.

qi-gong psychotic reaction

Fundamental Feature: Acute, time-limited episode with dissociative, paranoid, or other psychotic or nonpsychotic symptoms that may occur after participation in Chinese folk health-enhancing practice of *qi-gong* ("exercise of vital energy").

Cultures: Chinese

DSM-Related Disorders: Included in the *Chinese Classification of Mental Disorders,* Second Edition (CCMD-2).

rootwork

Fundamental Feature: Cultural interpretations that ascribe illness to hexing, witchcraft, sorcery, or the evil influence of another person. "Roots," "spells," or "hexes" can be "put" on others, causing emotional and psychological problems. The "hexed" person may fear death until "root" has been "taken off," usually by a "root doctor."

Symptoms: Generalized anxiety and gastrointestinal complaints (e.g., nausea, vomiting, diarrhea), weakness, dizziness, the fear of being poisoned, and sometimes fear of being killed ("voodoo death").

Cultures: Southern United States among African Americans and European Americans, and in Caribbean societies. Known as *mal puesto* or *brujeria* in Latino societies.

sangue dormido ("sleeping blood")

Fundamental Feature: Pain, numbness, tremor, paralysis, convulsions, stroke, blindness, heart attack, infection, and miscarriage.

Cultures: Portuguese Cape Verde Islanders (and immigrants from there in the United States).

shenjing shuairuo ("neurasthenia")

Fundamental Feature: Hysterical and mental fatigue, dizziness, headaches, other pains, concentration difficulties, sleep disturbance, and memory loss.

Symptoms: Gastrointestinal problems, sexual dysfunction, irritability, excitability, and various signs suggesting disturbance of the autonomic nervous system.

Cultures: China

DSM-Related Disorders: Mood or Anxiety Disorder. Included in the *Chinese Classification of Mental Disorders,* Second Edition (CCMD-2).

shen-k'uei (Taiwan); shenkui (China)

Fundamental Feature: Anxiety or panic symptoms with somatic complaints with no physical cause.

Symptoms: Dizziness, backache, fatigability, general weakness, insomnia, frequent dreams, and complaints of sexual dysfunction (such as premature ejaculation and impotence). Symptoms are attributed to excessive semen loss from frequent intercourse, masturbation, nocturnal emission, or passing of "white turbid urine" believed to contain semen.

Cultures: Chinese folk label.

shin-byung

Fundamental Feature: Anxiety and somatic complaints (general weakness, dizziness, fear, anorexia, insomnia, gastrointestinal problems), with subsequent dissociation and possession by ancestral spirits.

Cultures: Korean.

spell

Fundamental Feature: Trance state in which individuals "communicate" with deceased relatives or with spirits. Can be associated with brief periods of personality change. Spells not considered medical events in folk tradition but may be misconstrued as psychotic episodes in clinical settings.

Cultures: African Americans and European Americans from the southern United States.

susto ("fright," or "soul loss")

Fundamental Feature: Folk illness attributed to frightening event that causes the soul to leave the body and results in unhappiness and sickness. Individuals experience significant strains in key social roles. Symptoms may appear from days to years after the fright is experienced. Extreme cases may result in death. Ritual healings are focused on calling the soul back to the body and cleansing the person to restore bodily and spiritual balance.

Symptoms: Appetite disturbances, inadequate or excessive sleep, troubled sleep or dreams, feeling of sadness, lack of motivation to do anything, and feelings of low self-worth or dirtiness. Somatic symptoms include muscle aches and pains, headache, stomachache, and diarrhea.

Cultures: Latinos in the United States, Mexico, Central America, and South America. Susto is also referred to as *espanto, pasmo, tripa ida, perdida del alma,* or *chibih.*

DSM-Related Disorders: Major Depressive Disorder, Posttraumatic Stress Disorder, and Somatoform Disorder

taijin kyofusho

Fundamental Feature: Phobia resembling Social Phobia in DSM-IV. This syndrome refers to an individual's intense fear that his or her body, its parts or its functions, displease, embarrass, or are offensive to other people in appearance, odor, facial expressions, or movements.

Cultures: Japan.

DSM-Related Disorders: Social Phobia. Included in Japanese diagnostic system for mental disorders.

zar

Fundamental Feature: Experience of spirits possessing an individual.

Symptoms: Persons possessed by a spirit may experience dissociative episodes that can include shouting, laughing, hitting the head against a wall, singing, or weeping. Individuals may show apathy and withdrawal, refusing to eat or carry out daily tasks, or may develop a long-term relationship with the possessing spirit. Not considered pathological locally.

Cultures: Ethiopia, Somalia, Egypt, Sudan, Iran, and other North African and Middle Eastern societies.

DIFFERENTIAL DIAGNOSIS

Differential diagnosis is not done as such with culture-bound syndromes, but the clinician should use a rule-out process in any evaluation involving significant cultural differences. Also important are a careful review of the role of culture in the presentation of symptoms, the meaning of the symptoms to the person, and the degree of understanding of the disorder. The culture-bound syndromes listed in the DSM-IV should be ruled out, as well as other possible cultural explanations for the behavior and symptoms. The clinician should also review the "Other Conditions That May Be a Focus of Clinical Attention" section, specifically the conditions Religious or Spiritual Problem (V62.89) and Acculturation Problem (V62.4) (p. 685). These conditions should be considered in relation to cultural factors to determine which condition or syndrome best explains the person's symptoms and behavior.

RECOMMENDED READING

Mezzich, J. E., Kleinman, A., Fabrega, H., and Parron, D. L. (1996). *Culture and Psychiatric Diagnosis: A DSM-IV Perspective.* Washington, DC: American Psychiatric Press.

Tseng, W. and Streltzer, J. (1997). *Culture and Psychopathology: A Guide to Clinical Assessment.* New York: Brunner/Mazel.

REFERENCES

American Psychiatric Association (1994). *Diagnostic and Statistical Manual of Mental Disorders,* Fourth Edition. Washington, DC: American Psychiatric Association.

Frances, A., First, M. B., and Pincus, H. N. (1995). *DSM-IV Guidebook: The Essential Companion to the* Diagnostic and Statistical Manual of Mental Disorders. Washington, DC: American Psychiatric Association.

Mezzich, J. E., Kleinman, A., Fabrega, H., and Parron, D. L. (1996). *Culture and Psychiatric Diagnosis: A DSM-IV Perspective.* Washington, DC: American Psychiatric Press.

Bibliography

Ainsworth, M. D., Blehar, M. C., Waters, E., and Wall, S. (1978). *Patterns of Attachment: A Psychological Study of the Stranger Situation.* Hillsdale, NJ: Lawrence Erlbaum Associates.

Alexander, F. G. and Selesnick, S. T. (1966). *The History of Psychiatry: An Evaluation of Psychiatric Thought and Practice from Prehistoric Times to the Present.* New York: The New American Library.

Akiskal, H. S. and Cassano, G. B. (1997). *Dysthymia and the Spectrum of Chronic Depressions.* New York: Guilford.

American Psychiatric Association (1980). *Diagnostic and Statistical Manual of Mental Disorders,* Third Edition. Washington, DC: American Psychiatric Association.

American Psychiatric Association (1992). *DSM-IV Options Book.* Washington, DC: American Psychiatric Association.

American Psychiatric Association (1993). *American Psychiatric Association Practice Guidelines for Eating Disorders.* Washington, DC: American Psychiatric Press.

American Psychiatric Association (1994). *Diagnostic and Statistical Manual of Mental Disorders,* Fourth Edition. Washington, DC: American Psychiatric Association.

American Psychiatric Association (1994). *DSM-IV Sourcebook,* Volume 1. Washington, DC: American Psychiatric Association.

Andreasen, N. C. (1994). *Schizophrenia: From Mind to Molecule.* Washington, DC: American Psychiatric Press.

Attwood, T. (1998). *Asperger's Syndrome: A Guide for Parents and Professionals.* London: Jessica Kingsley.

Barkley, R. A. (1990). *Attention Deficit Hyperactivity Disorder: A Handbook for Diagnosis and Treatment,* Second Edition. New York: Guilford.

Barkley, R. A. and Benton, C. M. (1998). *Your Defiant Child: Eight Steps to Better Behavior.* New York: Guilford.

Barkley, R. A., Edwards, G. H., and Robin, A. L. (1999). *Defiant Teens: A Clinician's Manual for Assessment and Family Intervention.* New York: Guilford.

Barton, W. E. (1987). *The History and Influence of the American Psychiatric Association.* Washington, DC: American Psychiatric Press.

Beck, A. T. (1967). *Depression: Causes and Treatment.* Philadelphia, PA: University of Pennsylvania Press.

Beck, A. T. and Emergy, G. (1985). *Anxiety Disorders and Phobias: A Cognitive Perspective.* New York: Basic Books.

Brown, L. S. and Ballou, M. (1992). *Personality and Psychopathology.* New York: Guilford.

Caplan, P. J. (1995). *They Say You're Crazy: How the World's Most Powerful Psychiatrists Decide Who's Normal.* New York: Addison-Wesley.

Cassidy, J. and Shaver, P. R. (1999). *Handbook of Attachment: Theory, Research, and Clinical Applications.* New York: Guilford.

Chess, S. and Thomas, A. (1996). *Temperament: Theory and Practice.* New York: Brunner/Mazel.

Cohen, S. (1998). *Targeting Autism: What We Know, Don't Know, and Can Do to Help Young Children with Autism and Related Disorders.* Berkeley, CA: University of California Press.

Czerniewska, P. (1992). *Learning About Writing: The Early Years.* Malden, MA: Blackwell.

Davison, G. C. and Neale, J. M. (1990). *Abnormal Psychology.* New York: John Wiley.

Denburg, E. V. and Choca, J. P. (1997). *Interpretive Guide to the Millon Clinical Multiaxial Inventory.* Washington, DC: American Psychological Association.

De Silva, P. and Rachman, S. (1998). *Obsessive-Compulsive Disorder: The Facts,* Second Edition. New York: Oxford University Press.

Edgerton, J. and Campbell, R. J. (1994). *American Psychiatry Glossary.* Washington, DC: American Psychiatric Association.

Ewen, R. B. (1998). *Personality: A Topical Approach.* Mahwah, NJ: Lawrence Erlbaum Associates.

Fauman, M. A. (1994). *Study Guide to DSM-IV.* Washington, DC: American Psychiatric Association.

First, M. B., Spitzer, R. L., Gibbon, M., and Williams, J. B. W. (1997). *Structured Clinical Interview for DSM-IV Axis I Disorders (SCID-I), Clinical Version.* Washington, DC: American Psychiatric Association.

First, M. B., Gibbon, M., Spitzer, R. L., Williams, J. B. W., and Benjamin, L. (1997). *Structured Clinical Interview for DSM-IV Axis II Disorders (SCID-II).* Washington, DC: American Psychiatric Association.

First, M. B., Frances, A., and Pincus, H. N. (1995). *DSM-IV Handbook of Differential Diagnosis.* Washington, DC: American Psychiatric Association.

Flannery, D. J. and Huff, C. R. (1998). *Youth Violence: Prevention, Intervention, and Social Policy.* Washington, DC: American Psychiatric Press.

Fletcher, P. and MacWhinney, B. (1996). *The Handbook of Child Language.* Malden, MA: Blackwell.

Frances, A. (1995). *DSM-IV Audio Review.* Washington, DC: American Psychiatric Press.

Frances, A. and First, M. B. (1998). *Your Mental Health: A Layman's Guide to the Psychiatrist's Bible.* New York: Scribner.

Frances, A., First, M. B., and Pincus, H. N. (1995). *DSM-IV Guidebook: The Essential Companion to the* Diagnostic and Statistical Manual of Mental Disorders. Washington, DC: American Psychiatric Association.

Frances, A. and Ross, R. (1996). *DSM-IV Case Studies: A Guide to Differential Diagnosis.* Washington, DC: American Psychiatric Press.

Galanter, M. and Kleber, H. D. (1999). *Textbook of Substance Abuse Treatment.* Washington, DC: American Psychiatric Press.

Gay, P. (1998). *Freud: A Life for Our Time.* New York: Norton.

Gordon, R. A. (1999). *Eating Disorders: Anatomy of a Social Epidemic.* Malden, MA: Blackwell.

Greenberg, G. S. and Horn, W. F. (1991). *Attention Deficit Hyperactivity Disorder: Questions and Answers for Parents.* Champaign, IL: Research Press.

Hall, H. V. and Pritchard, D. A. (1996). *Detecting Malingering and Deception.* Boca Raton, FL: CRC Press.

Hauri, P., Sanborn, C., Corson, J., and Violette, J. (1988). *Handbook for Beginning Mental Health Researchers.* New York: The Haworth Press, Inc.

Henggeler, S. W., Schoenwald, S. K., Borduin, C. M., Roland, M. D., and Cunningham, P. B. (1998). *Multisystemic Treatment of Antisocial Behavior in Children and Adolescents.* New York: Guilford.

House, A. E. (1999). *DSM-IV Diagnosis in the Schools.* New York: Guilford.

Ingersoll, B. (1988). *Your Hyperactive Child: A Parent's Guide to Coping With Attention Deficit Disorder.* New York: Doubleday.

Kagan, J. (1984). *The Nature of the Child.* New York: Basic Books.

Kamphaus, R. W. and Frick, P. J. (1996). *Clinical Assessment of Child and Adolescent Personality and Behavior.* Boston, MA: Allyn and Bacon.

Kaplan, H. I. and Sadock, B. J. (1998). *Synopsis of Psychiatry: Behavioral Sciences/Clinical Psychiatry,* Eighth Edition. Baltimore, MD: Williams and Wilkins.

Karls, J. M. and Wandrei, K. E. (1994). *Person-In-Environment System: The PIE Classification System for Social Functioning Problems.* Washington, DC: National Association of Social Workers.

Keefe, R. S. E. and Harvey, P. D. (1994). *Understanding Schizophrenia: A Guide to the New Research on Causes and Treatment.* New York: Free Press.

Kennedy, J. A. (1992). *Fundamentals of Psychiatric Treatment Planning.* Washington, DC: American Psychiatric Press.

Kessler, R. C., McGonagle, K. A., Zhao, S., Nelson, C. B., Hughes, M., Eshleman, S., Wittchen, H. U., and Kendler, K. S. (1994). Lifetime and 12-Month Prevalance of DSM-III-R Psychiatric Disorders in the United States. *Archives of General Psychiatry,* 51(1), 8-19.

Kirk, S. A. and Kutchins, H. (1992). *The Selling of the DSM: The Rhetoric of Science in Psychiatry.* Hawthorne, NY: Aldine de Gruyter.

Kozloff, M. A. (1998). *Reaching the Autistic Child: A Parent Training Program.* Cambridge, MA: Brookline Books.

Kutchins, H. and Kirk, S. A. (1995). Should DSM Be the Basis for Teaching Social Work Practice in Mental Health? No! *Journal of Social Work Education,* 31(2), 159-168.

Kutchins, H. and Kirk, S. A. (1997). *Making Us Crazy: DSM: The Psychiatric Bible and the Creation of Mental Disorders.* New York: Free Press.

Lewis, M. and Volkmar, F. (1990). *Clinical Aspects of Child and Adolescent Development,* Third Edition. Philadelphia, PA: Lea and Febiger.

Lynn, S. J. and Rhue, J. W. (1994). *Dissociation: Clinical and Theoretical Perspectives.* New York: Guilford.

Mash, E. J. and Terdal, L. G. (1997). *Assessment of Childhood Disorders,* Third Edition. New York: Guilford.

Mezzich, J. E., Kleinman, A., Fabrega, H., and Parron, D. L. (1996). *Culture and Psychiatric Diagnosis: A DSM-IV Perspective.* Washington, DC: American Psychiatric Press.

Miklowitz, D. J. and Goldstein, M. J. (1997). *Bipolar Disorder: A Family-Focused Treatment Approach.* New York: Guilford.

Millon, T. (1997). *The Millon Inventories: Clinical and Personality Assessment.* New York: Guilford.

Millon, T. and Davis, R. (1995). *Disorders of Personality: DSM-IV and Beyond,* Second Edition. New York: Wiley.

Morrison, J. (1994). *The First Interview: Revised for DSM-IV.* New York: Guilford.

Morrison, J. (1995). *DSM-IV Made Easy: The Clinicians' Guide to Diagnosis.* New York: Guilford.

Morrison, J. (1997). *When Psychological Problems Mask Medical Disorders: A Guide for Psychotherapists.* New York: Guilford.

Morrison, M. R. and Stamps, R. E. (1998). *DSM-IV Internet Companion.* New York: Norton.

Mueser, K. T. (1994). *Coping with Schizophrenia: A Guide for Families.* Oakland, CA: New Harbinger.

Olin, J. T. and Keatinge, C. (1998). *Rapid Psychological Assessment.* New York: Wiley.

Othmer, E. and Othmer, S. C. (1994). *The Clinical Interview Using DSM-IV,* Volume 1: *Fundamentals.* Washington, DC: American Psychiatric Association.

Othmer, E. and Othmer, S. C. (1994). *The Clinical Interview Using DSM-IV,* Volume 2: *The Difficult Patient.* Washington, DC: American Psychiatric Association.

Pliszka, S. R., Carlson, C. L., and Swanson, J. M. (1999). *ADHD with Comorbid Disorders.* New York: Guilford.

Putnam, F. W. (1997). *Dissociation in Children and Adolescents: A Development Perspective.* New York: Guilford.

Rapoport, J. L. and Ismond, D. R. (1996). *DSM-IV Training Guide for Diagnosis of Childhood Disorders.* New York: Brunner/Mazel.

Ray, O. (1995). *Drugs, Society, and Human Behavior.* New York: McGraw-Hill.

Reite, M., Ruddy, J., and Nagel, K. (1997). *Concise Guide to Evaluation and Management of Sleep Disorders,* Second Edition. Washington, DC: American Psychiatric Press.

Roazen, P. (1985). *Helen Deutsch: A Psychoanalyst's Life.* New York: Doubleday.

Robinson, D. J. (1999). *Disordered Personalities,* Second Edition. Port Huron, MI: Rapid Psychler Press.

Samuels, S. K. and Sikorsky, S. (1998). *Clinical Evaluations of School Aged Children,* Second Edition. Sarasota, FL: Professional Resource Press.

Satcher, D. (2000). *Mental Health: A Report of the Surgeon General.* Washington, DC: U.S. Government Printing Office.

Seeman, M. V. (1995). *Gender and Psychopathology.* Washington, DC: American Psychiatric Press.

Shirar, L. (1996). *Dissociative Children: Bridging the Inner and Outer World.* New York: Norton.

Shorter, E. (1997). *A History of Psychiatry: From the Era of the Asylum to the Age of Prozac.* New York: Wiley.

Spitzer, R. L., Gibbon, M., Skodol, A. E., Williams, J. B. W., and First, M. B. (1995). *DSM-IV Casebook.* Washington, DC: American Psychiatric Association.

Stein, M. T., Rapin, I., and Yapko, D. (1999). Challenging Case: Selective Mutism. *Developmental and Behavioral Pediatrics,* 20(1), 38-41.

Steinberg, M. (1995). *Handbook for the Assessment of Dissociation: A Clinical Guide.* Washington, DC: American Psychiatric Press.

Stone, M. H. (1997). *Healing the Mind: A History of Psychiatry from Antiquity to the Present.* New York: Norton.

Swinson, R. P., Antony, M. M., Rachman, S., and Richter, M. A. (1998). *Obsessive-Compulsive Disorder: Theory, Research, and Treatment.* New York: Guilford.

Torrey, E. F. (1995). *Surviving Schizophrenia: A Manual for Families, Consumers, and Providers.* New York: HarperPerennial.

Triolo, S. J. (1998). *Attention Deficit Hyperactivity Disorder in Adults.* Philadelphia, PA: Accelerated Development.

Tseng, W. and Streltzer, J. (1997). *Culture and Psychopathology: A Guide to Clinical Assessment.* New York: Brunner/Mazel.

Underwood, G. and Batt, W. (1996). *Reading and Understanding: An Introduction to the Psychology of Reading.* Malden, MA: Blackwell.

Vance, H. B. (1998). *Psychological Assessment of Children: Basic Practices for School and Clinical Settings.* New York: Wiley.

Van der Kolk, B. A., McFarlane, A. C., and Weisbeth, L. (1996). *Traumatic Stress: The Effects of Overwhelming Experience on Mind, Body, and Society.* New York: Guilford.

Wicks-Nelson, R. and Israel, A. C. (1997). *Behavior Disorders of Childhood,* Third Edition. Upper Saddle River, NJ: Prentice-Hall.

Williams, J. B. W. and Spitzer, R. L. (1995). Should DSM Be the Basis for Teaching Social Work Practice in Mental Health? Yes! *Journal of Social Work Education,* 31(2), 148-158.

Wodrich, D. L. (1997). *Children's Psychological Testing: A Guide for Nonpsychologists,* Third Edition. Baltimore, MD: Brooks.

Yingling, L. C., Miller, W. E., McDonald, A. L., and Galewaler, S. T. (1998). *GARF Assessment Sourcebook: Using the DSM-IV Global Assessment of Relational Functioning.* New York: Brunner/Mazel.

Video/Audio/Electronic Resources

Diagnosis According to the DSM-IV (1994). New York: Newbridge Communications. 1-800-347-7828.

DSM-IV Audio Review (1995). Washington, DC: American Psychiatric Association. 1-800-368-5777.

DSM-IV Video Case Reviews (1996). Washington, DC: American Psychiatric Association. 1-800-368-5777.

DSM-IV Videotaped Clinical Vignettes (1995). New York: Brunner/Mazel. 1-800-825-3089.

Electronic DSM-IV Plus. Version 3.0 (1999). Washington, DC: American Psychiatric Association. 1-800-368-5777.

Highlights of the DSM-IV (1996). Washington, DC: American Psychological Association. 1-800-374-2721.

Video Review of Psychiatry (1999). New York: Specialty Preparation, Inc. 914-738-6911.

Index

Page numbers followed by the letter "v" indicate visuals.

HAWORTH Social Work Practice in Action
Carlton E. Munson, PhD, Senior Editor

WOMEN SURVIVORS, PSYCHOLOGICAL TRAUMA, AND THE POLITICS OF RESISTANCE by Norma Jean Profitt. (2000).

THE MENTAL HEALTH DIAGNOSTIC DESK REFERENCE: VISUAL GUIDES AND MORE FOR LEARNING TO USE THE DIAGNOSTIC AND STATISTICAL MANUAL (DSM-IV) by Carlton E. Munson. (2000). "A carefully organized and user-friendly book for the beginning student and less-experienced practitioner of social work, clinical psychology, or psychiatric nursing . . . . It will be a valuable addition to the literature on clinical assessment of mental disorders." *Jerrold R. Brandell, PhD, BCD, Professor, School of Social Work, Wayne State University, Detroit, Michigan and Founding Editor,* Psychoanalytic Social Work

HUMAN SERVICES AND THE AFROCENTRIC PARADIGM by Jerome H. Schiele. (2000). "Represents a milestone in applying the Afrocentric paradigm to human services generally, and social work specifically. . . . A highly valuable resource." *Bogart R. Leashore, PhD, Dean and Professor, Hunter College School of Social Work, New York, New York*

SOCIAL WORK: SEEKING RELEVANCY IN THE TWENTY-FIRST CENTURY by Roland Meinert, John T. Pardeck and Larry Kreuger. (2000). "Highly recommended. A thought-provoking work that asks the difficult questions and challenges the status quo. A great book for graduate students as well as experienced social workers and educators." *Francis K. O. Yuen, DSW, ACSE, Associate Professor, Division of Social Work, California State University, Sacramento*

SOCIAL WORK PRACTICE IN HOME HEALTH CARE by Ruth Ann Goode. (2000). "Dr. Goode presents both a lucid scenario and a formulated protocol to bring health care services into the home setting. . . . This is a must-have volume that will be a reference to be consulted many times." *Marcia B. Steinhauer, PhD, Coordinator and Associate Professor, Human Services Administration Program, Rider University, Lawrenceville, New Jersey*

FORENSIC SOCIAL WORK: LEGAL ASPECTS OF PROFESSIONAL PRACTICE, SECOND EDITION by Robert L. Barker and Douglas M. Branson. (2000). "The authors combine their expertise to create this informative guide to address legal practice issues facing social workers." *Newsletter of the National Organization of Forensic Social Work*

SOCIAL WORK IN THE HEALTH FIELD: A CARE PERSPECTIVE by Lois A. Fort Cowles. (1999). "Makes an important contribution to the field by locating the practice of social work in health care within an organizational and social context." *Goldie Kadushin, PhD, Associate Professor, School of Social Welfare, University of Wisconsin, Milwaukee*

SMART BUT STUCK: WHAT EVERY THERAPIST NEEDS TO KNOW ABOUT LEARNING DISABILITIES AND IMPRISONED INTELLIGENCE by Myrna Orenstein. (1999). "A trailblazing effort that creates an entirely novel way of talking and thinking about learning disabilities. There is simply nothing like it in the field." *Fred M. Levin, MD, Training Supervising Analyst, Chicago Institute for Psychoanalysis; Assistant Professor of Clinical Psychiatry, Northwestern University, School of Medicine, Chicago, IL*

CLINICAL WORK AND SOCIAL ACTION: AN INTEGRATIVE APPROACH by Jerome Sachs and Fred Newdom. (1999). "Just in time for the new millennium come Sachs and Newdom with a wholly fresh look at social work. . . . A much-needed uniting of social work values, theories, and practice for action." *Josephine Nieves, MSW, PhD, Executive Director, National Association of Social Workers*

SOCIAL WORK PRACTICE IN THE MILITARY by James G. Daley. (1999). "A significant and worthwhile book with provocative and stimulating ideas. It deserves to be read by a wide audience in social work education and practice as well as by decision makers in the military." *H. Wayne Johnson, MSW, Professor, University of Iowa, School of Social Work, Iowa City, Iowa*

GROUP WORK: SKILLS AND STRATEGIES FOR EFFECTIVE INTERVENTIONS, SECOND EDITION by Sondra Brandler and Camille P. Roman. (1999). "A clear, basic description of what group work requires, including what skills and techniques group workers need to be effective." *Hospital and Community Psychiatry* (from the first edition)

TEENAGE RUNAWAYS: BROKEN HEARTS AND "BAD ATTITUDES" by Laurie Schaffner (1999). "Skillfully combines the authentic voice of the juvenile runaway with the principles of social science research."

CELEBRATING DIVERSITY: COEXISTING IN A MULTICULTURAL SOCIETY by Benyamin Chetkow-Yanoov. (1999). "Makes a valuable contribution to peace theory and practice." *Ian Harris, EdD, Executive Secretary, Peace Education Committee, International Peace Research Association*

SOCIAL WELFARE POLICY ANALYSIS AND CHOICES by Hobart A. Burch. (1999). "Will become the landmark text in its field for many decades to come." *Sheldon Rahan, DSW, Founding Dean and Emeritus Professor of Social Policy and Social Administration. Faculty of Social Work, Wilfrid Laurier University, Canada*

SOCIAL WORK PRACTICE: A SYSTEMS APPROACH, SECOND EDITION by Benyamin Chetkow-Yannov. (1999). "Highly recommended as a primary text for any and all introductory social work courses." *Ram A. Cnaan, PhD, Associate Professor, School of Social Work, University of Pennsylvania*

CRITICAL SOCIAL WELFARE ISSUES: TOOLS FOR SOCIAL WORK AND HEALTH CARE PROFESSIONALS edited by Arthur J. Katz, Abraham Lurie, and Carlos M. Vidal. (1997). "Offers hopeful agendas for change, while navigating the societal challenges facing those in the human services today." *Book News Inc.*

SOCIAL WORK IN HEALTH SETTINGS: PRACTICE IN CONTEXT, SECOND EDITION edited by Toba Schwaber Kerson. (1997). "A first-class document . . . It will be found among the steadier and lasting works on the social work aspects of American health care." *Hans S. Falck, PhD, Professor Emeritus and Former Chair, Health Specialization in Social Work, Virginia Commonwealth University*

PRINCIPLES OF SOCIAL WORK PRACTICE: A GENERIC PRACTICE APPROACH by Molly R. Hancock. (1997). "Hancock's discussions advocate reflection and self-awareness to create a climate for client change." *Journal of Social Work Education*

NOBODY'S CHILDREN: ORPHANS OF THE HIV EPIDEMIC by Steven F. Dansky. (1997). "Professional sound, moving, and useful for both professionals and interested readers alike." *Ellen G. Friedman, ACSW, Associate Director of Support Services, Beth Israel Medical Center, Methadone Maintenance Treatment Program*

SOCIAL WORK APPROACHES TO CONFLICT RESOLUTION: MAKING FIGHTING OBSOLETE by Benyamin Chetkow-Yanoov. (1996). "Presents an examination of the nature and cause of conflict and suggests techniques for coping with conflict." *Journal of Criminal Justice*

FEMINIST THEORIES AND SOCIAL WORK: APPROACHES AND APPLICATIONS by Christine Flynn Salunier. (1996). " An essential reference to be read repeatedly by all educators and practitioners who are eager to learn more about feminist theory and practice: *Nancy R. Hooyman, PhD, Dean and Professor, School of Social Work, University of Washington, Seattle*

THE RELATIONAL SYSTEMS MODEL FOR FAMILY THERAPY: LIVING IN THE FOUR REALITIES by Donald R. Bardill. (1996). "Engages the reader in quiet, thoughtful conversation on the timeless issue of helping families and individuals." *Christian Counseling Resource Review*

SOCIAL WORK INTERVENTION IN AN ECONOMIC CRISIS: THE RIVER COMMUNITIES PROJECT by Martha Baum and Pamela Twiss. (1996). "Sets a standard for universities in terms of the types of meaningful roles they can play in supporting and sustaining communities." *Kenneth J. Jaros, PhD, Director, Public Health Social Work Training Program, University of Pittsburgh*

FUNDAMENTALS OF COGNITIVE-BEHAVIOR THERAPY: FROM BOTH SIDES OF THE DESK by Bill Borcherdt. (1996). "Both beginning and experienced practitioners . . . will find a considerable number of valuable suggestions in Borcherdt's book." *Albert Ellis, PhD, President, Institute for Rational-Emotive Therapy, New York City*

BASIC SOCIAL POLICY AND PLANNING: STRATEGIES AND PRACTICE METHODS by Hobart A. Burch. (1996). "Burch's familiarity with his topic is evident and his book is an easy introduction to the field." *Readings*

THE CROSS-CULTURAL PRACTICE OF CLINICAL CASE MANAGEMENT IN MENTAL HEALTH edited by Peter Manoleas. (1996). "Makes a contribution by bringing together the cross-cultural and clinical case management perspectives in working with those who have serious mental illness." *Disability Studies Quarterly*

FAMILY BEYOND FAMILY: THE SURROGATE PARENT IN SCHOOLS AND OTHER COMMUNITY AGENCIES by Sanford Weinstein. (1995). "Highly recommended to anyone concerned about the welfare of our children and the breakdown of the American family." *Jerold S. Greenberg, EdD, Director of Community Service, College of Health & Human Performance, University of Maryland*

PEOPLE WITH HIV AND THOSE WHO HELP THEM: CHALLENGES, INTEGRATION, INTERVENTION by R. Dennis Shelby. (1995). "A useful and compassionate contribution to the HIV psychotherapy literature." *Public Health*

THE BLACK ELDERLY: SATISFACTION AND QUALITY OF LATER LIFE by Marguerite Coke and James A. Twaite. (1995). "Presents a model for predicting life satisfaction in this population." *Abstracts in Social Gerontology*

BUILDING ON WOMEN'S STRENGTHS: A SOCIAL WORK AGENDA FOR THE TWENTY-FIRST CENTURY edited by Liane V. Davis. (1994). "The most lucid and accessible overview of the related epistemological debates int he social work literature." *Journal of the National Association of Social Workers*

NOW DARE EVERYTHING: TALES OF HIV-RELATED PSYCHOTHERAPY by Steven F. Dansky. (1994). "A highly recommended book for anyone working with persons who are HIV positive. . . . Every library should have a copy of this book." *AIDS Book Review Journal*

INTERVENTION RESEARCH: DESIGN AND DEVELOPMENT FOR HUMAN SERVICE edited by Jack Rothman and Edwin J. Thomas. (1994). "Provides a useful framework for the further examination of methodology for each separate step of such research." *Academic Library Book Review*

CLINICAL SOCIAL WORK SUPERVISION, SECOND EDITION by Carlton E. Munson. (1993). "A useful, thorough, and articulate reference for supervisors and for 'supervisees' who are wanting to understand their supervisor or are looking for effective supervision." *Transactional Analysis Journal*

ELEMENTS OF THE HELPING PROCESS: A GUIDE FOR CLINICIANS by Raymond Fox. (1993). "Filled with helpful hints, creative interventions, and practical guidelines." *Journal of Family Psychotherapy*

IF A PARTNER HAS AIDS: GUIDE TO CLINICAL INTERVENTION FOR RELATIONSHIPS IN CRISIS by R. Dennis Shelby. (1993). " A welcome addition to existing publications about couples coping with AIDS, it offers intervention ideas and strategies to clinicians." *Contemporary Psychology*

GERONTOLOGICAL SOCIAL WORK SUPERVISION by Ann Burack-Weiss and Frances Coyle Brennan. (1991). "The creative ideas in this book will aid supervisors working with students and experienced social workers." *Senior News*

SOCIAL WORK THEORY AND PRACTICE WITH THE TERMINALLY ILL by Joan K. Parry. (1989). "Should be read by all professionals engaged in the provision of health services in hospitals, emergency rooms, and hospices." *Hector B. Garcia, PhD, Professor, San Jose State University School of Social Work*

THE CREATIVE PRACTITIONER: THEORY AND METHODS FOR THE HELPING SERVICES by Bernard Gelfand. (1988). "[Should] be widely adopted by those in the helping services. It could lead to significant positive advances by countless individuals." *Sidney J. Parnes, Trustee Chairperson for Strategic Program Development, Creative Education Foundation, Buffalo, NY*

MANAGEMENT AND INFORMATION SYSTEMS IN HUMAN SERVICES: IMPLICATIONS FOR THE DISTRIBUTION OF AUTHORITY AND DECISION MAKING by Richard K. Caputo. (1987). "A contribution to social work scholarship in that it provides conceptual frameworks that can be used in the design of management information systems." *Social Work*